D0848718

Psychosomatic Families

Psychosomatic Families

Anorexia Nervosa in Context

Salvador Minuchin

Bernice L. Rosman

Lester Baker

With the Collaboration of Ronald Liebman

HARVARD UNIVERSITY PRESS

Cambridge, Massachusetts, and London, England

10   9   8   7

This book is printed on acid-free paper, and its binding materials have
been chosen for strength and durability.

Library of Congress Cataloging in Publication Data

Minuchin, Salvador.
  Psychosomatic families.

  Includes index.
  1.   Anorexia nervosa.   2.   Medicine, Psychosomatic.
3.   Family psychotherapy.   I.   Rosman, Bernice L.,
joint author.   II.   Baker, Lester, joint author.
III.   Title.
[DNLM: 1.   Anorexia nervosa.   2.   Psychotherapy.
3.   Family. WM175 M668p]
RC552.A5M56   616.8'5   78-1742
ISBN 0-674-72220-5

To the first diabetic children
Karen, Patricia, and Deborah
who forced us to look at the critical role of the
family in psychosomatic disease

Acknowledgments

This book is the end result of ten years of research on families with psychosomatic children, supported by Grants NIMH 21336 and NIH AM 13518. The research on the children who were hospitalized in the Clinical Research Center of the Children's Hospital of Philadelphia as part of this study was supported by Grant NIH RR 240.

The authors of the book represent an interdisciplinary team: psychiatrist, pediatrician, and psychologist. Yet the contributions of these individuals represented far more than the sum of their areas of expertise. In the process of working together, we developed a system of differentiated but interdependent parts. The psychiatric input was enhanced by the contribution of Ronald Liebman, M.D., who wrote Chapter 10 and was the therapist for a number of the cases followed in the outcome study. Thomas Todd, Ph.D., and Leroy Milman, M.D., who completed the team, contributed greatly to the development of ideas contained in the book.

Many other colleagues, students, and teachers at the Philadelphia Child Guidance Clinic and the Clinical Research Center participated in the treatment of the families and in the research meetings creating the atmosphere of curiosity, excitement, and exploration that sustained us through the difficulties of the project. They helped us to crystallize our ideas and encouraged us in their presentation. Among them, we owe special thanks to Lynn Hoffman, who suggested the format of analysis that was used in the clinical chapters; Gottlieb Guntern, who read the manuscript and gave useful suggestions; Patricia Minuchin, Ph.D., who helped with the organization of the book and in other aspects of the writing; Fran Hitchcock, whose collaboration in the writing and editing was invaluable; Sherry Bell and Joyce Kobayashi, who carried out the follow-up study; and Marge Arnold, who patiently typed many drafts and redrafts of the book. We also want to thank Virginia LaPlante from Harvard University Press for her contribution to the finished work.

Another group of people who collaborated in our book, though anonymous, are the most significant contributors of all. They are the families we studied, who endured our uncertainty and groping and helped us to grow. To them go our warmest thanks.

The transcripts of therapeutic interviews appearing in this book have been edited to protect the privacy of the families involved. The family interviews have also been made into training videotapes, under the titles: "People Take My Voice," with commentary by Lynn Hoffman (Chapter 8); "Rescue Mission," edited by Gottlieb Guntern, M.D., with the assistance of Giovanna Todini, M.D., and David Heard, Ph.D. (Chapter 9); "The Priestman Family" (Chapter 10); and "The Menotti Family" (Chapter 11). Information concerning these videotapes is available from the Philadelphia Child Guidance Clinic, Two Children's Center, 34th and Civic Center Boulevard, Philadelphia, Pennsylvania 19104.

Contents

Figures

Tables

Psychosomatic Families

Perspectives on
Anorexia Nervosa

1 ————————————————————————————

At the age of fourteen, Deborah Kaplan developed the syndrome known as anorexia nervosa, or self-starvation. Typically, the illness seems to have begun when she decided to go on a diet in order to pursue a career as a model. At first she followed a normal reducing diet. But over a period of eighteen months she cut out more and more foods, until she was eating only apples, cottage cheese, and water. Her weight dropped from 110 pounds to 78 pounds, and amenorrhea developed. At the same time, Deborah's activity increased. Sometimes she would wake up at four or five in the morning and go out to walk for miles until it was time to leave for school. If confined to the house, she ran endlessly up and down the stairs. She continued to be a good student, as she always had been, but she withdrew almost entirely from the social activities of school and synagogue. Deborah's parents described her as a good girl. They were proud of her grades and her behavior. They could not explain her refusal to eat.

Finally, on her pediatrician's recommendation, Deborah was hospitalized in a children's facility that was researching family influences on psychosomatic syndromes in children. Rigorous medical workups ruled out the possibility of an organic cause for her refusal to eat, so Deborah and her family were referred to the psychiatric component of the team. The presenting problem was anorexia nervosa.

Anorexia nervosa is a psychosomatic syndrome characterized by both physical and psychological symptoms. It is potentially fatal, with reported mortality rates of 10–15 percent. The disease usually appears in middle class females, the percentage of male anorectics being very low. It generally starts during adolescence, though cases can also begin in preadolescence and in adulthood.[1]

There is some debate in the medical field concerning the exact components of the syndrome. In this study the disease is defined by both physical and psychological criteria. The physical symptoms include a loss of over 25 percent of the body weight as well as one or more of the following conditions: amenorrhea, hyperactivity, and hypothermia. The psychological symptoms include a pursuit of thinness, fear of gaining weight, denial of hunger, distorted body image, sense of ineffectiveness, and struggle for control.

As is usual in our practice, the first session held at the psychiatric clinic with the Kaplan family was planned to include lunch.[2] Present at the interview were Deborah, her parents, and her seventeen-year-old brother, Simon. When Deborah was earlier negotiating with the dietitian at the hospital, she had ordered a hot dog, peas, milk, and cottage cheese, to be sent over on a tray for lunch. The family and the therapist ordered sandwiches during the session. But when Deborah's tray arrived, she refused to eat. Consequently, the therapist instructed the parents to take over the task of getting their daughter to eat while he was out of the room.

MINUCHIN: I will be watching through the one-way mirror. I will come back shortly. I want you to negotiate with Debbie. Otherwise she will die. She is starving herself to death. I don't want that to happen. And she is your daughter. (*He exits.*)

MOTHER: Deborah, do you want to finish this half of my sandwich? It is very good.

DEBORAH: Dad, I told you last night that I didn't like it. But I tried it.

FATHER: Are you talking to me? I told you that you are going to have to eat everything. When you get up to a certain weight, you can pick your own shots, but right now, we are negotiating for your survival, like Dr. Minuchin said. Your life. It is important that you eat.

DEBORAH: The dietitian was up here, and she asked me what I wanted to eat.

MOTHER: You are old enough to understand. Dr. Minuchin was just in here. And before you came to the hospital, I told you that you were going to die. Do you know what that means, Deborah? You are going to *die*! You have a beautiful life ahead of you—you are only fifteen! Deborah, this contains protein—

FATHER: Deborah, how many doctors have told you that you are *not* a dietitian? Now wipe out of your mind what those things contain, and just eat them.

MOTHER: Let her finish eating. I think she is going to try to eat.

DEBORAH: I was talking to a real dietitian here. She told me to order what *I* wanted. And she said that cottage cheese is a very good source of protein, and I don't have to eat all that—

MOTHER: You have been losing weight ever since you went on cottage cheese and apples. Doesn't that mean anything? You have to start to gain. Do you understand what that means? You have to order milk shakes, cakes, pies—

DEBORAH: I don't like that stuff! I don't want it!

FATHER: Your life is involved, and you have to eat. Listen, Deb, don't grasp onto what a dietitian says or what a doctor says and use that as an excuse. To me, cottage cheese is a side order. Just a dish—

DEBORAH: Look at you.

FATHER: What's wrong with me? I weigh just what I should weigh. I wish to hell you looked like me. Deb, eat what's on your tray.

DEBORAH: I don't like this!

FATHER: But eat it.

DEBORAH: No! No! I don't care. You can shove it down my throat! I'll get sick, and I *will* die.

MOTHER: Well, why didn't you order something else then? Another kind of food?

DEBORAH: Because I ordered cottage cheese! And they said they would give me meat three times a day, if I wanted it.

FATHER: You *have* to eat meat three times a day.

DEBORAH: No, no, no! You know a growing girl eats what she wants. Oh, golly, you *make* me eat it!

MOTHER: A normal growing girl eats certain nourishing foods, and then she eats other things that she likes as well. You are starving your body.

DEBORAH: I am *not* starving it! My pulse went up. Everything is going up.

MOTHER: Then why are you losing weight? Over two pounds since yesterday, a half-pound the day before that. You have got to eat more. You have got to start to gain, because you are going to die, Deborah! You won't have another chance. You have only one chance, right now.

DEBORAH: I won't die.

MOTHER: You will.

FATHER: Dr. Minuchin said today you can get out of here at 88 pounds. I am not worried about that. I know that you are going to eat, and you are going to eat well, because if you want to get out of this hospital, you are going to eat. And you are going to put plenty of weight on. But the thing is this, Deborah. You are starting out on the wrong foot, and you are acting wrong. I cannot understand the difference in you between last night and this afternoon. Last night you told me, "Dad, I am going to *try*. I am going to eat."

MOTHER: Wait a minute, Abe.

DEBORAH: I ate the peas instead of apples. And this morning I asked them to bring me tea instead of milk.

FATHER: But I told you last night that *whatever* anybody gives you is not poison. It is food. It is not going to hurt you.

DEBORAH: I can't eat that much! You have to remember that I am—

MOTHER: Deborah, you don't have to eat that much. But eat food that will help to put weight on you. You don't even have to eat that much of that, but certain types of food are necessary . . .

In this family, a pattern repeats endlessly. Mother pleads, Deborah refuses, Father enters with a firm demand, Mother intervenes to soften Father's demand, Mother pleads, Deborah refuses, and so on. Each repetition increases the intensity of the pleading, defying, and demanding, but nothing is resolved. The pattern only continues.

To the therapist observing the situation, it seemed that whenever the three family members came close to a decision, one of them would react in a way that deflected conflict resolution, returning the triad to the static repetition of an endless pattern. The parents, in particular, seemed to nullify each other's efforts. Consequently, the therapist re-entered the room after half an hour and asked the mother if she could help Deborah better alone. Mrs. Kaplan nodded, so the therapist took Mr. Kaplan and his son with him to the observation room behind the one-way mirror.

MOTHER: Deborah, I want you to eat. After you get your certain weight back, you can eat anything you want. Deborah. Deborah!

DEBORAH: Why doesn't Dad get a sandwich? Why don't you get one?

MOTHER: Because Dad has enough meat on him, and he is not in the hospital like you are. You are in the hospital, Deborah. You are here for a reason. You are here because you have to eat. You have to eat. There is no way out. Deborah, could you live if you stopped breathing?

DEBORAH: Did I stop breathing?

MOTHER: No, but you had better start eating. It is the same thing as breathing. I eat enough all day.

DEBORAH: You don't eat the right foods!

MOTHER: No, but I eat enough—I don't have to eat the right foods! I am fully grown. I never left a piece of food. How could I eat and watch you starve? Hold your breath. See how long you can hold your breath. Food is like air! You didn't touch your milk or your beef.

DEBORAH: Okay, I will finish the beef. But I'll get sick and vomit all over.

MOTHER: I promise you, you won't get sick.

DEBORAH: I don't want it! You force everything on me. Everything I ever did! You have always forced me!

MOTHER: I have never forced you. Deborah, from day to day we don't know whether you are going to survive. You are losing weight so rapidly. I mean, you are an intelligent girl. I don't see why you can't reason this thing out. The only way to go home is to eat. Let me see you start eating again, and see how far you go. Then we'll discuss it further.

DEBORAH: No, no, no! I'll be defeated!

MOTHER: Well then, be defeated. And I lost my appetite! Because you have never known me to leave anything. Start eating the hot dog now. You said you were going to. Go ahead.

DEBORAH: No, no, no! After I finish that, you will start all over again. I don't want to eat any of it! What did you eat before you came up here?

MOTHER: I eat all day long, Deborah. I eat a tremendous meal at dinner.

DEBORAH: Coffee! Mints!

MOTHER: I eat a tremendous meal! I'm not in the hospital. You are. Am I underweight, or are you? Yes, I should be in a hospital—

a mental institute, that's where I should be. Because that's where you are going to put me! Now go ahead and eat. I said, go ahead and eat. Start wherever you want, and—

DEBORAH: I am not going to finish it!

MOTHER: Let's see how far you go. You know, Deborah, I am desperate. Do you know what being desperate is?

DEBORAH: Yes, I do know.

MOTHER: Suppose you were me, and I were you. Would you let your little girl starve to death? Would you?

DEBORAH: I wouldn't force her.

MOTHER: If she were going to die, you wouldn't force her? If she were going to die?

DEBORAH: I—no! She wasn't going to die.

MOTHER: Oh no, honey. You know she's going to die because she's not eating. You know she's going to die. Now what would you do in that case? Would you feed her, or let her do what she wants?

DEBORAH: I would let her eat vegetables and protein. This isn't going to kill me.

MOTHER: What kind of nonsense is that? You are starving! You are starving to death! Why do you think we are all here? This is no picnic. Your father can't do any business. Your father is losing the business! Do you understand that? Now start to eat, because we may not be sitting here tomorrow, because you'll be dead. Start to eat!

DEBORAH: I don't want it!

MOTHER: Start to eat now! Start to eat right now! (*She is screaming.*) Right now! Because every minute means something to you. To all of us. Start to eat, Deborah!

DEBORAH (*crying*): I don't want it!

MOTHER: You've got to!

DEBORAH: I don't want it!

Exhausted, Mrs. Kaplan burst into tears. The therapist, who had come back into the room with the other family members, suggested that she sit down and that Mr. Kaplan help Deborah to eat. This time the therapist remained in the room. Mrs. Kaplan continued to weep silently.

FATHER: All right, Deborah. Now I'm not going to play any games with you. And I'm not going to leave this room unless they carry me out bodily unless you finish everything that's on that tray. Now, you want my love. You want to walk the dog with me. You're going—

DEBORAH: I don't want your love! I don't want anything.

FATHER: Deborah, you can throw that hot dog on the floor, but by the time I leave this room, you're going to eat that hot dog.

DEBORAH: You can try, but I don't want it!

FATHER: Deborah, you can talk all you want, but—

DEBORAH: I don't want to talk. Now leave me alone! You are always making me do things I don't want to do. You always force me!

FATHER: Deborah, listen to me. You say that I yell loud? You yell louder than I do. Now listen to me.

DEBORAH: This is not going to get me anyplace.

FATHER: This is going to get you plenty of places. But you're not going to be able to do things you want to in life unless you feel a little better. I don't want to talk about the rest of your life. Right now you'll finish what's on that tray. And I mean every morsel! You understand? Because if you had a little more flesh on you, I'd beat the shit out of you! Do you understand what you've done to this family? Now you eat every goddamn thing that's on that tray! And if you don't, you're not going to leave this room until you do. Now start eating! I'm going to give you three minutes to eat it, and if you don't start, you're going to find it in your ears and your eyes and down your mouth and everywhere else! Now you start eating! I'm not playing any games with you. Because we're past the game-playing stage. I lost my goddamn business and everything else. I lost my wife, and I lost my family because of you. And goddamn it, I'm not going to play any more games with you! Now you eat! Now come on. That's not poison.

DEBORAH: It is poison. Did you try it?

FATHER: All right. I'll eat a little of it. (*He takes a bite of the hot dog.*) Now, is this poison?

DEBORAH: I tried it! (*She sobs hysterically.*)

FATHER: This is good food, and you eat it. Deborah, don't pull that shit on me. Now eat it! If I thought it would kill you, I wouldn't let you eat it. Don't you tell me about cottage cheese and protein. You're no goddamn doctor. Now eat it! Or you'll find milk all over your hair and your body and on your— (*Still sobbing, Deborah takes the hot dog and crushes it.*) Now I told you I'm going to give you a couple of minutes, and then I'm going to feed you myself. Because eventually you're going to get fed with a tube down your stomach anyway. Look at your body, and look at your arms. Now come on, start to eat it. Start to eat! And don't be like a two-year-old baby and make a big fuss out of eating a stupid hot dog. A lot of kids wish to hell they had a hot dog for lunch.

DEBORAH: Well, give it to them!

FATHER: I'm not going to give it to them, I'm giving it to you! And I'm not wasting any food, either. Now Deborah, don't put me in a position where I'm going to get violent, goddamn it. You eat the food, or you're not going to see me in this goddamn hospital again. I don't care if they carry you out of here on a stretcher. Now you eat it. Come on, eat the goddamn hot dog! Deborah, if you don't eat this hot dog, you're going to be sorry.

DEBORAH: I don't want it! (*She crumbles the mush in her hands.*)

FATHER: You eat it! Don't you destroy it, or I'll get you ten more. Now you eat it!

DEBORAH: I don't want it! Look at it! It's ugly!

FATHER: Eat that hot dog! I'm not leaving this place, I swear to God, until you eat it. Eat it! And drink this milk. And eat the peas. I don't mean leave it. Eat that hot dog! God damn you! You son of a bitch! You eat the goddamn hot dog! I told you to eat it! (*He takes the crushed hot dog and shoves it into Deborah's mouth. She resists, and is smeared with food. The therapist intervenes, telling Mr. Kaplan to stop. Mr. Kaplan sits down, visibly exhausted and ashamed of his failure.*)

These three members of the Kaplan family are all seriously troubled individuals. But when one watches the family together, it is the futility of the triad's interactions that impresses the most. The family repeats stereotyped transactions, no matter how many times they prove ineffective. There is no resolution or closure, and no escape. The Kaplans are trapped in a Sisyphean pattern.

Deborah demonstrates the hopelessness and helplessness common to anorectics. "You force everything on me. Everything I ever did," she cries. Her refusal to eat the hot dog is a pathetic assertion of self against her conviction that she has always given in and that she will always be made to give in. This is a classic component of anorexia nervosa.

At the same time, Deborah displays an impressive ability to resist her parents' combined and separate efforts. She seduces them into peripheral issues with great skill, and at times takes on an almost parental stance herself. She feels helpless, but she is far from powerless.

Mrs. Kaplan is desperate. But she is equally incompetent. She is a woman who has devoted her life to being a good wife and mother in accordance with her values. But her futile reasoning, her mindless repetition of ineffective interactions, and her inability to resist Deborah's red herrings all lend credence to her hints that she is part of the problem.

The intensity of the father's authoritarian statements is impressive. But so is their lack of effect. He presents a clear demand, but he always undercuts his own position by a long monolog that delays the necessity to act. If one ignores the noise, his pain becomes apparent. But equally apparent is his inability to give a simple command.

In this family, Deborah is labeled the problem. She suffers from anorexia nervosa, and her illness occupies center stage. "I lost my goddamned business and everything else. I lost my wife, and I lost my family, because of you," the father shouts. To the family, all events and transactions are intermingled with Deborah's terrifying and mysterious refusal to eat. The professionals concur, and the case is labeled "anorexia nervosa." But when these three members of the Kaplan family are seen together, anorexia nervosa seems equally valid as a diagnosis of the family system.

Our work with anorexia nervosa began as a search for more effective models of treating psychosomatic illnesses in children. In the course of ten years of research, we have broadened the scope of both diagnosis and therapy by taking the current conflicts of the anorectic and her family into account. Our paradigm, a systems model, explores the past influence of family members on the development of symptoms. But it also explores the influence of family members on the maintenance of those symptoms in the present. The model delineates, and therefore opens to therapeutic change, aspects of the family members' behavior that currently constrain the anorectic child as well as the other family members and maintain the anorexia syndrome.

Linear and Systems Frameworks

In our study of anorexia nervosa, we found it useful to organize the various approaches to diagnosis and treatment of this disease into two main conceptual models. The first, which we call the linear model, encompasses all the approaches that focus on the individual patient: medical, psychodynamic and behavioral. The second, the systems model, builds on the work of the linear approaches, but goes beyond them to look at the patient in context.

The linear model has governed most efforts to understand anorexia nervosa through the 300-year history of the illness. Until recently, an investigator describing Deborah Kaplan's case would have presented material relating only to her. The case report would have included the kind of feelings she expressed in the interview segment: her sense that she is controlled and helpless, that she is dependent and incompetent, and that her parents run her life. The conflicts between Deborah and her parents might have been described, but they would not have been deemed significant in therapy. Therapy would have focused on Deborah alone.

The linear approach to anorexia nervosa has led to a number of valuable insights into the inner life of the patient and her fantasies around food and eating. But it has also seriously restricted the observation of the syndrome. Diagnosis, and therefore therapy, have tended to zero in on the individual, to the exclusion of the contextual components of the anorexia syndrome. The result has been a treatment outcome that, even with the best practitioners, attains a cure rate of no better than 70 percent, and seems to average a cure rate of 40–60 percent.[3]

The systems model analyzes the behavior and psychological makeup of the individual by emphasizing the continuity of the influences that family members have on each other from the earliest life of the child through the present moment. This model affirms the significance of the individual family member's psychological experience. The individual within the system has large areas of autonomy where he or she transcends the system. But the systems model also requires the observation of how and to what extent interpersonal transactions govern each family member's range of behavior. The systems model thus has a wider lens than the linear. It looks at the individual, but also at the individual in context. Treatment governed by this conceptual model has proven to be 86 percent effective in the fifty-three cases followed up over a period of almost eight years.

The history of the diagnosis and treatment of anorexia nervosa is one of these evolving medical concepts. Approaches to anorexia have changed in response to a general trend to include more and more of the patient's context in the study and treatment of psychosomatic illness—a change in mental health concepts that has followed the same general shift in Western civilization's conceptualization of man. In our time, we have learned that man is a wary traveler on Spaceship Earth, dependent on her dwindling resources. The study of man apart from his circumstances—man as a hero—is being replaced by a view of man as influenced by his context. This change can be traced in the history of anorexia nervosa.

The Medical Model

The first identification of anorexia nervosa is generally credited to an English physician, Richard Morton, who reported on two cases in 1689. His clinical description then included amenorrhea, hyperactivity, and the loss of weight commonly regarded as components of the syndrome today:

> Mr. Duke's Daughter, in St. Mary-Axe, in the year 1684, in the eighteenth year of her age . . . fell into a total suppression of her Monthly Courses from a multitude of Cares and Passions of her Mind. From which time her Appetite began to abate . . . She wholly neglected the care of herself for two full years, till at last being brought to the last degree of Marasmus . . . and thereupon subject to frequent Fainting Fits, and apply'd herself to me for Advice.
> I do not remember that I did ever in all my practice see one, that was conversant with the Living so much wasted . . . (like a Skeleton only clad with skin).

Morton treated this patient with "aromatic bags" applied to the stomach, "bitter medicines," and "antihysterick waters." She seemed to improve, "but being quickly tired with Medicines, she begged that the whole Affair might be committed again to Nature. Whereupon, consuming every day more, she was after three months taken with a Fainting Fit, and died."[4]

The characteristics noted by Morton occur again and again in descriptions of anorexia nervosa. Two hundred years later, W. W. Gull presented a similar picture:

> Miss A., age 17, was brought to me in 1866. Her emaciation was very great. It was stated that she had lost 36 pounds in weight . . . She had amenorrhea for nearly a year . . . Slight con-

stipation. Complete anorexia for animal food and almost complete anorexia for everything else. Abdomen shrunk and flat, collapsed . . . The condition was one of simple starvation . . .

Occasionally for a day or two the appetite was voracious, but this was rare and exceptional. The patient complained of no pain, but was restless and active. This was in fact a striking expression of the nervous state, for it seemed hardly possible that a body so wasted could undergo the exercise which seemed agreeable. There was some peevishness of temper and a feeling of jealousy. No account could be given of the exciting cause.[5]

E. C. Lasègue, who was working in France at about the same time, described the syndrome in terms similar to Gull's.[6] Both suggested a psychological basis for the disease, as had Morton. Lasègue considered it a hysterical phenomenon.

Early investigators noted the influence of the family in anorexia nervosa. J. Naudeau, writing in 1789, attributed an anorectic's death to the influence of her mother.[7] Lasègue, describing anorectics in 1873, observed: "This description . . . would be incomplete without reference to their home life. Both the patient and her family form a tightly knit whole, and we obtain a false picture of the disease if we limit our observation to the patients alone."[8]

These early investigators were medical men. They considered "nervousness" to be causative in anorexia nervosa, but they did not explore this component, just as they did not explore the patient's context. They postulated that the patient's body was responding to unspecified psychological causes, and they explored and treated the organic responses without attempting to differentiate or treat the psychological causes.

Even today investigators apply the same model in the study of anorexia. Research into the possible etiologic role of cerebral, pituitary, and hypothalamic factors is being conducted. Metabolic and hormonal changes seen in patients with anorexia nervosa are being explored. In these investigations, treatment programs are confined to drug therapy with amitriptyline, cyrporheptadine, dilantin, and L-dopa.[9] But the medical model, as Theodore Lidz pointed out, "could not encompass the interrelationship between mind and body, or between the stresses of interpersonal relations and physiologic activities. Psychiatry . . . focused increasingly upon man's development as a social being, reluctantly abandoning animal models to concentrate on man's uniqueness among animals."[10]

The Psychodynamic Model

Anorexia nervosa was early recognized as a psychosomatic syndrome. In fact, according to E. Weiss and O. S. English, it was "one of the clinical syndromes perhaps most responsible for bringing the medical profession to believe that there may be a psychological background for certain physical diseases.[11] Under the influence of psychiatry, particularly of Freud's ideas, in the twentieth century, many investigators in the field of psychosomatic medicine shifted from a concern for somatic manifestations to a concern for the psychological underpinnings of those manifestations.

By the 1930s, the aim of psychosomatic studies was to explore the interrelationships between the psychological and physiological aspects of all bodily functions and to integrate somatic and psychotherapy. The aim was broad, but predictably, the field still showed a tendency to splinter along the lines drawn by its dual nature. On the one hand, there was the tradition of W. B. Cannon, later built upon by H. Selye and H. G. Wolff, which emphasized the physiological concomitants of psychological states.[12] On the other hand, there was the tendency, which has more relevance to anorexia studies, to focus on the psychic components of psychosomatic syndromes.

Psychodynamic investigators were interested primarily in the psychodynamic profiles of patients with specific psychosomatic diseases. The chronological sequence in which Freudian concepts were given specific application to psychosomatic disease reflected a widening inclusion of man's context in psychiatric thinking. H. F. Dunbar, having noted marked similarities in the personality traits of patients with certain psychosomatic diseases, considered that the personality profiles derived from those traits were the important factor in the etiology, prognosis, and therapeutic approach to the diseases.[13] Franz Alexander and his coworkers broadened this formulation to include three other factors that they considered etiologic in specific psychosomatic diseases: organ system vulnerability, genetic or acquired; psychological patterns of conflict and defense; and the immediate situation of the individual at the time of the development of the disease.[14] Roy R. Grinker went still further, regarding the patient as embedded in his social context and emphasizing the need for a system orientation in exploring psychosomatic syndromes.[15]

Under the influence of the early psychodynamic thinking, the study of anorexia nervosa became the search for a specific psychodynamic of the illness. W. Patterson Brown suggested that the ingestion of food symbolized impregnation.[16] J. V. Waller, R. M. Kaufman, and F. Deutsch agreed that in anorexia "psychological factors have a certain specific constellation centering around the symbolization of pregnancy fantasies involving the gastrointestinal tract." They were impressed by the "oft repeated pattern of emphasis on food, alternate over and under eating." The alternation of overeating with disgust for food represented to them a shift in the dynamic conflict. In the first instance, the impregnation fantasy was gratified. In the second, the ensuing guilt and anxiety forbad the intake of food. The amenorrhea and constipation of anorexia nervosa were also viewed as reflecting the pregnancy fantasy.[17]

For a time, psychodynamic theory took precedence over empirical findings. Cases exhibiting the classic symptoms of anorexia—loss of weight, lack of appetite, amenorrhea, and hyperactivity—were not considered anorexia if the psychodynamics of the case did not fit the schema. A presentation by J. H. Masserman was challenged because his descriptions of the dynamics of the case did not include pregnancy fantasies.[18] The specificity theory was becoming a Procrustean bed.

Eventually the theory of a one-to-one correlation between the psychodynamic and the psychosomatic was challenged even in psychoanalytic circles, and more varied explanations appeared. Helmut Thoma described the case of Henrietta A., a nineteen-year-old secondary school girl, who was admitted to the hospital with a diagnosis of anorexia nervosa and underwent 289 sessions of psychoanalysis spread over two years:

> Torn between her inability to be a boy and her dislike of being a girl, she bolstered up her confidence with a new ideal of sexuality . . . By denying "dangerous" aspects of the outside world and by repressing her drives, the patient eventually attained a state of the ego that was free from anxiety . . .
>
> In the anorexia itself, the following psychogenetic processes are discernible. (a) avoidance of realistic drive satisfaction. (b) the fending off of receptivity ("something comes into me") because the unconscious is linking nourishment with impregnation. Revulsion and vomiting are related to the sexual defense. (c) oral satisfaction is connected unconsciously with destruction and killing. Therefore, eating is restricted or is fraught with guilt.[19]

For E. I. Falstein, S. C. Feinstein, and I. Judas the possible psychodynamic sources of anorexia had become almost unlimited: "Eating may be equated with gratification, impregnation, intercourse, performance, growing, castrating, destroying, engulfing, killing, cannibalism. Food may symbolize the breast, the genitals, feces, poison, a parent, or a sibling."[20]

As psychosomatic studies pulled away from the specificity theory, it became possible to bring more of the components of anorexia and of the patient's context into the field of observation. In fact, all models of investigation were responding to the change in world view that saw man increasingly as an acting and reacting member of a social context. More and more, the patient's context was being included as a significant variable in concepts of psychosomatic illness. The locus of pathology, however, was still described as internal. "External" stresses were seen as impinging upon the individual, and the individual remained the focus of diagnosis and treatment.

By the 1950s the various trends in psychosomatic medicine had merged into a conceptual model that linked together the three components of stress, emotion, and illnesses in a linear, causal relationship (fig. 1).[21] This model is like a large funnel. Many factors are recognized as significant in the exploration and treatment of psycho-

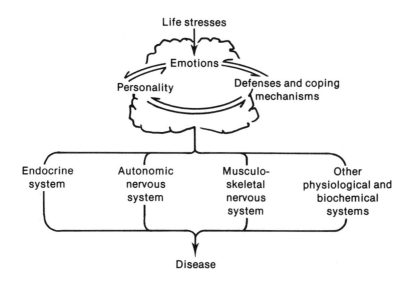

Figure 1. Linear model of psychosomatic disease.

somatic disease, but ultimately they all converge on the individual, who is presumed to be the passive target of their effects.

Much research was focused on fleshing out this model. Sophisticated studies were made on the mechanisms by which the physiological mediating systems were involved in disease, on differentiation of the various kinds of life stress, and on the relevance of personality profiles and psychodynamic patterns. However, the impact of this research was disappointing. Clinical psychosomatic research had not kept pace with developments in other fields of medicine, Engel charged, and experts in psychosomatic medicine had failed to deliver much more than platitudes and largely untestable hypotheses. In particular, he pointed out, the impact of increased understanding had not been reflected by more effective methods of therapy.[22]

The linear model itself was increasingly questioned. Engel specifically rejected the linear concept of psychosomatic etiology, arguing that the pathogenesis of disease involved a series of negative and positive feedbacks.[23] I. A. Mirsky defined psychosomatic medicine as an approach to man which emphasizes that "every level of organization, from the social to the molecular, is involved in the predisposition, and precipitation and the perpetuation of the various clinical derangements that plague man in his society."[24] Grinker too called for a broader viewpoint: "It has become the contemporary task of biological science, advanced by the borrowing of field theory from physics, to study integration in a more sophisticated manner than as a simple relationship between parts . . . Often the psychosomatic field has been sharply broken into fragments . . . [But] today we have come to realize that both the genetic and the transactional approach require for analysis and synthesis the concepts of a field theory.[25]

Hilde Bruch, one of the foremost investigators of anorexia nervosa, also called for a more comprehensive framework for study: "Fascinating as it [is] to unravel the unconscious symbolic motivation, the why of the disturbed eating patterns, the great diversity itself [suggests] the question of how it has been possible for a body function as essential and basic as food intake to develop in such a way that it could be misused so widely in the service of nonnutritional needs."[26] In attempting to devise a broader framework, Bruch hypothesized that something had gone wrong in the anorectic patient's early experiential and interpersonal processes, warping her ability to identify hunger correctly and to distinguish hunger from other states of bodily need or emotional arousal. More specifically, "if confirmation and reinforcement of his own initially rather undifferentiated needs and impulses have been absent, or have been contradictory or inaccurate, then a child will grow up perplexed when trying to differentiate between disturbances in his biological field and emotional and interpersonal experiences, and he will be apt to misinterpret deformities in his self-body concept as externally induced. Thus he will become an individual deficient in his sense of separateness, with diffuse ego boundaries, and will feel helpless under the influence of external forces."[27]

Bruch's work is a serious attempt to encompass the contextual components of anorexia, which have been acknowledged by many investigators. But the boundaries of her exploration are still determined by the linear paradigm. Although she explores the interpersonal, chiefly the interactions between the mother and child, her focus remains on the past, and on the internalization of the interpersonal as an intrapsychic phenomenon. The interactions of patient and family in the here and now are still outside the focus.

Consider Bruch's report of a patient called Gail, who was twenty-one and had been under psychiatric treatment for anorexia nervosa for nearly ten years:

> Her absolute insistence on remaining at this magic weight of 96 pounds led to her dominating the household with enforced rituals. Her parents were forced to shop three times a day because she would not permit food in the home between meals. Any food left over after a meal had to be thrown away, since she feared that she might succumb to the compulsion of eating it and thereby spoil her magic weight ... In order to study, she had to have absolute quiet around the home and her parents were not allowed to be there when she worked ... After one of her hospitalizations her behavior was so violent that her parents moved out into a furnished room, the address of which they kept a strict secret [from Gail] ... It was arranged that Gail and her parents would not communicate directly, but that all messages would go through the social worker, who would also see the parents regularly.[28]

Gail's tragedy was not an individual matter. It was a tragedy involving at least three people, interacting in the present, victimizing and being victimized, enmeshing and seeking escape. However, the diagnosis over ten years of treatment was still individual. Consequently, the treatment of choice was individual therapy, a choice resulting in years of enormous stress for Gail, her parents, and undoubtedly the therapists as well.

The same restrictive organization of data affects the work of many other investigators who observed their patients' family contexts and reported on the family's influence on the syndrome and the syndrome's impact on the family.[29] They described the precipitating factors of anorexia nervosa in family terms, such as marital conflict, the return of a long-absent parent, or a death in the family. Nevertheless, the main thrust of their etiological investigation was to search for the fantasies connected with eating disturbance. Here again, the individual framework created a Procrustean bed. Current conflicts in the family, though well observed and clearly described, were still presented as recurrences of conflicts in the patients' early childhood. The ongoing influence of current circumstances stayed outside the focus. Whereas psychodynamically oriented investigators consistently described anorexia nervosa in terms that should have logically directed their attention to the family context, they continued to deal with the individual patient alone.

The Behavioral Model

In the history of anorexia nervosa, the medical and psychodynamic models have been the two major linear governing concepts. In the past decade, a third approach, operant conditioning, has been added to this conceptualization and treatment of anorexia. Behaviorists interpret the patient's context as a set of contingencies that need to be controlled.

In contrast to psychodynamic investigators, behavioral theorists are much less interested in the origins of processes than in the development of instrumentalities for changing those processes. As Leonard P. Ullman explained, "the behavioral therapist looks at what people are doing, not why they are doing it, in order to design a program that will reinforce behavioral change and extinguish pathological behavior." To the behavioral therapist, Ullman further remarked: "a person's difficulty is his behavior in reaction to situations, and . . . this behavior is the result of previous and current reinforcing stimuli and is not symptomatic of some deeper underlying discontinuity with normal functioning that must be dealt with prior to the emitted behavior . . . In evaluating a situation, the behavior therapist must shift from the traditional why questions to what questions. He must ask: What is the person doing? Under what conditions are these behaviors emitted? . . . What other behaviors might the person emit?[30]

John Paul Brady and Wolfram Rieger, when using behavioral therapy in the treatment of anorectics, approached the syndrome as an eating phobia: "Eating generates anxiety, and their failure to eat represents avoidance. In other words . . . cessation of eating after ingesting a very small portion of a meal (or removing it from the body by self-induced vomiting) is reinforced by anxiety reduction. From such an analysis, two treatment procedures suggest themselves: deconditioning the anxiety associated with eating, and/or shaping eating behavior . . . by making access to powerful reinforcers contingent on eating."[31] Such a precise, clear analysis makes it possible for the behaviorist to create a milieu for the hospitalized patient in which appropriate contingencies are developed. Because the hospital context can be controlled, behavior in this environment can be changed.

Unfortunately, the focus on the individual's dysfunctional learning has handicapped the behavioral therapist in drawing appropriate conclusions from his own data. Once the patient has achieved the desired weight gain in the hospital, she is commonly returned to her unchanged environment, which of course is not controlled by the behavioral therapist. It is not surprising, therefore, that in a large percentage of cases the improvement is not sustained after the patient has been discharged from the hospital.

Only the barest outline of the history of anorexia nervosa has been presented here. There are cases in the literature reporting cures by the use of methods ranging from frontal lobotomy to conversion to Christian Science. But most of the methods reported effective in some cases have been reported ineffective in others. In many reports, it is impossible to derive even an estimate of results. Where results are given, the success rate attains a level no higher than 70 percent.

In any other field, such a disappointing outcome would certainly call the procedures used into question. Unfortunately, investigators of anorexia nervosa have demonstrated, to a startling degree, the blinders imposed on the scientist by his conceptual model. Practitioners maintain their previously learned paradigms as though they were causes to be defended, not hypotheses to be tested.

Thomas S. Kuhn, in examining this tendency of researchers to cling to existing models and to resist change, contended that the scientist's vision is severely restricted because, "to an extent unparalleled in most fields, they have undergone similar educations and professional initiations; in the process they have absorbed the same technical literature and drawn many of the same lessons from it. Usually the boundaries of that standard literature mark the limits of a scientific subject matter." Much of the success of the scientific community in fact derives from its willingness to defend its shared assumptions—or "normal science," in Kuhn's terminology —"if necessary at considerable cost. Normal science, for example, often suppresses fundamental novelties because they are necessarily subversive of its basic commitments." But, Kuhn suggests, when the profession "can no longer evade anomalies that subvert the existing tradition of scientific practice—then begin the extraordinary investigations that lead the profession at last to a new set of commitments, a new basis for the practice of science."[32] His formulation bears considerable relevance to the history of anorexia nervosa.

The Systems Model

Today, many investigators are beginning to include in their formulations the interdependence of parts in a social context. The governing framework for their approach is the systems model. This model posits a circular movement of parts that affect each other (fig. 2). The system can be activated at any number of points, and feedback mechanisms are operative at many points. The activation and regulation of the system can be done by system members or by forces outside the system.

In the linear model, the behavior of the individual is seen as sparked by others. It presumes an action and a reaction, a stimulus and a response, or a cause and an effect. In the systems paradigm, every part of a system is seen as organizing and being organized by other parts. An individual's behavior is simultaneously both caused and causative. A beginning or an end are defined only by arbitrary framing and punctuating. The action of one part is, simultaneously, the interrelationship of other parts of the system.

The systems model postulates that certain types of family organization are closely related to the development and maintenance

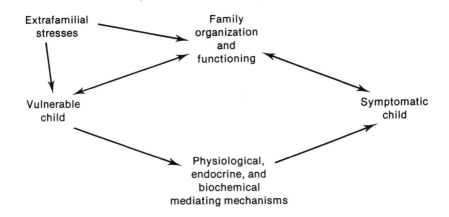

Figure 2. Open systems model of psychosomatic disease.

of psychosomatic syndromes in children, and that the child's psychosomatic symptoms in turn play an important role in maintaining the family homeostasis. Anorexia nervosa is defined not only by the behavior of one family member, but also by the interrelationship of all family members.

This model challenges our everyday experience. We all tend to experience ourselves as the unit of our lives. When psychiatry, therefore, deals with transactions among people as introjects in the individual's experience, it is merely validating the common reality. The systems model demands a quantum jump: acceptance that dependency and control, attraction and aggression, symbiosis and avoidance, are more than introjects. They are interpersonal interactions in the present. The psychological unit is not the individual. It is the individual in his significant social contexts.

Nowhere is the truth of this modern challenge demonstrated more clearly than in the studies of psychosomatic medicine. It seems to violate common sense that the contraction of a child's bronchiole is regulated by sequences of transaction between other family members. Or that a diabetic patient's ketoacidosis is affected by the way his parents request his allegiance. Or that an anorectic's not eating is controlled by the way the anorectic and her parents transact the issues of control. Nevertheless, our findings clearly indicate that, when significant family interactional patterns are changed, significant changes in the symptoms of psychosomatic illness also occur.

The change to a systems paradigm results in a different observational frame. Instead of observing and studying the anorectic
child alone, we look at the feedback processes by which the family
members and the anorectic constrain and regulate each other's
behavior. In therapy, we look at the transactions among family
members that sustain the anorectic syndrome, and we work to
change those transactions. Anorexia nervosa becomes more than
Deborah's not eating. It is the way the Kaplan family behaves.

The Psychosomatic Family

2

Mental health practitioners do not, as a rule, deal with issues of life and death. If a patient suffers a psychotic breakdown, or if there are bickering and unhappiness in a family, the therapist can take his time in unraveling these mysteries of life. But when a therapist deals with a seriously disturbed psychosomatic patient, he suddenly enters a more dramatic arena. The psychosomatic diabetic, the severely asthmatic child, or the cachectic anorectic are children whose lives are in danger.

We were drawn into the field of psychosomatic medicine, not by any fixed philosophical bent, but by the severity of the clinical problems posed by patients who came under our care. Like many other projects in psychosomatic medicine, ours grew out of a disappointment with the therapeutic results of individually oriented approaches. New ideas in the mental health field, highlighted by our own observations, encouraged us to broaden our focus to include extraindividual components of the psychosomatic process which had always been peripheral to the individual concept frameworks.

Early Explorations on Diabetes

The patients who first forced us to question the methods for studying and treating the relationship between psyche and soma were diabetic children who had undergone unusually numerous hospitalizations for diabetic acidosis. Such hospitalization should be an infrequent occurrence in a diabetic child's life. Acidosis may be one of the initial, presenting symptoms in a child with previously undiagnosed diabetes. But it is rare for a diabetic child to be rehospitalized for acidosis once treatment has begun, primarily because the child and the family, after having learned to recognize the early warning signals for impending acidosis, can treat it correctly at home by administering supplemental doses of insulin. Repeated bouts of diabetic acidosis are therefore distinctly unusual and are generally thought to be avoidable.

But unlike children with "normal" diabetes, these children did not respond as expected to an optimal medical regimen. They continued to suffer from medically inexplicable attacks of acidosis. As a result, they were virtually crippled by their disease, requiring repeated hospitalizations—as often as ten to fifteen times per year—to correct life-threatening diabetic acidosis. The initial approach to these children was to hospitalize them once more in order to evaluate thoroughly any organic factors that might be responsible for the repeated bouts of acidosis, to reeducate the child and the family in acting early to prevent diabetic acidosis, and to look for any other complicating factors. The children were placed on what was considered an optimal diabetic regimen, which would prevent repeated hospitalizations.

During this hospitalization no complicating organic factors were found that might explain the repeated bouts of acidosis. The children and their parents were given intensive diabetic education. The pediatric team was therefore taken aback when, following the children's discharge, the previous pattern of hospitalization persisted. This outcome was particularly striking because these children had been easy to take care of while in the hospital and their diabetic control had been excellent.

Because of the fortuitous referral of three diabetic girls in close succession, it seemed that there was always one girl in the hospital recovering from acidosis, one on the way to the emergency room for treatment, and one on the telephone reporting that things at home were sliding inexorably downhill. The most baffling aspect of their cases was the repeated observation that these children did not respond as expected to insulin administered at home. One of the girls, whose daily insulin requirement was 30 units, received over 500 units of insulin at home within an eighteen-hour span. The insulin, which had been administered to the child by the mother, was later checked and found to have full biologic potency. Nevertheless, the child still had to be admitted to the hospital because of diabetic acidosis. In the hospital, following correction of her acidosis, she once again required only 30 units of insulin to achieve satisfactory control of her diabetes.

The three girls were much alike. All were in early adolescence and appeared quiet, gentle, and pleasant. They were model patients, often helping the nurses to care for the younger children on the wards. Their families appeared stable, helpful, concerned, and eager to follow instructions. In the traditional medical model, the absence of organic factors suggested that the disorder be considered functional, or of psychogenic origin. Psychiatric consultation was therefore obtained, and the children were entered into therapy.

Although different individually oriented psychiatrists saw each child, the psychiatric formulations of the problems in each case were similar: the patients had difficulty in handling "stress," they tended to internalize anger, and they were somewhat immature in their ability to cope with difficult situations. It therefore seemed that these children had a major psychosomatic component to their disease in the most literal sense, that is, an emotional arousal of their psyche causally and directly led to a decompensation of their diabetic state. While it was clear that emotions were not the cause of the diabetes, it was becoming more and more evident that emotions and emotional arousal were the key to the repeated bouts of acidosis.

The girls were begun on individual psychotherapy oriented toward defining personality issues and reducing "stress factors." The families were involved only in the sense that they were told to be extremely gentle in their handling of the children and to be careful not to add any further stress at home.

But the weekly therapy sessions had no obvious impact on the hospitalization patterns, for the bouts of acidosis continued. Consequently, the children were sent to an intermediate care facility associated with the acute care hospital, where individual therapy sessions were continued. Again, no problems with diabetic control were encountered while the children were institutionalized. This result was viewed as corroboration of the formulation which held that these children had a low threshold of response to stress.

The therapeutic endeavors at this time were shaped by the linear model of psychosomatic disease. The child was viewed as a "container and carrier" of the disease. External stresses and the child's personality profile were viewed as the key factors. Consequently, an effort was made to treat the patient on an individual basis, in order to make her understand and express her emotions more appropriately and to help her acquire better coping capacities. Some attempt was also made to reduce external stressful situations.

The importance of the family was recognized, but only in a non-specific manner. The striking difference between the ease of diabetic control in the hospital and the impossibility of diabetic control in the home led to the conclusion that the family environment was somehow noxious. The child was viewed as the passive recipient of external stress—a victim of her environment. The resulting therapeutic decision was to separate the child from the family—to perform, in the old phraseology, a "parentectomy." In each case, the bouts of ketoacidosis reappeared when the child was returned home.

Because of this lack of therapeutic success, a new pediatric-psychiatric team composed of the authors was set up. The psychiatric members of the team, who came from a background of family therapy, set out to investigate the role of the family in the child's illness and, equally important, to explore the function of the child's illness in the family.[1] The pediatric members of the team set as their task the study of the mediating mechanisms by which emotional arousal could be translated into diabetic acidosis. In the end, these two areas of investigation merged, when it was shown that the emotional arousal of the child and its metabolic consequences are best documented within the family context.

The Metabolic Studies

For a child with diabetes to go into acidosis, there must be a preceding rise in the concentration of free fatty acids (FFA) found in the blood. These acids are the substrates or "building blocks" from which the liver produces the excessive amounts of ketone bodies that give rise to the disease of ketoacidosis. Previous observations in the field of psychophysiology had shown that free fatty acids can also serve as a marker for emotional arousal.[2] In the diabetic child there is thus a measure which at one and the same time reflects emotional arousal and signals the advent of the psychosomatic symptom. As researchers, we therefore began to set up experimental situations in which changes in FFA were used to document the relationship between emotional arousal and psychosomatic crisis.

At this time, the physiological studies continued to be shaped by the linear framework. We wanted to assess the role of psychological stress in the control of the child's diabetes. We knew that free fatty acids were both a marker for emotional arousal and a metabolic intermediary for the production of excessive amounts of ketones, and that they could therefore be viewed as a key link in the sequence through which emotional arousal can be mediated into diabetic acidosis. A series of interviews to explore and document this sequence was designed. The families of the children involved were informed as to the nature and purpose of the interviews and gave their informed consent for the children's participation.

Two interviews compared FFA levels in the diabetic child under both nonstressful and stressful conditions. The stressful interview was designed to elicit the child's anger but at the same time to inhibit her repression of this emotion—a design based on the classic linear model of psychosomatic disease. A third interview tested the effects of a beta-adrenergic blocking agent on the emotional arousal as measured by a rise in the FFA sequence. A beta-adrenergic blocking agent does not interfere with emotional arousal but will ultimately block the release of free fatty acids. The results of these experiments were impressive. Emotional arousal in the stressful interview was accompanied by a dramatic rise in the concentration of free fatty acids, which if sustained could have quickly led to diabetic acidosis in the child. These metabolic consequences were, however, almost completely aborted in the third interview with the introduction of the blocking agent.

This indication that the physiological consequences of emotional arousal can be altered by the use of beta-adrenergic blocking agents led to long-term therapeutic trials of beta-adrenergic blockade in the affected children. The early results of this therapy were encouraging. Longer experience, however, has indicated that the beta-adrenergic blockade approach is not a panacea. A psychosomatic crisis in children with diabetes can break through the beta blockade, just as insulin's effectiveness can be inhibited.[3]

These experiments represented an attempt both to analyze the mediating pathways by which emotional arousal is converted to diabetic acidosis, and to gain more specific information about "stress," or exactly what it is that can produce disease in these children. The research was still constrained within the linear model, the family environment being viewed as one of several noxious factors impinging upon the child. Then one of our patients caused us to re-evaluate this thinking.

The child in question had averaged one hospitalization every three weeks for diabetic acidosis for a period of two years. Despite weekly sessions with a psychiatrist, oriented around individual personality and coping issues, no change had been seen in the pattern of her admissions. It was then decided to take the child and her family into family therapy.

We as family therapists tried an approach diametrically opposed to the tack taken by the psychiatrist who had previously treated this child. Instead of assuming a supportive role to shield her from stress, we deliberately induced family crises. The strategy was designed to actualize hidden conflicts in the session, to help the family deal with them, and to help the child engage in these conflicts as an autonomous individual.

The therapy sessions, often quite dramatic, were accompanied by a change in the pattern of hospital admissions. The child, having previously been admitted for acidosis every three to four weeks, now entered the hospital in acidosis every week. The family sessions were held on Tuesday afternoon; the child was regularly admitted some time between Monday evening and Tuesday evening. During these difficult weeks, when both pediatricians and psychiatrists were responding to each episode of acidosis at no matter what time it occurred, the pediatric-psychiatric team was forged. The psychiatrists felt free to continue this interventionist approach because of the backup support of the pediatrician, and the pediatrician was reassured by seeing the psychiatrists' commitment to the patient during bedside family therapy sessions held in the middle of the night after the acute acidosis had been corrected with intravenous fluids and insulin.

After several months of family therapy, major changes were observed in the family and in the child's role in her family. In particular, the parents were able to initiate and negotiate conflicts without involving their daughter. Concomitant with these changes, the pattern of hospitalizations was broken.[4] This case has now been followed up for nine years. During that time, the child has not once been hospitalized for inexplicable ketoacidosis.

As we reviewed the research and treatment results in the diabetic children, it became more and more apparent that we were witnessing two sides of the same coin. Emotional arousal could produce elevations of plasma free-fatty-acid concentration which, in turn, could lead to ketoacidosis. In addition, the more these children were seen in therapy that involved and changed their families, the more apparent it became that arousal was related to the family in specific, testable ways.

Development of a Clinical Model

While working with diabetics, we began to study and treat children with asthma whose clinical course was far more severe than could be accounted for by the organic disease. At about the same time we also began seeing cases of anorexia nervosa.

From the beginning, we considered these three groups to represent different instances of psychosomatic illness. We distinguished however, between "primary" and "secondary" psychosomatic disorders. In the primary disorders, a physiological dysfunction is already present. These include metabolic disorders like diabetes and allergic diathesis such as that found in asthma. The psychosomatic element lies in the emotional exacerbation of the already available symptom. Thus, a child with diabetes who has recurrent bouts of ketoacidosis triggered by emotional arousal can be considered a "psychosomatic diabetic." Likewise, a child with asthma whose recurrent and severe attacks represent an exacerbation of the underlying disorder in response to emotional rather than physiological stimuli can be termed a "psychosomatic asthmatic." In no way does this imply a psychological etiology for the original disease. In the secondary psychosomatic disorders, no such predisposing physical dysfunction can be demonstrated. The psychosomatic element is apparent in the transformation of emotional conflicts into somatic symptoms. These symptoms may crystallize into a severe and debilitating illness like anorexia nervosa.

Symptom choice may thus be differently determined in these two instances. We questioned whether patients with primary or secondary disorders might also differ in terms of their family dynamics and organization. However, as we worked in therapy with the families of the children with these different psychosomatic presenting problems, we began to realize that certain transactional patterns seemed to be characteristic of all the families. The family of a psychosomatic diabetic functioned in significant ways very like the family of an anorectic or a psychosomatic asthmatic. But the functioning of these "psychosomatic families" differed markedly from the functioning of the families of normal diabetics who came into therapy for other problems. Continued immersion in family therapy sessions permitted us to sharpen these observations and, as our experience grew, to generalize from family to family, until we finally evolved an exploratory model of the psychosomatic family.

Four characteristics of overall family functioning emerged from our observations. No one of these characteristics alone seemed sufficient to spark and reinforce psychosomatic symptoms. But the cluster of transactional patterns was felt to be characteristic of a family process that encourages somatization. The four family characteristics are enmeshment, overprotectiveness, rigidity, and lack of conflict resolution.

Enmeshment refers to an extreme form of proximity and intensity in family interactions. It has implications at all levels: family, subsystem, and individual. In a highly enmeshed, overinvolved family, changes within one family member or in the relationship between two members reverberate throughout the system. Dialogs are rapidly diffused by the entrance of other family members. A dyadic conflict may set off a chain of shifting alliances within the whole family as other members get involved. Or one family member may relay messages from another to a third, blocking direct communication.

Subsystem boundaries in enmeshed families are poorly differentiated, weak, and easily crossed. This situation results in the inadequate performance of subsystem functions. For instance, the spouse relationship is subordinated to carrying out parental functions. Or parental control of children is ineffective. When boundaries are crossed, children may act inappropriately parental toward parents or siblings. Or a child may join or be enlisted by one parent against the other in decision making.

On an individual level, interpersonal differentiation in an enmeshed system is poor. In all families, individual members are regulated by the family system. But in enmeshed families the individual gets lost in the system. The boundaries that define individual autonomy are so weak that functioning in individually differentiated ways is radically handicapped. Excessive togetherness and sharing bring about a lack of privacy. Family members intrude on each others' thoughts and feelings. All these problems of enmeshment are reflected in the family members' poorly differentiated perceptions of each other and, usually, of themselves.

The overprotectiveness of the psychosomatic family shows in the high degree of concern of family members for each others' welfare. This concern is not limited to the identified patient or to the area of illness. Nurturing and protective responses are constantly elicited and supplied. Family members are hypersensitive to signs of distress, cueing the approach of dangerous levels of tension or conflict. In such families, the parents' overprotectiveness retards the children's development of autonomy, competence, and interests or activities outside the safety of the family.

The children in turn, particularly the psychosomatically ill child, feel great responsibility for protecting the family. For the sick child, the experience of being able to protect the family by using the symptoms may be a major reinforcement for the illness.

Rigid families are heavily committed to maintaining the status quo. In periods when change and growth are necessary, they experience great difficulty. For example, when a child in an effectively functioning family reaches adolescence, his family can change its rules and transactional patterns in ways that allow for increased age-appropriate autonomy while still preserving family continuity. But the family of a psychosomatically ill child insists on retaining the accustomed methods of interaction. Issues that threaten change, such as negotiations over individual autonomy, are not allowed to surface to the point where they can be explored. Even when coming into therapy, these families typically represent themselves as normal and untroubled, except for the one child's medical problem. They deny any need for change in the family. Such families are highly vulnerable to external events, such as changes in occupation or loss of kin. Almost any outside event may overload their dysfunctional coping mechanisms, precipitating illness.

The rigidity and overprotectiveness of the psychosomatic family system, combined with the constant mutual impingements characteristic of pathologically enmeshed transactional patterns, make such families' thresholds for conflict very low. Usually a strong religious or ethical code is used as a rationale for avoiding conflict. As a result, problems are left unresolved, to threaten again and again, continually activating the system's avoidance circuits.

Each psychosomatic family's idiosyncratic structure and functioning dictate its ways of avoiding conflict. Often one spouse is an avoider. When the nonavoider brings up areas of difficulty, the avoider manages to detour confrontation that would lead to the acknowledgement of conflict and, perhaps, its negotiation. Or one spouse simply leaves the house when the other tries to discuss a problem.

Many psychosomatic families deny the existence of any problems whatsoever, see "no need" ever to disagree, and are highly invested in consensus and harmony. Other psychosomatic families disagree openly, but constant interruptions and subject changes obfuscate any conflictual issue before it is brought to salience. Family members quickly mobilize to maintain a manageable threshold of conflict. They achieve this control through position shifts or distractive maneuvers that diffuse issues. Whether the families with psychosomatically ill children avoid or diffuse, an inability to confront differences to the extent of negotiating resolution is characteristic of all such families. Normal families are able to disagree.

These are the four general structural and functional characteristics that were identified as typical of families with psychosomatic children. However, while they are descriptive of a stress-inducing family context for a vulnerable child, the identification of these characteristics alone would not have moved us from a linear to a systems explanation for the etiology and maintenance of the psychosomatic child's symptom. It was the observation of the circularity of feedback that necessitated the move to a new order of explanation.

Viewed from a transactional point of view, the patient's symptom acquired new significance as a regulator in the family system. More specifically, it became apparent that the key factor supporting the particular symptom was the child's involvement in parental conflict. This factor, then, is the fifth characteristic of a psychosomatic family.

Within the psychosomatic family context, the symptomatic child is involved in parental conflict in particular ways. Parents unable to deal with each other directly unite in protective concern for their sick child, avoiding conflict by protective detouring. Or a marital conflict is transformed into a parental conflict over the patient and her management. In some families, the child is recruited into taking sides by the parents, or intrudes herself as a mediator or helper. The effectiveness of the symptom bearer in regulating the internal stability of the family reinforces both the continuation of the symptom and the peculiar aspects of the family organization in which it emerged.

In our therapeutic work with psychosomatic families, there

emerged characteristic patterns of conflict-related behavior that involved the child. Families may move from one to another of these patterns over time, but one tends to predominate. The three conflict avoidance patterns of involvement that we identified were triangulation, parent-child coalition, and detouring.

In the first two patterns, triangulation and parent-child coalitions, the spouse dyad is frankly split in opposition or in conflict, and the child is openly pressed to ally with one parent against the other. In triangulation, the child is put in such a position that she cannot express herself without siding with one parent against the other. Statements that impose a choice, such as "Wouldn't you rather do it my way?" are used in the attempt to force the child to take sides. In a parent-child coalition, the child tends to move into a stable coalition with one parent against the other. The role of the excluded parent varies according to the degree that he or she tries to disrupt the coalition.

In the third type of pattern, detouring, the spouse dyad is ostensibly united. The parents submerge their conflicts in a posture of protecting or blaming their sick child, who is defined as the only family problem. In some families, the parents require the children to reassure them that they are good parents or to join them in worrying about the family. The parents occasionally vacillate between their concern for the sick child and their exasperation over the burdens that she imposes by "not trying to help herself." In most cases, parental concerns absorb the couple, so that all signs of marital strife or even minor differences are suppressed or ignored.

These three patterns of involvement are not themselves family classifications. They describe transactional sequences that occur in response to family conflict. Such sequences, which often occur in effectively functioning families, are within the wide range of methods that families use to cope with conflict. However, the families in the normal range can shift to other modes of conflict confrontation and negotiation. The families with a psychosomatically ill child enact maladaptive sequences again and again. Because they are usually operating under conditions of stress and tension, the child is frequently involved in the role of conflict defuser.

Verification of the Model

The development of the exploratory model in the context of the family therapy sessions was exciting, and it helped us greatly in organizing our thinking. But in order to test the validity of this model, it was necessary to conduct a more formal study. Special techniques had to be developed to permit the collection of quantifiable data in a behavioral domain comparable to a therapeutic interview.

In order to take a more rigorous look at the first four characteristics hypothesized as being typical of psychosomatic families, we developed a standardized interview that enabled us to analyze each family as it carried out a series of family tasks. This approach required us to operationalize our concepts by identifying specific behavioral referents for them in each task. It also allowed us to compare psychosomatic with nonpsychosomatic and normal families, for whom therapy material would have been unavailable or noncomparable.

The observations told us little about such factors as intrapsychic dynamics, individual psychopathology, or the strengths and weaknesses of individual family members. These aspects of functioning, though real, could have been studied through other types of assessment, such as questionnaires, projective tests, and individual interviews with each family member. However, those other tests would not have enabled us to evaluate the family relationships, which require direct observation of the family in action.

Similarly, in order to explore our hypotheses about the involvement of the child in parental conflict, we designed a family diagnostic interview which recreated a conflict situation in the family and opened the ensuing family transactions to observation. This broadening of the observational field not only provided the needed data but also fostered the emergence of new data and new aspects of what was being seen. We were also able to assess physiological indicators of emotional arousal directly, via FFA markers, in this experimental family stress context.

Altogether, forty-five families were involved in the research, all of whom were studied prior to therapy. The three psychosomatic groups who participated included eleven families with anorectic children, nine families with psychosomatic diabetic children, and ten families with asthmatic children. There were two control groups: seven families with normal or nonpsychosomatic diabetic children, and eight families with diabetics whose illness was under good medical control but who had been referred for behavioral problems.

In all the psychosomatic cases, frequent and severe symptoms that could not be explained on any organic basis were present. The diagnosis of psychosomatic was always made by the pediatrician, who indicated that there were no organic or physiological reasons for the difficulty of medical management.

The two control groups of diabetic children were studied in order to compare them with the psychosomatic children. The normal diabetic children were included because they shared with the psychosomatic patients a serious chronic illness, with all that this entails for the family. The behavioral diabetic children provided a useful comparison, first because they were identified as psychiatric patients, similar in this respect to all three psychosomatic groups, and second because they were behavioral deviants, unlike the psychosomatic diabetics and asthmatics but similar to the anorectics from a functional point of view.

The Family Task

The family task administered in our study was an elaboration of the Wiltwyck Family Task, which involves engaging the family in a series of interactive tasks that they administer and carry out by themselves.[5] This technique has the advantage of enabling the researcher to study the family in a quasi-natural situation without the shaping of an interviewer. The questions are recorded on a tape, which the family members start and stop by themselves. They seat themselves as they wish. They answer or not; they understand or avoid. In short, they make it their own family task.

Each family was asked in succession to make up a menu together, to discuss a family argument, to describe what pleased and displeased them about other family members, to make up stories about family pictures, and to put together a color forms design (for complete protocol, see Appendix A). Two siblings were requested to join with the identified patient and parents in carrying out this procedure in order to get a more comprehensive view of the family. All of the transactions were videotaped and, subsequently, counted, rated, and scored by independent raters.

A major task for the experimenters was to operationalize the concepts of enmeshment, overprotectiveness, low tolerance for conflict, and rigidity so that they could be assessed in the family's transactions around carrying out the task. Enmeshment, for example, was scored at three levels: family, subsystem, and individual-interpersonal. Information from the task items was utilized within each of these areas. The scores at the family level reflected the family functioning as a whole. To evaluate this area, the pattern of communications was examined. The extent to which people acted as communication go-betweens was measured, as was the distribution of the spoken transactional sequences to, through, and around certain family members. Shifting alliances, defined as arbitrary and alternating switches of support from one member to another, were rated as an index of overall family enmeshment. All of these factors were seen as indicators of the excessive interdependence of family members.

The assessment of enmeshment at the subsystem level focused on the clarity of boundaries between the parents and the children. First, the quantity, effectiveness, and unity of the parents' executive behavior in controlling the family in the process of performing the task were objectively rated and counted. Secondly, both cross-subsystem alliances, such as parent and child versus parent, particularly in relation to executive activities, and the executive dominance of one parent as compared to the other were examined, because these factors were considered to reflect the weakening of subsystem boundaries. Finally, individual-interpersonal differentiation was reflected in the degree to which individualized percepts and expectations of other family members emerged in each one's likes and dislikes, and in the extent to which family members "read each other's minds" or answered for another person.

An overview, however, of the behavioral definitions, quantitative data, and analyses is all that is needed here; a more detailed report is given elsewhere.[6] Although the trends reported here are descriptive and clinical in tone, they represent formal categories whose reliabilities and significance levels have been established. *The results are presented so as to contrast the anorectic group with the two other psychosomatic groups (asthmatic and diabetics) on the one hand, and with the control groups (behaviorals and normals) on the other.*

Normal families differed most from the others on the indices of enmeshment, being particularly strong on clear subsystem boundaries and having a higher degree of interpersonal differentiation. While behavioral problem families showed poor parental executive functioning in terms of effectiveness, the anorectic and other psychosomatic families were most deficient in parent-child subsystem differentiation. A child, for example, would run the task or consult with one parent about what to advise the other parent. In these families there was more imbalance within the parental subsystem, so that one parent would do most of the executive work, directing activities and managing the family, while the other parent joined the child in responding to this management. On the interpersonal level family members were intrusive and tended to be global in expressing their percepts of other family members. For example, instead of saying what they liked or disliked about husband or son, mothers would say, "I like it when we're all happy together," or "I'm unhappy when the kids fight."

On a family level, all of the dysfunctional families, both psychosomatic and behavioral, showed a skew or uneven distribution in the speaking pattern. But the anorectic and other psychosomatic families were most likely to have members who acted as mediating go-betweens. For example, in one family all of the members spoke only to the mother, while she, the most talkative, communicated with all of them. In other families the members passed messages back and forth through one another. In sum, whereas some of the behavioral families were enmeshed according to the criteria, and some of the normals showed occasional enmeshed behavior, the anorectic and psychosomatic families as a group were more outstanding in this multifaceted dimension.

Overprotectiveness was assessed behaviorally, both by counting instances of nurturant-protective or protectiveness-eliciting behavior, and by analyzing the content of the family argument and of other items for protective themes. The behavioral measures were the more definitive in distinguishing the normal diabetic families from the anorectic and psychosomatic groups. For example, crying by a parent, child, or sibling occurred only in the psychosomatic families, as did concern about hunger and physical comfort.

The evaluation of conflict avoidance and diffusion was more complex, requiring consideration of the making of simple decisions in addition to the handling of arguments and real conflicts. Normal families were able to both agree and disagree more, just as they were able to consider more alternatives. Occasionally they denied having any arguments or "fights," but they were able to state issues clearly and to resolve them in some satisfactory way. The behavioral families tended to diffuse an unresolved conflict, but they were more able to express conflict directly than the psychosomatic groups. Some anorectic families agreed on everything instantly, denied or suppressed any mention of conflicts, or took advantage of the anorectic child's noncompliance with the meal-planning task to skip through the interview or focus only on her. Other anorectic families went on and on about poorly defined arguments, which they then rejected as unsuitable for the task. In this area, as in the assessment of protectiveness, the transactional behavior was more discriminating between the groups than was the content of their task responses.

The final characteristic, rigidity, was the most difficult to define in terms of family task performance. We have begun to look at the extent to which alliance patterns, namely the ways in which the family members group themselves with regard to such matters as making choices and supporting decisions, are flexible and develop in relation to functional or objective tasks and topics rather than being fixed or bound regardless of the issue. For example, a mother in a functional family supported her daughter's food suggestion in making up a menu but united with her husband around setting a family rule. In the dysfunctional families, it seemed that alliances usually ended up in fixed patterns. For example, a father who started out supporting someone in the family on an issue would always shift, ending up in support of a particular daughter, regardless of whatever position she embraced. However, further operationalizing of this factor in family interaction is necessary.

The Family Diagnostic Interview

While the family task provided the opportunity to study the four structural characteristics of the family for a time-limited period, it did not usually reveal the way in which the vulnerable child was used to detour conflict. The family was in control of the situation and could to a large extent avoid stress or conflict. The family diagnostic interview was therefore designed in order to assess simultaneously the child's involvement in parental conflict and the physiological effects of parental conflict on the child's disease.

The idea of this interview was to bring about conflict between the parents, based on issues that were idiosyncratic to each family. A therapist would exacerbate the conflict beyond the family's usual threshold of tolerance and then, when the conflict was at its height, bring the child into the situation. The triadic interaction could be evaluated for both its psychological content and the physiological consequences.

The interview was also employed to verify a theory we had formulated during family sessions about the development of a psychosomatic crisis. We hypothesized that it consists of two phases, which encompass both psychological and physiological components. In the "turn on" phase, a situation produces emotional arousal in the child, which in turn triggers physiological responses. At some later point there is a time for "turn off," with a return of the physiological responses toward baseline levels. A psychosomatic crisis could therefore be related to the exaggerated nature of the physiological responses in the turn-on phase, or it could be due to difficulties in the turn-off phase. The family diagnostic interview, by eliciting idiosyncratic family conflict and involving the child in parental conflict, enabled us to study the physiological responses of the child to her emotional arousal in both the turn-on and turn-off phases.

An important feature of the interview was the combination of naturalistic observation with the experimental manipulation of family variables. The identified patient was seen in a significant natural context: she was in a transactional situation with her parents, interacting around issues selected by her parents and particular to that family. It was possible not only to understand the individual patient's experience and behavior better, but also to evaluate her parents' experience of her, as well as the ways in which the three family members regulated each other's behavior. At the same time the experimental format permitted the manipulation of the idiosyncratic family variables—such as to increase the intensity of the conflict by handicapping escape, by supporting one member against another, or by prolonging the duration of the conflict—even though the family members evolved its content by themselves. Unfortunately the complexities of developing the experimental situation did not permit the inclusion of siblings, as was possible in the family task.

The format of the family diagnostic interview was standardized to comprise three stages. In stage one the parents were seated in an interview room, with the child in an observation room behind a one-way mirror. Heparin locks (intravenous blood sampling units) had earlier been inserted in the arm of each family member, after which there had been a half-hour equilibration period. During the interview the arm attached to the unit was allowed to rest on a table behind a screen. The lab personnel remained out of sight behind this screen, where they could draw blood samples unobtrusively. After the parents had been seated, the psychiatric interviewer told them to discuss a family problem, and then left.

After half an hour the interviewer returned, for the start of stage two. Using the technique of supporting one spouse against the other, he attempted to exacerbate, or in some families to elicit, family conflict around the issues that they had chosen. At the end of another half-hour, the interviewer brought the child into the interview room, launching stage three. The therapist asked the parents and the child to help each other decide how they should change. After this stage, which lasted half an hour, the interview proper was terminated. The family was taken to a comfortable office in which to relax. After this period of turn off and rest, a debriefing was held with the family in order to make sure that the interview had no undesirable consequences.

During each stage of the interview, including the rest period, blood samples were taken, from which FFA levels were subsequently calculated. All of the interviews were videotaped for content analysis of the interactions. Thus we were in a position to analyze both the transactional and the physiological sequences in parallel. The videotaped interviews were rated in the same manner as the family task videotapes, that is, by independent, "blind" raters according to criteria developed by the researchers.

Transactional Results

Our purpose during the first two stages of the interview was to find out how the parents dealt with conflictual issues when the child was not physically present, even though they knew that the child could see and hear their discussion. The behavior of the spouses was rated along three dimensions: activity level—who talked and how much; conflict initiation—who raised conflictual issues and how frequently; and conflict level—the intensity and degree of mutual confrontation by the spouses. It was important to determine whether all of the children were being exposed to equally stressful situations with their parents before we could evaluate their involvement. The question was whether the control group children, both normals and behaviorals, were exposed to the same degree of overt conflict between their parents.

We found, on the average, that spouse couples from all five groups were very similar in activity level and initiation of conflict. However, levels of conflict were different. The parents of the normals conflicted more intensively than the others; that is, they were more persistent and mutually confronting. The parents of the psychosomatics, especially the anorectics, were the least involved in conflict. This experimental finding was consistent with our previous clinical observations of conflict avoidance in the psychosomatic families.

Important differences could also be seen in the way that the couples handled these conflictual discussions. The parents of the normal children were able to bring their own point of view into play and to listen to their spouses' view and acknowledge it. They seemed less concerned about the fragility of their spouses when they had to tell them something critical, and conversely, they were less likely to put down or otherwise invalidate the bad news that the spouse was imparting about them.

The parents of the psychosomatics, however, especially the anorectics, displayed a wonderful variety of conflict-avoiding techniques. Some couples enacted the stereotyped complementarity of a comedy team. The wife listed complaints about the husband, such as being too cold, unavailable to the children, or inconsiderate, and gave examples to back them up. He considered each one, and agreed: "You're right," "I can see that," "I know that's true." Each agreement deflated her, causing her to turn to a new subject. Joking, evasion ("I don't remember that," "So what?" "That's your problem"), collapse (crying), or rationalizing were other methods used by a parent to tune out a complaining spouse and keep the level of conflict low. Other couples worked together earnestly searching for problems, but then agreed that the problems discussed did not exist in their families.

During the first stage of the interview we also scrutinized the content of parental conversations to determine whether it was focused on parental-marital issues or revolved around the children. Child-focused conversations were characterized by either protective concerns or criticisms of the child's behavior. Parental-marital issues were reflected in spouse interchanges about each other as spouses or as parents. A content analysis of the parental dialogs revealed that while the parents of the normal and behavioral diabetic children spent more time on parental-marital issues than the others, the parents of the psychosomatic children talked more about their protective concerns for their children.

For example, one couple in the normal group engaged in a hot and heavy discussion of the way the family finances were handled, since in their views of family budgeting the husband was an "ant" and the wife a "grasshopper." Another couple, the parents of a behavioral diabetic, argued about the discipline of the children, the mother insisting that the father was too lax and the father objecting to the mother's inconsistent punishment. Another father in the behavioral diabetic group attacked his wife's housekeeping, while she complained of his late hours and insufficient time at home.

In contrast, the parents of the anorectic and other psychosomatic children spent much more of their time alone ruminating about their children, the siblings as well as the patients. For example, one couple in the anorexia group divided their worries between the sick child, the brother who ate too much, and the sister who they thought "might destroy her life" because she was silly and had poor judgment. Other parents' concerns were tinged with complaints about the child for causing so much worry, for taking advantage of the family, and for manipulating others through the illness.

The first stage of the interview was supposed to elicit typical family conflict issues in the physical absence of the child. As it turned out, the ways that the parents of the psychosomatic children avoided spouse issues by detouring through a concern for their children in this first stage anticipated some of the child-involved behaviors that would develop in the third stage.

In the second stage of the interview the psychiatric interviewer developed or exacerbated the conflict issues that had emerged during the first half-hour. Differences of behavior between the spouses, such as how active each one was and how each initiated or handled conflict, provided important clues about the role that each spouse played in the avoidance of conflict. This information was used by the interviewer in deciding whom to ally with or whom to press in order to enhance the conflict. The results of these efforts to raise the level of conflict were successful; that is, while the normals continued their conflicts at the same level of intensity as before, the previously avoiding parents of the psychosomatics were stimulated to engage more directly, more intensely, and more persistently, to the same degree as the normals. Thus the children in all the groups were exposed to similar degrees of conflict between their parents as they observed them through the one-way mirrors.

The third and last stage of the interview provided a unique opportunity to test directly for child involvement in parental conflict by bringing the child into the heated-up parental context. The effect of the child's entry on the spouses' behavior toward each other revealed a significant pattern. The parents of the normal and behavioral diabetic children continued to interact with each other as well as with the child during this period. In the psychosomatic groups, spouse interaction ground to a halt and parental attention focused almost exclusively on the child. In the anorectic group, nine of the eleven parent pairs spoke to each other less than ten minutes during this half-hour. Thus the use of even this gross measure supported the hypothesis of parental detouring through the child.

The triadic interactions among parents and children were much more difficult to score than the interactions of the couple alone. Although the ratings that were devised—parents' involvement with child and child's involvement with parents—were fairly simple to count and categorize, they may not do justice to the feedback system in operation. The sequence in which the results are reported should not suggest a linear causal sequence in the real behavior of the family. Parental involvement and child involvement alternated in cyclical patterns. Furthermore, the expression "involvement of the child" should always be interpreted in the passive and active voice at the same time; that is, the child is both involved *by* and involved *in* the parental conflict.

Certain patterns of involving the child emerged when parental conflicts became open and explicit. These included the parents pressing the child to express opinions, triangulating the child by trying to recruit him as an ally, and covertly or openly allying with the child against the other parent. In one anorectic's family, for example, the father had criticized his wife as a cold, unloving mother. When the child appeared, she was bombarded by the parents to tell whether she agreed or not, and whether she would like her mother to be different. Another mother recruited her daughter to join her in aggravation over the father's long work hours. In one family with a son who was an athletic prodigy, the father and mother quarreled over pushing the child and involved him in deciding who was right. Some parents encouraged the child to complain about the other parent's discipline. The parents of the psychosomatic children engaged in this kind of behavior to a significantly greater extent than the parents of the normal or behavioral diabetics. And the anorectics' parents attempted to involve their children more than anyone else in the sample.

A pattern of behavior was observed in the children with respect to their parents which complemented the parents' efforts to involve the child. It included the formation of alliances or coalitions with one parent against the other, extreme distress when caught in the parents' involving maneuvers, or the initiation of conflicts between parents. All such behavior reflected the child's involvement in parental conflict.

Children who were highly involved in coalitions or who were intrusive in the parents' concerns often showed signs of tension or stress, even though their involvement seemed self-initiated rather than elicited by their parents. An asthmatic boy, self-appointed protector of his mother against his father, began to wheeze audibly during the interview. A diabetic girl who criticized her parents' marriage and urged her father to complain that his wife was not demonstrative enough cried as she said her parents' drab life was her fault. The anorectic children were rated as the most highly involved in their parents' conflicts, significantly more than the normal or behavioral diabetics. They were similar to the other psychosomatic children, who were also highly involved, but again the reactions of the anorectics were the most extreme.

These findings provided observable support for the first two pathogenic patterns, triangulation and coalition, posited in the psychosomatic family model, by revealing the role of the child as a mediator of parental conflict. They also confirmed the third pathogenic family pattern, protective detouring. In detouring families, conflict could be avoided altogether by shifting attention to and amplifying protective and nurturant concerns for family members, particularly the patient. The pattern included the parents showing protective concern toward the children, the children protecting their parents, and parents and children eliciting protective behavior from each other. Again the anorectics' families were very similar to the families of other psychosomatics, all of whom gave and elicited much more protection than the normal and behavioral diabetic family members did.

These findings provided substantial support for our ideas both about the ways psychosomatic children are involved in parental conflict and about the complimentarity and mutuality of parent and child in maintaining this involvement. While the protective patterns may superficially appear more benign than the involvement patterns, both types serve to reinforce the psychosomatic symptoms of the child in the service of the family homeostasis. The impingement and intrusions of the child into the parental domain via self-involvement or inappropriate protective-protection-eliciting behavior are as dysfunctional as the parents' stress on the child through inappropriate involvement or overprotective control. Furthermore, these observations confirmed that our model of psychosomatic family organization, derived from our clinical work, was applicable across the varieties of psychosomatic illness, both primary and secondary, and nonspecific with respect to the particular symptom of disorder.

Physiological Results

The FFA results obtained from the blood samples taken during the course of the family diagnostic interviews made it possible to match the physiological assessment with the concurrent family interactional patterns. However, the FFA results were necessarily restricted to the three groups with diabetic children. Although we did look at FFA changes during experimental situations in patients with asthma and with anorexia, such changes do not play the same role in the pathophysiological events leading to those diseases as they do in diabetic children. FFA is not related to an asthmatic attack; indeed, there are many physiological reasons to believe that free fatty acids are peripheral to the sequence of events through which emotional arousal is mediated into an asthmatic attack. Similarly, free fatty acids do not lie in any straight line between the psyche and the somatic event in anorexia nervosa. It is only in diabetes that this direct link exists, and it is in this group that there is physiological evidence providing strong support for our hypotheses of psychosomatic disease. In the diabetic children, FFA are simultaneously markers and intermediaries in the metabolic sequence that leads to the psychosomatic symptom. In addition, the diabetic, by virtue of the absence of insulin, allows amplification of the FFA response, so that it can be seen at its most dramatic.

The FFA data on the three groups of diabetic children during the course of the family diagnostic interview clearly showed that the psychosomatic group differed sharply from the two other groups of diabetic children in at least two respects. There was a major difference in the response to the parental conflict that the child was viewing through the one-way mirror (fig. 3). FFA responses in the psychosomatic group were exaggerated, much different from the two other groups. In addition, during the recovery period, the FFA in the psychosomatic children remained elevated, whereas the FFA levels in the two control groups of diabetic children returned toward baseline levels. These data provided physiological evidence that psychosomatic diabetic children have an exaggerated turn-on in response to family conflict, as shown by FFA, and that their ability to turn off following their involvement in family conflict is seriously impaired. Yet control studies carried out earlier with these children showed no intrinsic physiological difference between the psychosomatic children and the control groups. The abnormalities in the psychosomatic diabetics could be demonstrated only within the family context.

The physiological evidence also supported the hypothesis that the psychosomatic symptom plays a role in family homeostasis (fig. 4). The FFA levels of the index child were plotted along with those of the parent whose arousal during the interview was most pronounced. Focus on stages three and four of the interview—the period of family conflict when the child was present and the recovery phase—revealed in the psychosomatic group a crossover phenomenon. The parent whose FFA indicated that he or she was emotionally aroused showed a decrease when the child was brought into the situation. In contrast, the child's FFA continued to rise when he or she was brought into the situation and did not return toward the baseline during the recovery period. The physiological measurement showed that the presence of the child decreased the parent's emotional arousal, at the cost of a continued rise in the child's arousal, propelling him toward disease. The sustained arousal of FFA during the recovery period attested to the maintenance of the pattern in the face of unresolved family conflict.

The importance of these physiological observations cannot be overemphasized. Physiological evidence could be shown to support family psychological hypotheses. The abnormalities of FFA, demonstrable only in the setting of the family, are completely consistent with the hypothesis that emotional arousal in these children is related to family conflict and will produce a somatic consequence.

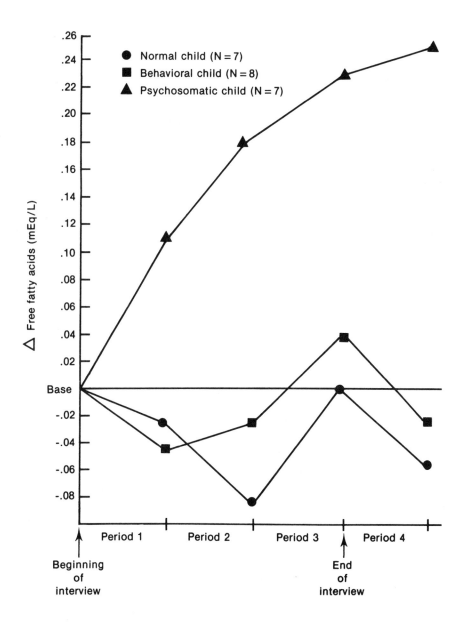

Figure 3. Changes in FFA levels of diabetic children during family interview.

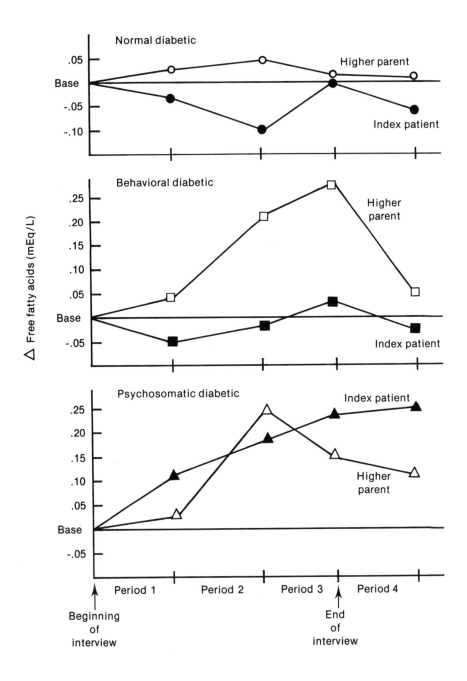

Figure 4. Medians of parent with higher FFA response and index patient.

In addition, the crossover phenomenon strongly supports the hypothesis that the illness plays a role in these families. Parental arousal can be alleviated by the participation of the child, but only at the expense of symptom maintenance.

Although these physiological derangements could not be demonstrated in either the psychosomatic asthmatics or the anorectics, therapeutic observations of such patients have validated the generalizability of these hypotheses, as have the strikingly successful therapeutic results. Another validation is the similarity of interactional characteristics, as quantified by the content analysis of the family diagnostic interview and the family task.

Implications of the Research

In scientific explorations, significant phenomena emerge in relation to a given point of view. It is not only the interpretation of events that differs from one worker to another, but the very selection of the events to be studied as well as of the methods of study. This is particularly the case when a shift is occurring from conventional to novel conceptual models. The different kinds of data that result inevitably continue to reinforce and to shape the underlying conceptualizations in a given direction.

Our work with psychosomatic children is a case in point. As our thinking shifted from a linear to a circular model, our methods of study changed. Instead of focusing on the child's psychological or physiological vulnerability alone, we looked at the child in the family context. When we did so, new data emerged whose import was dramatic for theory and hardly less significant for treatment.

Our first opportunities to collect important information about the psychosomatic child in the family context came in family therapy sessions. During these interviews the therapists were able to observe the patient, parents, and siblings interacting together, to examine the family members' responses to interventions that probed the strength or direction of interactional patterns, and to follow sequences of interaction over a period of time. Our therapeutic orientation, which required that interventions be made in the interpersonal rather than intrapersonal system, broadened the field of observation and thereby fostered the emergence of new kinds of data. Some of it was rather startling to observe firsthand. For example, a girl who had hitherto presented herself as helpless and hopeless, dominated and invaded by her mother, could now be seen as tyrannically manipulating her intimidated parents. A father whose dearest wish was to have his child eat and grow healthy again could be seen as undercutting his wife's efforts in this direction.

The evaluation of these patterns proved invaluable in understanding anorexia nervosa. Since most studies of anorexia have been undertaken from an individual framework, the information gathered tells only about the experience or personality of the individual patient during the anorectic period, although it may involve a reconstruction of the etiologically significant events seen through her eyes. The information derived from such studies of the identified patient can only be about her alone, as is true also of formulations about the anorectic's interpersonal relationships.

But because the formal research designed to test our hypotheses about family transactional patterns was derived from a systems model, the unit of study was no longer the child. It was the transactional pattern. What we were observing and evaluating were cyclical or sequential patterns of behavior in these families, patterns which both maintained and were maintained by the psychosomatic behavior of a child.

These patterns are not causal chains. It is difficult to grasp the notion of a pattern as the cause of psychosomatic problems because one is so accustomed to thinking of causality in terms of events that occur in chronological order. It is much easier to think of parental pathology or psychophysiological mediating mechanisms as converging on the individual, thereby causing the pathology. In a systems view, however, the chain of events cannot be seen as causally related. Perhaps the nearest metaphor is a melody or a musical pattern. The notes E and B may follow C, and they must follow C to produce a certain pattern. Yet one would not say that C has caused E and B.

Our research had important implications for therapy. Having characterized pathological transactional patterns, we were able to explore ways to change the sequence pattern. The advantage, however, of the systems model goes beyond the precise delineation of the causal sequences. It brings many new factors into the equation, so that the therapeutic points of entry are geometrically increased.

The Anorectic Family

3

The title of this chapter is, of course, incorrect. Anorexia, "loss of appetite," is a term that can describe only the behavior of the identified patient, not the behavior of a family.

We can coin a new word, albeit an uncomfortable one—"anorexogenic"—to describe families that produce children with anorexia. But we would still remain within a linear framework, attributing causality to the family and making the anorectic child a helpless victim.

The term anorectic family is intended to posit the dilemma of the systems thinker caught in a field in which words reflect descriptions of individuals. We are attempting to describe the interpersonal transactions that organize the behavior of family members in dysfunctional patterns—the feedback circularity by which family members constrain each other. We are attempting to describe the multiple determination of symptoms, the multiplicity of symptoms, and the symptoms carried by different members. We are attempting to describe the identified patient as an active participant in a process in which there are no victimizers or victims, only family members involved in the small details of everyday living. But trapped by words, we end up with an incorrect label: the anorectic family.

To understand and describe the anorectic family required that we integrate our assumptions about psychosomatic families into a larger theoretical framework, one that conceptualizes the nature of the transactions organizing the behavior of members of normally functioning families. Examination of the relationship between a model of normal families and the anorectic family highlights the dysfunctional patterns of behavior. These aspects of anorectic family functioning are then easier to observe in vignettes drawn from treatment sessions with such families.

The Functions of a Family

Both our observations of families and our selection of the variables to be investigated were organized according to an implicit model of functioning families. It is not easy to give a thumbnail sketch of this underlying model; the field of family study, like that of individual study, has developed few clear descriptions of normal functioning. In both fields, it has always been easier to describe the pathological.

We nevertheless found it useful to postulate that every human being's sense of identity depends, in large measure, on the validation of self by a reference group. One of the most important reference groups is the family, or a family substitute. The family's validation is vital for all family members, but is particularly important for children who are undergoing the fluid processes of identity formation. Two characteristics—autonomy and belonging—are vital in human identity. And it is within the family that children develop a sense of themselves as autonomous individuals, who belong to and can depend on a certain group. The way that the family functions, therefore, has enormous implications for individual development. Family transactional patterns form the matrix of psychological growth.

Many patterns of family functioning are compatible with healthy development. Although some forms may appeal more than others, families with widely differing value systems, child-rearing practices, and ways of organizing space, time, and roles offer reasonable environments for child growth.

The easiest way to conceptualize a family system is to picture it as having a beginning in time when two people join with the purpose of forming a family.[1] Since each partner has grown up in his or her own family, each one has his or her own cognitive map and role expectations for human interaction. Each assumes that people will communicate using certain rules. Each assumes that certain values are true. Both partners' paradigms must be retained, so that each person can retain a sense of self. But the two paradigms must also be reconciled, so that a life in common becomes possible.

In the process of reconciling their paradigms, the spouses develop new transactional patterns. These patterns may represent compromises, or they may embody unresolved differences. But in either case the new transactional patterns become familiar, and then preferred. A spouse unit has been formed.

Consider, for instance, the parents of an anorectic patient who were discussing an unsatisfactory sexual relationship. They mentioned one of their transactional patterns which had existed for as long as they could remember in their thirty years of marriage: the wife always closed the door before they had intercourse. The husband explained that the wife closed it when she wanted sex, which made him unhappy because he felt that he should initiate the act. The wife countered that she rarely initiated the act, and that she closed the door only when she saw that the husband wanted sex. The husband insisted that she in fact did initiate, for whenever the wife looked at him in ways which indicated that she was wondering if he wanted sex, he indicated that he did, and then she closed the door.

The therapist asked in which other areas of life the same process occurred. Naturally, the couple described their transactions around food. When they went out to eat, the husband "initiated" the transaction by asking his wife to choose a restaurant. She said that he should choose. He stopped the car and said that he would not start it again until she made a decision. She named a restaurant, where they went and got a table. Then the wife asked, "Did I guess right?"

A child born into such a family learns a particular way of punctuating experiences. She also learns to accommodate kaleidoscopically.[2] She is her father's daughter and her brother's sister and, in general, she and her grandfather clear the table after supper. She belongs to these people. At the same time, her participation in different roles in different patterns and in different family subsystems develops her early sense of autonomy. Within the structure that gives her a sense of belonging, the child has many transactional choices to make. The wider her range of possible choices, the greater her experience of freedom.

From her earliest years, the child experiments with different segments of her biopsychological potential. Some aspects of her personality are reinforced by transactions within the family. Other aspects are discouraged or restricted. As a result of this feedback, certain ways of being fall into disuse and become less available to the child. Other types of input and response, encouraged by the family, become familiar and easily available. These familiar ways of being tend to become identified as the self.

As the child grows, her way of being comes into contact with other social groups. In the extrafamilial world she experiments with the patterns she has learned in the family. She uses the patterns developed in the parental and sibling subsystems to approach relationships with other people of differing power. She uses the patterns she has seen in the adult subsystems to approach a relationship with peers.

She also experiments with extrafamilial inputs and values. At first these are transmitted through the family. Later they are experienced more directly, on an individual level. But the child's sense of herself as part of the world is still mediated by her family, and her responses to the extrafamilial continue to be validated or disqualified by the reactions of the family. The family remains the group that must ensure her very survival, providing for her physical and psychological needs and protecting her from danger and disease.

Identity grows slowly, building on the many interactions within the family and the extrafamilial that define for the child who she is and how she fits in. Her sense of interaction changes as she grows, since she is herself a changing organism with changing needs, interests, and capacities. In the process, she organizes her experience in increasingly complex ways. But well into adolescence, the family system is the primary workshop of growth. The way it functions affects and even defines the progress of the child.

Subsystems

The family carries out its functions by differentiating into subsystems. Subsystems can be formed by generation, by sex, and by interest or function. They may include one member, a dyad (such as the spouse subsystem), or more members (such as the sibling subsystem). Subsystems may be temporary and changeable, such as those that are built around shared projects or passing alliances. But three more enduring subsystems typical of the Western family have particular relevance to child growth: the spouse, the parental, and the sibling subsystems.

The subsystem of husband and wife has its own boundary and, by definition, does not include the child. Nonetheless, the functioning of this system is vital for the child's growth. Any major dysfunction in the spouse subsystem reverberates throughout the family, affecting all its members. Children may be either scapegoated or co-opted into an alliance by one spouse as the couple experiences conflict and dissatisfaction in its own relationships.

The spouse subsystem models for the child the nature of intimate relationships, at least as expressed in visible daily interaction. The child identifies with the parent, often assuming a particular behavior seen in an influential adult even if it is not immediately workable or rewarded. The spouse subsystem also provides models of transaction between man and woman. The child sees patterns for expressing affection, for relating to each other when one or both partners are externally stressed, and for dealing with conflict. Such models become part of the child's schema at some level, to be explored in intimate subsystems later in life.

The parental subsystem, which may include grandparents or parental children, carries out the familiar child-rearing functions of nurturance, guidance, and control. But many other aspects of the child's development are affected by interactions within this subsystem. Here the child establishes basic patterns of relating and interacting in situations of unequal power. He learns how to communicate what he wants, and what to expect from people who have greater resources and strength. He learns whether he will be supported in his needs and how conflicts can be resolved. He learns what behavior must be controlled, and from the nature of the controlling transactions he derives a general conception of authority as either rational or arbitrary. His sense of adequacy in dealing with authority is shaped by how he is heard by his elders and by the system's capacity to respond to him in relevant, age-appropriate terms. As the child grows and his needs change, the patterns of functioning must change as well. The parents must shift to more moderate forms of guidance and relinquish authority as the child signals the increasing capacity for decision-making and self-control.

Just as there are one-parent families with no spouse subsystem, there are families with only one child. However, in families with more than one child, the sibling subsystem has an importance which has not always been recognized in psychological theory. Siblings form the first peer group. Within this context, children support, isolate, scapegoat, and teach each other. They develop patterns for negotiating, cooperating, and competing. They learn how to make friends and allies, how to save face while submitting, how to acquire skills, and how to achieve recognition for skills.

Children take different positions in this constant interplay, and the process furthers both their sense of belonging to a group and their sense of alternatives and individuation within a system. The training involved in exercising interpersonal skills at different levels with the sibling subsystem will be significant as the child moves out into extrafamilial peer groups, such as the classroom society and, later, the world of work.

Boundaries

Two particular attributes of family structure are crucial in its functioning: the nature of the boundaries that define its various subsystems, and the capacity of the system to change in response to changed conditions. The boundaries of a subsystem are the rules defining who participates in its transactions, and how. One boundary of the parental subsystem, for example, is defined when a mother tells her older child, "If your brother is riding his bike in the street, tell me, and I will stop him." Another boundary establishing the role of a parental child is defined when the mother tells the children, "Until I get back from the store, Andy is in charge."

Every family subsystem has specific functions and makes specific demands on its members. The development and exercise of skills in these subsystems depends on freedom from undue interference. The function of boundaries is to protect that necessary differentiation. For example, the development of skills for negotiating with peers, learned among siblings, depends on a salutary neglect. Parents must know how to monitor and mediate while allowing the sibling subsystem to function much of the time on its own.

The composition of a subsystem is not nearly as significant as the clarity of the subsystem boundaries. A parental subsystem that includes a grandparent, for instance, may function quite well as long as the lines of responsibility and authority are clearly drawn.

The clarity of family subsystem boundaries is a useful parameter for the evaluation of family functioning. All families can be conceived of as falling somewhere along a continuum whose poles are the two extremes of diffuse boundaries, or enmeshment, and overly rigid boundaries, or disengagement. The enmeshed family is a system which has turned upon itself, developing its own microcosm. There is a high degree of communication and concern among family members, boundaries are blurred, and differentiation is diffused. Such a system may lack the resources necessary to adapt and change under stressful circumstances. At the opposite extreme, the disengaged family has overly rigid boundaries. Communication is difficult, and the protective functions of the family are handicapped.

Most families have enmeshed and disengaged subsystems, varying according to function and developmental level. Mother-children subsystems are often enmeshed while the children are small, even to the point of excluding the father. Yet in the same family, the father may take a more engaged position with the older children. The parental subsystem moves from an enmeshed to a disengaged style as the children grow and begin to separate from the family.

Enmeshment and disengagement do not imply qualitative differences between the functional and dysfunctional. They are terms referring to a transactional style. However, operations at the extremes do indicate areas of possible pathology.

The disengaged system tolerates a wide range of individual variation in family members. But at the extreme end of the continuum, stresses in one family member do not cross inappropriately rigid boundaries. Only a high level of individual stress can reverberate strongly enough to activate the family supportive system. At the enmeshed end of the continuum the opposite is true. Stress in an individual member reverberates strongly, and is swiftly echoed in other subsystems. But at the extreme, individual autonomy may be severely curtailed.

Both extreme types of relating may cause problems when family adaptive mechanisms must be evoked. The highly enmeshed family responds to any variation with excessive speed and intensity. The disengaged family tends not to respond, even when response is necessary. The parents in an enmeshed family may become quite upset when a child does not eat dessert. The parents in a disengaged family may not respond to a child's delinquent behavior.

Change in a Family

One of a family's most important tasks is to maintain the continuity that protects its members' sense of belonging. At the same time, the family must meet continual demands for change. The way in which it responds to change is the other key element in the family structure.

The most obvious and inevitable source of disequilibrium comes from the growth of family members. Children, in particular, move rapidly through developmental stages. Small children may be content to accompany their parents on weekends. But a nine-year-old may want to stay and play with a friend on Sunday afternoon. And an adolescent may want to attend a weekend rock concert with friends, taking her new driver's license and the family car.

Eventually, the growth of the children must be met with change in the organization of daily life, a process that involves time and discomfort at best. The whole family must cope with the resulting sense of loss and strangeness. Parents find themselves being shut out of confidences and secrets, letting go of cherished family traditions, and ceding authority that they could themselves exercise more efficiently. At some point they must face the implications of their children's growth for their own sense of self. Children may find that their new autonomy means a loss of ease and protection.

The pressure for change also comes from extrafamilial sources. A parent changes jobs. The family moves. There is a school strike. Both internal and external pressures for change continually strain the family system.

But the disequilibrium produced is an essential factor in the growth and development of a family, just as it is of an individual. In time, new transactional patterns become necessary. As these new patterns are accepted, they will become familiar, and then preferred.

Alternate patterns remain possible, but the system tends to maintain itself within preferred ranges, thereby maintaining continuity. Deviations that approach the system's threshold of tolerance elicit counterdeviation responses. They re-establish the accustomed ranges of behavior until change again becomes unavoidable.

If a family is not changing, that is a sign of rigidity, unhealthy in itself. Some families respond to demands for even the most necessary change by increasing the rigidity of transactional patterns. Although the preferred patterns have become inadequate, they are stubbornly maintained. Such a system can become pathogenic. Family members no longer experience their system as a supportive, growth-fostering network. It becomes a cage. Responses that are no longer viable are still strongly reinforced by a closed system's overutilized counterdeviation mechanisms. The exploration of alternatives is closed. Responses become stereotyped and straitened. Family members are trapped.

The Anorectic System

The family is the matrix of identity. In the family, the child learns how to "punctuate the flow of experience," as Gregory Bateson put it.[3] The child's punctuation determines her reality. The anorectic child has grown up in a family operating with highly enmeshed patterns. As a result, her orientation toward life gives prime importance to proximity in interpersonal contact. Loyalty and protection take precedence over autonomy and self-realization. A child growing up in an extremely enmeshed system learns to subordinate the self. Her expectation from a goal-directed activity, such as studying or learning a skill, is therefore not competence, but approval. The reward is not knowledge, but love.

In our observation, a child who has learned to relate in highly enmeshed patterns can become an anorectic if certain other processes are also present in the family. The anorectic family, for example, is typically child-oriented. The child grows up carefully protected by parents who focus on her well-being. Parental concern is expressed in hypervigilance of the child's movements and intense observation of her psychobiological needs. Since the child experiences family members as focusing on her actions and commenting on them, she develops vigilance over her own actions. Since the evaluation of what she does is another's domain, the child develops an obsessive concern for perfection. She is both extremely conscious of herself and keenly alert to other people's signals. She is a parent watcher. Her concern about her effect on others leads to a hesitation to initiate action and an increased dependency on parental approval.

The child is socialized to act as the family expects and feels great responsibility for not embarrassing the family in the eyes of the extrafamilial. Parental punishment for infractions is related to experience of guilt and shame. In this atmosphere, the child develops as a keen observer of intrafamilial operations, dependent on parental assessment and highly loyal to family values.

The child's autonomy is curtailed by the intrusive concern and overprotection of other family members. Large areas of her psychological and bodily functioning remain the subject of others' interest and control long after they should have become autonomous. This control is maintained under the cloak of concern, so that the child cannot challenge it. Since family members make their wishes known indirectly and unselfishly—"I want this because it is good for you"—disagreement and even initiative become acts of betrayal. The denial of self for another's benefit and family loyalty are highly valued. The concern for mutual accommodation without friction produces an environment in which differences are denied and submerged.

The anorectic child tends not to develop the skills necessary for dealing with her own age level. Her overinvolvement with her family handicaps her involvement with the extrafamilial world, causing a developmental lag. Concomitantly, she becomes overly skilled in observing and transacting with adults.

With the child's entrance into adolescence, she finds herself in a crisis. Her wish to participate with a group of peers conflicts with her orientation to the family. The normal adolescent individuates by beginning to view her parents with the expanded viewpoint created by contact with the extrafamilial. But the anorectic cannot see herself as separate. Instead of focusing more and more on the extrafamilial world, the anorectic turns her expanded viewpoint back into focusing on her parents. She tries to help and change them. This overfocus and the parents' response strengthen the boundaries that keep the child overinvolved with the family.

In anorectic families, the boundaries that keep family members overinvolved with each other and separated from the world are typically well defined and strong. The boundaries within the family, however, are often diffuse and weak. Often the boundary between the nuclear family and the families of origin is poorly drawn. One or both of the spouses maintains a strong affiliation with the family of origin. Conflicts belonging to the spouse subsystem may be maintained by this strong affiliation; a coalition across generations interferes with the development of mutual accommodation in the marriage.

This model of cross-generational coalition is copied in the nuclear family. The spouse who has maintained a close relationship with his or her parents may shift that affiliation to a child. Or the peripheral spouse may join with a child against the spouse-grandparent coalition. In either case, the distance between the spouses is maintained without violating the family's value for proximity, and the child is drawn into conflict-avoidance patterns.

Finally, it is characteristic of anorectic families, as well as of psychosomatic families in general, to focus on bodily functions. Many family members present somatic complaints. Such complaints can represent either bona-fide illness or merely general sensitivity to normal physiological processes. In families with an anorectic child, the entire family often has a special concern with such matters as eating, table manners, diets, and food fads.

In one anorectic family, the mother developed neuralgia whenever the anorectic's older sister went on a trip. In another family the grandmother was hypertense and required a special diet, while the mother was deeply involved with a diet group. In another family, the spouses bickered for twenty years about the father's table manners. In still another anorectic family the father was greatly concerned about nutrition, and conflicts around the table usually sparked a discussion of the nutritional value of the meal.

When the disequilibrium that is a part of life threatens the psychosomatic family, all family members are rapidly mobilized to protect the system, particularly by coercing those members whose need for change is threatening the status quo. The concern for somatic issues that is an element in the family culture may spark the anorectic symptoms in a child. Because these symptoms can be utilized in conflict-detouring patterns, the family unites in a concern for and protection of the child, thereby rewarding the symptoms. Although the parents and siblings may feel exploited by the demands of the sick child, they continue their controlling protection.

The symptom becomes imbedded in the family organization. The concentration on the sick child's symptoms maximizes her self-appraisal as a patient. Illness may become her identity card. Feeling both protected and scapegoated, the child approaches all interpersonal situations as a weak, incompetent person. If this process continues for a period of time, the child may be rendered incompetent in many areas of life functioning. Her dependent demands increase, and family members respond by increasing their protective control. Challenged by the chronicity, the unpredictability, and the life-threatening danger of severe psychosomatic illness, the family may establish a strong dependency on the pediatrician. No other problems can gain salience. Everything would be all right, they feel, if their daughter could just be well.

Related Linear Studies

This model of the anorectic family is not unique to us. Many investigators, including many psychodynamic investigators, have noted the same data. Mohammed Shafii, Carlos Salguero, and Stuart M. Finch, for example, reported on a family with two anorectic siblings.[4] Karen was eight when she developed anorexia. Two years later Bonnie, then twelve, developed the same symptoms. The authors described many elements of family interaction in the case that are similar to our own observations: " 'We are normal. The only thing is, we can't eat,' the girls' mother said . . . She frequently used the pronoun 'we' to describe her daughter's condition . . . The children were not referred to by their first name. Often they were called 'first one,' 'second one,' etc. . . . Everyone, including the mother, was expected to do exactly as the father said. All these characteristics are elements of the quality labeled enmeshment.

The investigators reported the father's revealing remark: "We stress in our children the virtue of living a God-fearing life and obeying and loving each other . . . We did not want them to play with kids in the neighborhood because they would be subject to bad influences and learn bad things. Everyone was kind to the others and got along fine with others. We did not allow any quarreling between the children." Such a comment conveys the overprotection and the fear of the extrafamilial that is typical of anorectic families.

According to the authors, the mother expressed her disagreement with her husband's dictatorial approach, but she never openly disagreed with him. Like other anorectic families, this family placed a high value on conflict avoidance. Hidden conflict between the parents may also have been indicated by the couple's total sexual abstinence since the birth of their fifth child. "For religious reasons," they did not use contraceptives.

The father further informed the doctors, "My daughters wanted to wear their hair different styles, but I told all of them that they must wear their hair in a short, straight, simple cut." He said that his wife liked the girls' hair to cover their ears, but that he liked it behind their ears, so sometimes, "I playfully tuck Karen's hair behind her ears." Both the hidden conflict and the fear of individuation common to anorectic families are apparent here.

Eating was an important issue in this family. "I was chubby in college," the mother reported, "and I decided to go on a diet. I lost 30 pounds . . . Since that time, I have been a very picky eater and, in essence, I have continued to be on a diet . . . I have encouraged the girls not to eat between meals and I have told them that the renunciation of food has some virtues . . . My husband chastises me about being on a diet, but it doesn't bother me." The father's second cousin died, apparently of anorexia, when they were both eighteen.

The authors of this report have described the hidden spouse conflict, the utilization of children to detour conflict, the coalition of mother and children against father, the overconcern with food, and many of the other family components of anorexia nervosa. Although their analysis dismisses these factors as not significant for therapy, the data are unquestionably there.

The Families Speak for Themselves

The model presented here is the summation of research data from the total sample. It is an abstraction composed of the similarities among anorectic families—a collage of superimposed similarities, in which differences are overshadowed. It shows the statistically significant measures—the differences that are really different. But clinicians find themselves dealing not with abstract generalities, but with people. Therefore, it is useful to see the different ways in which different families deal with each other. The enmeshment, the overprotection, the involvement of the child in parental issues—all these factors are expressed in a language and style that are idiosyncratic to each family.

Many metaphors can describe enmeshment:

FATHER: We all congregate in our bedroom. And Steve will cuddle and scratch my back, and I'll scratch his back. And Mommy will be doing something, and Laura will be—
THERAPIST: Do you scratch her back also?
FATHER: Whose?
THERAPIST: Mom's.
FATHER: Mommy? No.

MOTHER: I don't like my back scratched.

FATHER: So I'll maybe massage the girls, their legs . . . Laura always enjoyed combing my hair. Or if I get dandruff and don't have time to wash my head, some of the girls will take the comb or brush and brush my hair out. Like last night I guess my head itched or something and I was too lazy to wash my head at that time. So I'd say, "Jill, comb my hair out." So we were cuddling. We always seem to cuddle, and so on, in our room, or I'll go to their room and cuddle, or what have you. So we're always doing something for one another . . . If I get a cramp in my leg, "Ooh, Jill, I got a cramp in my left leg. Ah, work it out for me." So Jill will put a little alcohol on it, or a hot cloth, and she'll massage me.

THERAPIST: Dad is describing a lot of nurturance going on between him and the kids. Where are you when all that happens?

MOTHER: Well, sometimes I'm just lying on the bed with them. Other times I'll just be doing needlepoint, or maybe I'll be going down to the kitchen and emptying the dishwasher, or heating up coffee.

THERAPIST: Daddy's a cuddler. He likes to cuddle. He likes the children to cuddle with him.

MOTHER: Yeah. He enjoys that at night.

THERAPIST: What about you? Are you a cuddler?

MOTHER: Am I? Ah, not as much as him, I guess. I don't know. I'm always busy in the house, it seems. I'm folding clothes and putting them away, or—

THERAPIST: Sometimes would you like him to drop the kids and be with you alone?

MOTHER: No. Absolutely not.

THERAPIST: Are there times when you say to the kids, "Okay you leave, because it is now time for me and Daddy alone"?

MOTHER: Never. Never!

THERAPIST: Do you leave the door of your room open?

MOTHER: Always. In fact, I don't even like the children to close theirs.

THERAPIST: Let me try to explore that area a little bit. This is a family that likes to be cuddled, and to close the doors is a little bit of an insult, a bit of an attack, because you are a bunched-in family.

FATHER: We like to think that.

THERAPIST: Yes. Maybe Mother also likes to think that, but

maybe not so much. You like to be rubbed more than she does. Isn't that so? What's your thinking, Mother, about this question of the closed doors? For your growing-up daughters.

MOTHER: Well, sometimes if Father hears them shut the door—maybe they'll have a friend over and they'll be up in the bedroom and they'll shut the door—Father will holler and say, "No closed doors! Tell them to leave the door open."

Closing doors is the metaphor used in another family:

DAUGHTER: I've talked with [her married sister]. She feels the same way. Why do you think she always ate in her room?

MOTHER: She was much older. She was already in college when she decided to eat her meals in her room. And when you're old enough to go to college, you can have meals in your room.

DAUGHTER: Why do you think she always kept the door closed?

MOTHER: Because she wanted privacy at her age: eighteen, nineteen, twenty, twenty-one, twenty-two. She was entitled to have her door closed. But not until you're eighteen!

DAUGHTER: I'm sorry that I can't keep my door closed. I'm sorry!

Hypervigilance is still another metaphor of enmeshment:

MOTHER: I am not home to watch you!

DAUGHTER: Well, that's what it feels like.

FATHER: You must have a guilty conscience or something.

DAUGHTER: No! You do watch me. Your room is right across from mine. I can't go up, I can't go down, I can't go anyplace.

MOTHER: You have to realize you're only fifteen. You can't have everything your own way. You have to be guided and supervised by your parents.

DAUGHTER: I have nothing my own way!

The anorectic is watched even when she is separated from her family:

MOTHER: When you went to Jean's party, her mother told me what you ate. She told me you ate fruit cup—

DAUGHTER: What did you do, check up on me?

FATHER: Yes.

DAUGHTER: I knew you would. I know you're checking up on me.

MOTHER: Because I'm concerned! And don't think she's not concerned. She said you were chewing, and she thought you were eating, but when she went over to see if you were eating, you were chewing gum the whole time, and your plate was the same way it had been given to you.

The anorectic's body seems to belong to the whole family:

FATHER: Why aren't you eating?

DAUGHTER: I haven't been hungry.

FATHER: Do the lumps in your tummy bother you?

DAUGHTER: Yes.

FATHER: Do you think it has anything to do with Mommy and Daddy?

Another seventeen-year-old anorectic complains: "Mother, I don't feel well. Am I going to throw up?"

Anorectic children are parent-watchers. They are also easily recruited to take sides in a spouse disagreement:

DAUGHTER: I don't think you respect Mom enough as a person. You look on her as someone who you come home to, but you don't really respect her personality. I think you consider yourself her superior.

FATHER: How do I treat her?

DAUGHTER: You analyze everything. Everything has to have a reason. That really upsets her.

FATHER: What happens when we argue?

DAUGHTER: Well, *you* never argue. You just sit there, feeling you're right, but not letting her know that.

MOTHER: How do you think I treat him?

DAUGHTER: You let him treat you like that. You accept your role as being just someone who cooks the dinner.

MOTHER: You don't think there's any love between us? Is that what you're trying to say?

DAUGHTER: Oh, no. I didn't say that. I just don't think that you mutually respect each other.

This fourteen-year-old anorectic describes her parents' interactions quite accurately. She pinpoints their complementarity: father's avoidance of conflict and silent undermining of mother; mother's nagging of father but accommodation to him. Although the daughter attacks her father for feeling superior to her mother, she clearly considers herself his equal. In this family the daughter is invited to enter the spouse subsystem and to criticize their relationship. Indeed, reading the transcript masked, one might assume that the daughter is a therapist.

Shortly after the preceding exchange, the father moves to rescue the mother from the girl's attack:

FATHER: Don't you think your mother takes care of her children well?

DAUGHTER: Very well.

FATHER: And has their interests at heart?

DAUGHTER: Very well.

FATHER: And commits a lot of time to their whims and wants?

DAUGHTER: I'm saying she does it too much.

MOTHER: What should I do? You mean I should say no?

DAUGHTER: I don't think you really understand each other. It seems that things that are important to you should be important to Mom, and you both should share problems. You should share the good things and the bad. If you really respected her as a person and considered her important—that she's a part of you and you're a part of her, then you would have told her about your job. Because it's hard on you having the tension, and it's hard on her when you're tense, and you should share the problems. The good and the bad.

The father discusses his job with his daughter, not his wife. In general, in this family, parent and child share issues that spouse does not share with spouse. The daughter is deeply involved in saving the marriage and the family, in which capacity she acts as her mother's advocate. But her participation, by protecting her mother, also undermines the mother's position in the family. The boundary that should delineate spouse subsystem transactions is almost nonexistent.

Cross-generation coalitions in the enmeshed family can take many forms:

DAUGHTER: I compare my mother to other wives, and when I compare her, she doesn't fit in. Other wives stock up on things, and they save coupons, and they save money. And I try to get her to save money, but in my opinion, she doesn't shop wisely.

THERAPIST: Do you talk with her about that?

DAUGHTER: Yeah. And she says, "Oh leave me alone. Stop nagging me."

MOTHER: She nags me! She leaves little lists all over the house. Shopping lists. She gave me one this morning at the breakfast table.

GRANDMOTHER: Well, there are some things that Janie and I think along the same lines. And one is where she says her mother is not neat. This is the issue. I've always been—well, right after supper, I clean up the dishes. *Then* I sit and read the paper. But Nancy is different.

DAUGHTER: She'll sit and read at the table!

GRANDMOTHER: The dishes can be on the table and the pots and pans in the sink. But Nancy will read her paper and relax. And then get back to them. Well, Janie and I—I don't know whether it is a good or bad trait, but this is the way we both are. She has a lot of my way of thinking.

In this extended family, a strong affiliation between grandmother and granddaughter has pushed the girl into a pseudomaturity. Instead of being treated like her mother's daughter, she is treated as her grandmother's partner. The mother is defined as incompetent, and grandmother and granddaughter take over her work.

Closely related to the enmeshment of anorectic families is their characteristic overprotection. An enormous concern for each other's well-being is usually coupled with a great fear of the outside world, as well as of disease, accident, or change. Overconcern permeates the family, from the smallest matters to the largest:

SIMON: Do you have a Kleenex?

FATHER: Use my handkerchief. Here. It's a clean handkerchief. Spread it apart.

THERAPIST: He's seventeen.

FATHER: But I'm going to have to use the handkerchief.

MOTHER (*passing a tissue to father*): Let him keep that one.

FATHER: All right.

THERAPIST: My goodness! Look how this family gets activated. Son wanted a handkerchief. So Father gave him his, Mother gave a Kleenex to Father, Daughter offered her handkerchief.

MOTHER: We have togetherness.

Protection is also an issue in the sibling system:

DAUGHTER (*to mother*): Whenever there is a fight, you always blame Judy. But it isn't always her fault. I remember one fight when we were little and it was Nancy's fault all the way. And when Judy finally hit Nancy, Judy really got it. And I ran upstairs and I was crying, saying that you were hitting Judy, stop hitting her.

The denial of self for others is used to avoid conflict:

THERAPIST: You are powerless in your family. Do you like that? Do you like being powerless?
MOTHER: It doesn't bother me. I always felt, even when I grew up, that the father was the head of the family. And if my mother didn't agree with him, she would say, "Go to your father." And if he said something, she would go along with it.
THERAPIST: That puts you in a strange position.
MOTHER: Yes, but I always felt that a house should be full of harmony. And where there is harmony, then the children grow up in harmony, not yelling and screaming at each other all day long.

Fear of disagreement or assertion is coupled with support for harmony:

FATHER: What would have happened if I had said, "No, Son, you can't do certain things"? And if I'd said, "No, Daughter, you can't go to modeling school"? Would they rebel against me and say to me, "Well, I'm going to go out and commit suicide"?

Rigidity is a difficult characteristic to illustrate in a dialog segment, because it reveals itself in repetition. Moreover every family system tries to maintain continuity. Deviations beyond a certain range automatically elicit mechanisms that restore the sense of the familiar, which is the only way that the continuity necessary for the family members' sense of belonging can be maintained. In the extremely enmeshed anorectic family, however, even the smallest deviations are swiftly and comprehensively restricted. As a result, individuals do not have the room to change and grow. In the family with no closed doors, for instance, the children are now fourteen, twelve, and eight. Nevertheless, even the fourteen-year-old is still expected to comb her father's hair. It seems impossible for the family to allow space for the independence proper to adolescence.

The anorectic symptom is maintained in a variety of ways. In this case different family members and different causes are suggested, but the message remains constant, that someone else owns your body:

FATHER: We are talking about things that involved you. What do you think? Why aren't you eating?
DAUGHTER: I haven't been hungry.
FATHER: Do the lumps in your tummy bother you?
DAUGHTER: Yes.
FATHER: Do you think it has anything to do with Mommy and Daddy—you know, anything we do or don't do for you?

Was it Mother?

MOTHER: Then it must have bothered you—what I was doing.
DAUGHTER: Yes.
MOTHER: Well, do you think that could have stopped you from eating as much?
DAUGHTER: I don't know. I was on a diet.

Was it sister?

FATHER: Did you want to lose more weight than Mary was going to lose?
MOTHER: Because Mary was making up a diet?
DAUGHTER: Yes, Mary has one too.
MOTHER: That's when you started cutting down on your food?
DAUGHTER: Yeah, I didn't get hungry any more.
FATHER: Did you want to lose weight?
DAUGHTER: Yes.
FATHER: Did you want to go to the hospital so everyone could come in and visit you?
DAUGHTER: No. I just wasn't getting hungry any more.

Another way of maintaining the symptom is for the father and mother to triangulate the anorectic:

FATHER: Are you going to try to eat?

DAUGHTER: Yes. Sometimes I just get full and I don't feel like eating, and that's why I don't eat that much.

FATHER: There are lots of things that we don't like to do that we have to do sometimes, that are good for us. Right now, yours is to eat.

DAUGHTER: Yeah.

MOTHER: Honey, I remember you telling me that you didn't want to eat because you had pains in your stomach.

Typically, the father insists on action and change, while the mother tries to find reasons to understand and therefore to justify the symptom. An implicit conflict between the spouses is expressed in this area:

FATHER: You're going to have to eat a lot. As much as they give you. You want to get your strength back, don't you?

DAUGHTER: Yes. But most of the time I don't get hungry and don't feel like eating. And when people make me, you know, then after that I just don't feel right. After I eat when I wasn't really hungry.

MOTHER: Now it's going to take time for you to get your body straightened out. But you've got to eat. You can't be expected to eat a whole lot at one time.

DAUGHTER: I know.

FATHER: Okay, you're going to have to eat, honey. That's all there is to it. If you want to get well, unless you want to spend the rest of your days in the hospital, you're going to have to eat. I think you are going to want to eat pretty soon. You want to get better, don't you?

DAUGHTER: Yeah, but sometimes I don't feel good.

MOTHER: But you'll start getting hungry once your system straightens out.

The pattern of symptom maintenance is quite clear. The daughter states that she is not hungry, the father insists that she has to eat, the mother qualifies the father's demands, the daughter complains, the father increases the intensity of his statement—and the pattern repeats:

FATHER: You know, even though you don't feel like eating all the time, try to eat what they give you.

DAUGHTER: I'll do it. I just don't like to eat when I'm not hungry.

FATHER: You told us that, honey. We know that. But you're going to have to, right?

MOTHER: She didn't just stop. You have to realize that she didn't just stop eating. It's not that her appetite just stopped like that.

FATHER: Um-hum.

MOTHER: She stopped gradually. She'd make herself half a sandwich for lunch when she went to school. When Mary went on the diet . . .

The father makes demands, but the mother disqualifies his statement by explaining the daughter's position and supporting her.

Autonomy is possible only by permission:

DAUGHTER: I still love grandmother. I mean for a while, I felt that you didn't want me to feel any love toward her, but I just can't turn that off.

FATHER: But we never said, even to your older sisters. "You can't do this, you don't go there."

DAUGHTER: Uh-huh.

FATHER: In fact we said the other way around to them, "You do what you want."

DAUGHTER: Right. Mom cleared it up. She told me that I'm allowed to feel how I want.

Only the artificial maneuver of taking our anorectic families and declaring them the anorectic family allows us the equally artificial framing which separates enmeshment from overprotection from conflict avoidance, and so on. These patterns are not self-contained units. In real life, or in the therapeutic system, they all intertwine.

Our dualistic way of punctuating reality forces us to frame things separately. We have not achieved a way of thinking that permits us to present feedback processes in all their complexity. We tend to see anorexia as the product of the system, instead of as one of its parts. What we have is an epistemological problem: where does the self end? We punctuate the child as separate from the father, the mother, the siblings. We talk as if the end product is the sum of each individual input. Similarly, when we talk about each family member's contribution to the system, with enmeshment being the result. But let us imagine as Bateson did, that we see a blind man with a cane in the street. Where is that self? Does it include the street? Does it include the cane? If you include the cane, would you cut it before it hits the street?

Bateson's self includes the self's context. Similarly, when we deal with the family, the concept of self must include the feedback processes by which each individual is activated and regulated by the other family members.

The difficulties of describing this process can move us to rely on a punctuation that makes each one of the family members an initiator. We then stop each self before it touches the other selves. But in systems thinking, that cannot occur. We must revamp our concepts of the boundaries of the self.

Blueprints for Therapy

4

The history of anorexia nervosa is an object lesson in the importance of point of view. The investigator's point of view, or governing concept, is his blueprint. It determines the selection of events to be studied and also the methods to be used. Data that are significant to the governing concept are highlighted. Other data are overshadowed or excluded. Identical observations thus yield radically different working formulations when they are organized according to different conceptual frameworks.

The context of the anorectic patient has been part of the data reported by investigators for the past two hundred years. But only since the 1950s have investigators with a systems orientation been looking at the anorectic in that context. And a great deal of research and therapy is still governed by individual concepts of anorexia.

As a result, we are now in a period in which at least two models of therapy coexist, around which the different theories and methods may be organized. They are the two conceptual frameworks that have characterized the study of anorexia nervosa, the linear and the systems. The linear model, which focuses on the individual, encompasses the psychodynamic, medical, and behavioral therapies. The systems model, which focuses on the individual, the context, and the feedback loops that connect them, leads to the contextual methods of therapy.

The two models are not sharply defined in practice. In fact, it is possible to find many common elements in the different points of view regarding anorexia nervosa and its treatment. Fifty years from now a medical historian may well point out how different theorists in this period built on each other's work and theories, translating other viewpoints into their own language in order to broaden their understanding and their therapeutic repertoires. Yet here it is important to take the opposite tack and to polarize differences. This format will distort, as polarization always does; but the oversimplification of the different frameworks may also serve to clarify the issues.

Paradigm Shifts

Through history the framework for the observation and thus the treatment of anorexia has expanded and changed. First there was the medical model, which addressed the different biological systems causing illness in the human organism. Then there was the psychosomatic approach, which examined the interrelationship of the patient's context, or life stresses, and the psychological and physiological mediating mechanisms. Finally the systems approach treated the patient and her context as an integrated whole. These changes of focus in the study and treatment of anorexia were not the result of any expansion in scientific knowledge. Rather they sprang from different conceptualizations of man and his position in the world.

Many studies of scientific paradigm-change concentrate on the relationship of belief systems to one another. But as Thomas S. Kuhn pointed out, major shifts in scientific paradigm are also discontinuous. Kuhn defined a scientific revolution as the process of working through a paradigm shift.[1]

Edgar A. Levenson argued in a similar vein: "When society changes . . . transformations shift, and the new system of relationships that emerges is not a lineal development from the past, but a new arrangement." Psychoanalysis, Levenson contended, has shifted with transformations in world view. As evidence of these shifts, he described three different models of psychoanalytic thinking: the energy paradigm, the communication paradigm, and the organismic paradigm. The shifts that these models incorporate are analogous to Kuhn's "scientific revolutions," in that they represent discontinuous changes in the basis for the practice of science.[2]

Don Jackson, one of the pioneers of family therapy, also discussed the discontinuity of theories: "One finds oneself . . . faced with certain conceptual watersheds, certain discontinuities between interactional data and individual theories." As an example of a "conceptual watershed," Jackson cited the term "individual therapy." "It is likely," he wrote, "that what we mean by the term individual when we take the family system into account may be quite different from what this term presently describes." In fact, from a systems viewpoint, there is no such thing as individual therapy. Intervention with an individual is, willy-nilly, a systems impingement. The therapist who works with an individual is making a one-way intervention into a family or some other natural group. He may not recognize the impact he has on the group, but it is there.[3] Thus investigators with different paradigms may use the same term with different meanings. "Individual therapy" describes one mode of intervention. But its implications in two different frameworks are quite different.

Psychotherapy is now in a period of scientific revolution or paradigm shift. Therapists seem at present to be working with mixed theories. As a result, systems thinkers, using old terms to explain new concepts, sometimes arrive only at global formulations. Psychodynamic clinicians, expanding their language to incorporate new meanings, may try to save old paradigms by creating complex elaborations, which serve only to confuse.

The difficulties of paradigm shift have handicapped the study and therapy of anorexia nervosa. Levenson's three models showing the shifts in psychoanalytic thinking offer an interesting structure for exploring this question. According to the energy paradigm (following Freud), man is a machine—a being run on energy. Like a machine, a man's mind can stop (fixation), be turned on again, and even go backward (regression). As Levenson described it, regression is the ultimate "mechanistic, clockwork image. One can go back, reverse the direction of movement—clearly an operation impossible in a time-oriented perspective. Moreover, since early events are cathexized (invested with energy), they remain inviolate in the timeless unconscious."[4]

The communication paradigm represents the first significant shift in psychoanalytic thinking. Levenson relates this model to cybernetics, the study of "patterns of signals by means of which information is transferred within a system." The emphasis of this model is not on "inexorable established clockwork machinery, but shifting patterns, never entirely the same twice."[5] H. S. Sullivan's attention to the interpersonal relationship of therapist and patient first opened up psychoanalysis to the influence of information and communications theory.

The organismic paradigm is "biological, not physical; it derives from the biological process that can be observed in living organisms." Psychiatry follows the systems theorist Ludwig von Bertalanffly in this paradigm shift. According to him, the organismic model views man as an "active personality system" involved in a web of relationships with his environment.[6]

The underlying concept for the energy paradigm, Levenson explained, is the work machine. The underlying concept for the communication paradigm is the electronic machine, and for the organismic model, which corresponds to the systems model, the underlying concept is the world as organization. All three models have been incorporated in psychoanalytic thinking.

But these shifts in conceptualization are mixed with adherence to traditional thinking. If this is the road, most therapists are stuck somewhere along it. The limitations of the linear model impose powerful constraints on the conceptualization, and therefore the therapy, of many present-day workers. For instance, Hilde Bruch, a psychodynamic therapist, trained in the interpersonal school, remains wedded to the mechanistic model when she deals with the locus of pathology. Her adherence to that model is evidenced by the significance that she attributes to the early mother-infant relationship. Repeatedly Bruch, as well as other psychodynamically oriented writers, report instances of therapy based on the attempt to explore the early relationship of mother and anorectic in transference, while the present mother-child relationship is excluded from the therapeutic field.

Bruch has encompassed the communication model in her descriptions of the process of regulation of the anorectic by her mother as well as of the therapeutic process. For example, she wrote: "the trend in biological inquiries [is] away from deterministic questions, away from reducing the complexities of . . . human behavior to simple parameters of isolated incidents of cause and effect . . . [which] in its very concept violates the true nature of the organism. Emphasis is increasingly on the constant feedback processes whereby parts and whole interact."[7] This statement clearly advances a communication tenet. Furthermore, Bruch has lately incorporated family therapy in her therapeutic procedures. But her writings indicate that while she may see all the members of the family together, her unit of intervention remains the individual.

This is a constraint imposed by the linear paradigm. Although the theoretical formulations may shift to encompass new ways of thinking, adherence to the previous concept prevents the acceptance of the implications of the broader point of view.

For instance, as described by Gerald Chrzanowski, "The construct of the participant observer, introduced by Sullivan, places the analyst-analysand contact in a novel light . . . It emphasizes the fact that the analyst as the observer, and the analysand as the observed, are both part of the same therapeutic field. Observing is a phenomenon that invariably modifies and alters what is being observed. In other words, the role of the analyst is such that epistemologically the notion of the mirror analyst or the concept of the analyst's neutrality is not viable. One cannot be outside of the field of one's observation . . . Accordingly, *participant observation includes significant aspects of the observer's personality in the emergence of therapeutically meaningful data.*"[8] This formulation clearly belongs in a communication paradigm. But this paradigm shift poses a philosophical problem, because the locus of pathology is still the intrapsychic. Change must take place in the patient's mind. "Reality," observed Jean Guillaumin, "exists psychoanalytically only to the extent it has first been detected and then worked through in the proper mental material of the patient."[9] But this concept of "reality" in the mind of the patient can find no common ground with Bertalanffly's "man as an active personality system."

The "mind" which is the target of psychoanalysis is different from the "mind" in a systems framework, which is located and regulated outside of the individual. As Bateson explained it: "Consider a man felling a tree with an axe. Each stroke of the axe is modified and corrected, according to the shape of the cut face of the tree left by the previous stroke. This self-corrective . . . process is brought about by a total system, tree-eyes-brain-muscles-axe-stroke-tree; and it is this total system that has the characteristics of . . . mind."[10] This sense of "mind" as the "total system" is the concept of organismic thinking. Psychodynamic thinking, with its emphasis on the primacy of the individual experience, has difficulty in encompassing extraindividual processes.

For the purpose of highlighting the different viewpoints imposed by the theoretical framework, we have framed four significant areas in the therapeutic process. The linear and systems models can be shown to differ in their approach to the unit of intervention, the locus of pathology, the therapist's role and scope, and the process of change.

The Unit of Intervention

Jay Haley argued that the choice of a unit of intervention imposes different theoretical constructs. Changing the unit from the individual to the dyad to the triad, he wrote, required discontinuous shifts, which required transformations of theory. These shifts might seem minor, but carried to their logical conclusion, they required "a revolutionary revision of clinical views."[11]

The contrasting arguments of Levenson and Haley offer an interesting framework for looking at therapy. If both are correct, one could logically expect that the shift of paradigms from the intrapsychic to the interpersonal, to man in his social structure, would result in changes in the unit of intervention. But it is typical of the present amorphous period that concepts of cause and the unit of intervention do not coincide. Therapists with an intrapsychic concept of the locus of pathology may intervene with a unit of two or more. Therapists with a systems framework may work with a unit of one.

For instance, Murray Bowen, a systems thinker, often selects as his unit of intervention only a part of the family system.[12] He may work with the healthiest or best motivated family member, using that individual as a change agent for the whole. Or he may instruct a patient in changing her relationship with her family of origin, expecting that these changes will resound throughout the system, changing its structure and, consequently, the changer. Or he may elect to work with the power centers. Thus he may see a symptomatic child only infrequently, concentrating his work on the parents, on the assumption that when the parents learn to keep their problems within the spouse subsystem, the child, freed from triangulation, will be able to develop and grow. Thus this system thinker frequently works with smaller units than the family. But such a therapeutic approach, which does not recognize the child's input in the family as a differentiated subsystem or his power to maintain system homeostasis or to facilitate change, would certainly not be correct in treating anorectics.

R. D. Laing, an existential thinker, has chosen the family as his unit of intervention. But in his formulation the family is the culprit.

It is the originator of the child's problem. Therefore, Laing's technique is to join with the child against the parents, increasing the polarization of the two. His therapy, therefore, loses two factors of significance in family therapy: recognition of the feedback from the child into the pathogenic system, and the chance to work with the unit as a whole to change it from a pathogenic to a growth-supporting system. His "family" interventions are actually oriented to "saving" the individual from the system to which he belongs.[13]

There are many examples of the overlapping of paradigms. A psychodynamically oriented family therapist may work with the whole family. But the goal is to change the introjects. Conversely, individual psychodynamic therapists, whose concepts of pathology and change are intrapsychic, may intervene massively in the system as a whole, in the name of "management."

Behavioral therapy was once directed exclusively toward the individual. Recently some behavioral therapists have begun to enlarge their unit of intervention. Once inclined to put the patient's natural environment outside the therapeutic field, some of them are beginning to teach the family how to decondition certain responses. In this case, family members are seen as producing the stimulus events that organize the patient's behavior. The target of behavioral intervention, however, is still the inside of the individual patient.

The systems therapist's unit of intervention, however, is always a subsystem. In a family session the therapist may see all members of a nuclear family and explore their patterns of mutual regulation. But he will include in his formulation the family's connections with the extended family and its spatial and social relationship to society. When the systems therapist works with an individual patient, his view of the patient and his therapeutic approach to that patient is related to the position of the patient as a subsystem of the family and of the social group. The true unit of intervention, for the systems therapist, is holistic. It is the individual in the web of significant relationships in which people interact.

The Locus of Pathology

The *psychodynamic view* of the locus of pathology today represents a collage of Levenson's three paradigms. The psychotherapist Mara Selvini-Palazzoli gave an overview of the situation when recounting her own twenty years of work with anorexia nervosa and detailing her corresponding movement from a psychoanalytical (energy) paradigm to an interpersonal (communication) paradigm and finally to a transpersonal, systems-oriented paradigm (organismic).[14]

When Selvini-Palazzoli regarded the locus of pathology as the anorectic individual, she described the development of anorexia as follows:

> The child's original experience with the primary object is a corporeal-incorporative experience . . . From the phenomenological point of view, the body is experienced as having all the features of the primary object as it was perceived in the situation of oral helplessness: "all powerful, indestructible, self-sufficient, growing, and threatening. . ." To the anorexic, being a body is tantamount to being a thing. If the body grows, the thing grows as well and the "person" starts to shrink.
>
> The ego defense which is thus built up is characterized by the rejection of the body as such and of food as a bodily substance. The pathological control of the body is effected by an attitude that I would describe as enteroceptual mistrust . . . It is as if the patient says to herself . . . "I must not pay any attention to [the body's] signals: hunger, fatigue or sexual excitement . . . I must differentiate myself from it, pretend that hunger speaks only for itself and hence is not worthy of my attention. I am here and the hunger is there. So let me ignore it."
>
> In this way though the patient feels and recognizes the body as her own, she treats it as if it were not.[15]

In this mechanistic conceptualization, the locus of pathology is internal. Anorexia nervosa is contained inside the patient. But concomitantly with this statement, Selvini-Palazzoli expressed a communication point of view about the locus of pathology, which grew out of her acceptance of the position that anorexia nervosa is a phenomenon of regulation between people:

> During infancy the ritual aspect of feeding takes precedence over the emotional relationship of the mother, who derives no pleasure from nursing the child; control prevails over tenderness and joy. Parental stimulation serves to stifle any of the child's own initiative . . . During the childhood and latency period, an insensitive parent constantly interferes, criticizes, suggests, takes over vital experiences and prevents the child from developing feelings of his own . . .
>
> It is thus—bound to a possessive mother who treats her as a mere appendage and never as an individual deserving uncritical support—that the patient enters adolescence.[16]

For Selvini-Palazzoli, the mechanistic and communication paradigms are not discontinuous but complementary: "The failure to detect, and the mistrust of, body signals may therefore spring from two sources: psychologically it may be due to the identification of the body with the bad object and its consequent rejection; neuropsychologically, it may be due to the maladministrations of an insensitive mother unable to recognize or satisfy her child's original needs."[17]

In the late 1960s Selvini-Palazzoli began to look at the patient in the context of her family. Her observations led her toward the systems view of the locus of pathology.

Behavioral therapy is defined as "the application of experimentally established principles of learning to overcome unadaptive learned habits."[18] Thus the behavioralist school, though profoundly different from the psychoanalytical schools, holds in common with them the assumption that the way to change the anorexia syndrome is to change internal characteristics. Both see the locus of pathology as internal.

Psychodynamicists have severely criticized the behavioral therapist on the grounds that modifying the present symptom does not modify the underlying pathology. Bruch wrote: "Proponents of behavior modification claim its superiority to other methods because the weight gain is achieved rapidly and also because it is fool proof . . . This claim is probably correct, but it contains the explanation why this method provokes such serious psychological damage. Its very efficiency increases the inner turmoil of the patients who feel tricked into relinquishing control over their bodies and their lives."[19]

The behavioral therapist acknowledges that his treatments are kept at the symptom level, but he contends that this is the correct approach. The symptom, the behavioralist argues, *is* the neurosis. In answer to Bruch's attack on behavioral therapy for anorectic patients, Joseph Wolpe claimed:

> If behavior therapy is to be applied to a case of anorexia nervosa, it must be guided by the information the behavioral analysis has established about the stimulus-response chains that culminate in the inhibition of eating (or the elicitation of vomiting). The behavioral analysis will also have probed all other revealed areas of behavioral disturbance whether these are related to anorexia or not. In most cases, unadaptive anxiety responses are at the heart of neurotic problems no

matter what the presenting picture. When the stimulus ante-
cedents have been identified, the anxiety-response habits are
tackled by an appropriate method—in many cases by system-
atic desensitization . . .

A treatment plan that does not eliminate unadaptive anxiety response habits is a failure even if it succeeds in controlling behavior that is secondary to them.[20]

The behavioralist, then, addresses the "unadaptive learned habits"
and "unadaptive anxiety response habits." But the locus of pathology is still in the patient.

The *systems model* holds that the formulations of the psychodynamicist and the behavioralist are each part of the answer. Anorexia
nervosa may well relate to early conflict, and there is unquestionably a tendency to continue accustomed responses in different environments. However, the current context is highly significant. The
individual's responses will change if the context changes significantly, and so will his experiences. Furthermore, if a symptom is
being sustained, the transactions of the individual with the family
members, or with other significant people, are reinforcing that
symptom.

To the psychodynamicist and the behavioralist, the locus of pathology is the patient. In the systems model, the locus of pathology
is the individual in context. The dysfunctional sequences that link
individual and context, regulating the utilization of the symptoms
by the system, are particularly significant.

The Therapist's Role and Scope

The *psychodynamic therapist* is oriented toward total personality
and psychological growth. Symptom remission is a byproduct of
total personality restoration. Treatment procedures, therefore, are
not specific, at least in theory.

The therapist who functions according to the energy paradigm is
interested in historical reconstruction in an atmosphere that encourages regression. The therapist does not intrude on the patient's
inner life. His task is simply to explore the truth; his goal is to
provide insight. Thus the therapist does not plan his interventions.
He responds to events only as they come out in the session.

The most significant healing interaction is the development of
transference. In the energy paradigm, transferential distortion, or
the projection onto the therapist of the patient's past, is the path-

way to insight. And insight is cure. Therapists of this persuasion, like almost all therapists dealing with anorexia nervosa, generally combine their approach with milieu therapy and medical management. But in this paradigm, the operations necessary to keep the patient alive are seen as secondary.

The therapist who conforms to the communication paradigm accepts the interpersonal nature of the therapeutic process. Bruch's advice to the therapist, for instance, relied on interpersonal concepts:

> For effective treatment it is decisive that the patient experience himself as an active participant in the therapeutic process. If there are things to be uncovered and interpreted, it is important that the patient makes the discovery on his own and has a chance to say it first . . .
>
> Psychiatry has paid a great deal of attention to the understanding of the disturbed language of patients . . . Less attention has been paid to what the patient hears when the psychiatrist talks to him . . .
>
> Interpretation . . . may mean the devastating re-experience of being told what he feels and thinks, confirming [the patient's] sense of inadequacy and thus interfering with his developing through self-awareness.[21]

In this position the therapist must respect the patient's present reality and her subjective experience. The therapist's authority may be challenged, and consensual validation is achieved by the patient in an exploratory partnership with a participant therapist.

But such a conceptualization does not go beyond the dyad. If the therapist involved the patient's parents, this technique would be considered to be "management" rather than "therapy." Writing as an analyst, Selvini-Palazzoli summarized the attitude: "Many therapeutically counter-productive and, hence, harmful reactions on the part of the parents are highly predictable and can therefore be mitigated by friendly preparatory talks. Thereafter, the therapist's dealings with the parents will be confined to occasional suggestions on how they should behave towards the patient and to fostering optimism and faith in the outcome even during the worst crisis."[22]

Bruch's approach also excludes parents from the therapeutic focus, although their input is recognized. Writing about obese children, Bruch noted: "I have been impressed with the intense involvement of these patients with their families, and how this close bond interferes with their developing a sense of separate identity. This is so glaring, even extreme, in some cases, that I cannot conceive of successful therapeutic work without changing the noxious interaction."[23] Yet she added: "I have not been able to convince myself that conjoint family therapy, which means seeing all members together for the whole treatment period, offers any advantage or is even feasible."[24]

It is difficult to understand how the same author could write such conflicting paragraphs. Bruch incorrectly defined conjoint therapy as always seeing all the family members, and she probably conceived of family therapy as working with the individual dynamics of each family member while all are in the room. In any case, her model of therapy stopped with the dyad.

The *behavioral therapist,* with a focus on the "what, not the why," is interested in symptom cessation.[25] Symptom removal comes as a result of creating conditions of reduced anxiety in the presence of threatening stimuli. The therapist's functions are therefore the exploration and mapping of the patient's behavior and the understanding of her subjective experience in order to develop a therapeutic procedure in which reward and punishment for desired and undesirable behavior can be engineered. While the behavioral therapist controls the environment of the patient in the hospital or acts in collusion with the patient's parents in outpatient therapy, he is nonetheless interested in the development of an affiliation with the patient and of a therapeutic partnership that encourages the patient to participate in the contract for behavioral change. These remarks refer specifically to operant conditioning therapy, since that is the prevalent behavioral treatment approach for anorexia.

If the patient does not improve, the behavioral therapist attributes this not to the patient's resistance but to the failure of incorrect or improperly developed procedures. The therapist therefore takes responsibility for the failure and changes the method. Such a therapist is goal-directed in the sense of searching for the enhancement of alternatives.

But even more than the psychodynamic therapist, the behavioral therapist sees himself as outside of the therapeutic system. He will organize the anorectic's milieu, producing contingencies designed to favor new behavior and corrective learning. But his therapeutic stance is that of the objective scientist.

Like some psychodynamic therapists, the behavioral therapist may work with the family. But family intervention is oriented toward the identified patient's behavior. Even when the behavioralist uses parents as reinforcers, the intervention is not oriented toward changing the parents' behavior.

The *systems or family therapist,* by contrast, sees himself as very much a member of the therapeutic system. He will change the system by participating in the interpersonal transactions that compose it. He is a strategist, oriented to the present. He is active and intrusive. He must participate in the family system to modify it.

The family therapist sees the family as programing the identified patient's behavior. But unlike the behavioral therapist, he also sees the identified patient as programing and controlling the other family members' behavior. Other family members, no less than the patient, must be freed of anorectic behavior.

To the family therapist, change comes in the formation of new family structures. The behavior of all members of the therapeutic system, family and therapist, can be a force for change. It is the therapist's responsibility to uncover more effective alternative transactional patterns in the therapeutic system and to foster their use.

The Process of Change

All therapeutic processes challenge reality as a prerequisite for change. The psychodynamic therapist postulates an expanded self. He teaches the patient that her psychological life is larger than her conscious experience, and helps her to recognize and accept the repressed parts of her reality. The behavioral therapist's relativistic concept sees the patient's reality as a mediated response to context. If the physical and social context changes so that different behaviors are rewarded, the patient's reality will change. The family therapist sees the patient's reality as a highly complex interaction of internal and external inputs. Change in any significant aspect of the patient's social ecology will in some way affect all the members of the system.

The *psychodynamic conceptualization* of the process of change is implicit in the treatment procedures of linear therapists. Mohammed Shafii, Carlos Salguero, and Stuart M. Finch, for example, in reporting the consecutive treatment of two young sisters—Karen, who developed anorexia nervosa at the age of eight, and Bonnie, who developed anorexia two years later at the age of twelve—described the children's psychopathology as being embedded in the family pathology. But they excluded the family input from consideration when planning the treatment. Karen was hospitalized for six months, then returned home with a recommendation for outpatient psychotherapy. Conjoint therapy for the parents was recommended. When Bonnie developed anorexia, she in turn was hospitalized and seen in individual exploratory psychotherapy three to four times per week. In therapy, the patients were able to express their feelings of hostility and aggression toward their parents in a transferential relationship with the therapists. The therapists' description of the treatment revealed their concept of the process of change:

> Karen began to verbalize her anger and hostility toward the milieu staff more directly and at the same time started eating more . . . Gradually she was able to express her anger toward her parents directly or by displacement in the transference situation . . . She became more spontaneous and outgoing and expressed aggressive and competitive feeling in play therapy and on the ward. After six months she left the hospital due to the insistence of her parents. She had returned to her normal weight . . . Bonnie was seen in intensive, individual exploratory psychotherapy three to four times per week. She developed a positive transference relationship with her male therapist early in the psychotherapeutic situation. She displaced the anger and resentment toward her parents in a passive-resistive way toward the ward and school staff. Gradually she was openly able to talk about her anger toward her authoritarian father and her submissive mother. She expressed envy toward her younger sister, Karen, who she felt was able to talk back to her parents and who was able to go to the public school and do most of the things she wanted to do.[26]

Treatment was unspecific. The therapists did not work with the symptoms because they were interested in total personality changes. Change, they indicated, occurred because of the girls' ability to get in contact with their feelings of anger at their parents in the relationship with the therapist and ward staff, and to work through these feelings. Treatment required their working indirectly with past feelings, projected in the present onto people other than the original target. According to this theory, when the patient is cured of the transference neurosis, her relationship with others, including her parents, will change. At this point the symptoms, ceasing to have a function, will disappear.

Unfortunately, the focus on the exploration of the relationship with significant figures in the past may bar fast recovery. Karen and Bonnie were hospitalized for many months. The financial cost of hospitalization and the psychological cost to the girls and their family were high. Happily, the treatment outcome was good. Both girls regained their normal weight. Five years after treatment, they were doing well at home and in school. The therapists, however, reported that they were standing by, ready to act should the girls' three siblings develop anorectic symptoms.

In this case the results of the psychodynamic strait-jacket are clear. The family components associated with the development of anorexia nervosa in two children were elucidated quite clearly, in terms that presented goals for family change. Yet the treatment of choice was to hospitalize the girls, one by one, and to work with them in isolation, while maintaining a sort of citizen's watch for signs of difficulty in three more siblings. It is one thing to park an ambulance at the bottom of a cliff. It is at once kinder and more efficient to place a guardrail at the top.

Furthermore, many anorectic adolescents develop chronic anorexia when treated with psychodynamic methods. It is possible that the concentration on affect, fantasy, and cognition around food maintains food as a major issue in interpersonal and intrapersonal transactions. The patient may begin to feel herself related to only in terms of being an anorectic, with the consequent development of secondary gains in this position and the further narrowing of interpersonal relationships. Her difficulty with interpersonal skills increases. She becomes isolated and finds herself attended to only as an invalid. Much of the poor outcome rate and the intransigence of the anorexia syndrome reported by psychodynamic therapists may actually be the unfortunate result of a treatment procedure that reinforces symptom maintenance instead of promoting change.

The *behavioral view* of the process of change was conveyed by John Paul Brady and Wolfram Rieger when describing an inpatient treatment program:

> 1. From the start, it is essential to obtain and record reliable daily weights under standardized conditions . . .
> 2. The patient should be observed for 3 or 4 days to obtain baseline weight data and knowledge of his daily habits. These

observations often suggest an adequate reinforcer for eating and hence weight gain. In general, behaviors that have a high frequency (high-probability behaviors) can be used contingently as reinforcers for less frequent behaviors . . . In our series this often proved to be vigorous physical activity, daily access to which was made contingent on weight gain . . .

3. Once a reinforcer is selected, the contingencies should be spelled out unequivocally to the patient, the nursing staff, and other relevant persons. The usual daily requirement is a minimum weight gain of ½ pound for access to the selected reinforcer . . .

4. If the patient gains weight consistently (with only occasional, small losses), the contingencies should be continued until weight is in the normal range. If he does not, a more potent reinforcer must be selected and tried in the same manner . . .

5. Confrontation and interaction with the patient over the issue of food, eating, or weight gain should be restricted to carrying out the contingencies described above . . . Parents and other visitors are also instructed not to discuss food, weight, or eating with the patient . . .

6. In general, the contingency should not involve the direct reinforcement of eating behavior . . . Rather, it is better to allow the patient to choose what he eats, when he eats, and how he eats. With the single requirement that he gain weight, this allows the patient maximum choice and freedom and facilitates his working out the issue of autonomy and independence in a more appropriate arena.[27]

For the behavioral therapist, man is an animal who learns. Behavior is learned in interaction with context, and it can be changed by changing the environmental input. The therapist engineers a set of contingencies that encourage the emission of more appropriate behavior and reward the behavior. As the patient increases her competence by repeated, rewarded performance, the new learning is stabilized and becomes self-rewarding. Insight about the change is unnecessary, though it may occur as a result of the change in behavior.

The behavioral therapist's linear view of people in context has produced interesting results in treatment. There is a very high rate of improvement in the hospital. Unfortunately, once patients are back in the real world, this success rate is not sustained.

To maintain her new learning, an anorectic patient would have to generalize her responses outside the therapeutic environment. This would be possible, theoretically, in a well-differentiated context. But the anorectic is part of an enmeshed family system that encourages belonging and family loyalty and proscribes separation. To expect the anorectic to maintain autonomous change in the face of an unchanged family system is unrealistic.

For the *systems therapist,* on the contrary, change occurs when there is a system transformation, which develops a new capacity among family members to select alternate ways of relating. Stereotyped dysfunctional relations are bypassed in favor of more adaptive patterns. In anorexia, symptom cessation is predicated on changes in the patterns by which family members regulate one another. In particular, the sequences that utilize the anorectic patient in conflict avoidance must be modified, to allow the direct expression of conflict and conflict resolution.

The activation of alternative patterns changes the family members' position vis-à-vis each other. As the new structure crystallizes, the experience of individual family members also changes.

Change must occur in the here and now. Linear therapies have focused on the significance of the past and the dominance of the past over the experience of the present. The systems clinician sees the present and past in a different figure-ground arrangement. The past is regarded as influencing the present. But it is also regarded as a creation of the present.

"The historian," wrote Arthur Schlesinger, Jr., "sees the past only as the flickering light of his own day picks out objects in the caverns of time: *new* light; *new* objects." The present, Schlesinger argued, creates, or at least reinvents, the past.[28] Ricardo Avenburg and Marcus Guiter presented a similar argument: "What was once history repeats itself somewhere else if it is preserved in our subjectivity because it is also present in other contexts . . . If an historical truth persists as psychical reality, it does so because it is still a material truth in some context."[29] Infantile sexuality, these psychoanalysts pointed out, acquires significance only when understood in terms of the adult neurosis.

With the systems model it is unnecessary to posit historical causes and to tease them out during the therapeutic process. The past, or the significant parts of the past, are contained in the present. The early mother-child relationship is embodied in the current patterns of mutual regulation in the family. A change in that pattern—a transformation in the present—will change the meaning and the influence of the past. To change the patterns is a way of introducing new light, picking out new objects in the "caverns of time."

Breaking the Constraints

Linear methods of treating illness are too restricted. Individual reality is more complex and more comprehensive than the aspects of it that the linear model highlights. The shortcomings of linear models are particularly apparent when the presenting problem is a dangerous psychosomatic illness. The cost of the constraints in terms of handicapping therapy is far too high.

Selvini-Palazzoli suggested that the linear practitioner's constraints are the result of an epistemological error: "I am referring explicitly to the common error of modern Western thought (and hence of psychiatry)—the idea that there is a self capable of transcending the system of relationships in which it forms part and hence of being in unilateral control of the system."[30] The systems model breaks this constraint.

The line between theory and dogma in this area is very thin. The systems model could carry the practitioner into rigidities that mirror the mistakes of linear therapists, denying the individual while enthroning the system. The input of the individual, who is also a shaper of circumstances, must be seen as part of the system's functioning.

The systems approach considers the individual as a member of a social group, usually the family. A functioning family is a system that provides its individual members with a supportive network. Within the range of that system's rules, however, individual members have a margin of choice. The anorectic family is a system that has closed down, increasing its demands for obedience to its rules. The freedom of choice of individual members has diminished to the point of psychological restriction. The goal of therapy is to facilitate the growth of a system that encourages the freedom to individuate while preserving the connectedness of belonging.

The jump to the systems model frees the therapist for the utilization of every school's insights and techniques. All techniques of individual therapy are available to the therapist, for the systems model does not abandon the individual. It recognizes, however, that the individual is in continuous dialog with the external, in the present. It broadens the approach, using a framework that is more complex than the linear models but which is, for that reason, more consonant with the complex reality of human experience.

Strategies for Change

5 ———————————————————————————

When an anorectic family comes into therapy, the index patient's parents and siblings almost invariably see themselves only as accompanying her. In their view, something has gone terribly wrong with this one child. They expect the therapist to work with her, believing that a cure will make it possible for them to return to the loving, happy family life they remember.

It is natural, though noteworthy, that the family follows the linear model in thinking about this illness. As they see it, the girl has become obsessed, and the parents cannot help her. They have passed through a long period of trying to deal with the problem, and have become convinced that they cannot solve it. They have tried everything they can think of—cajoling, scolding, coaxing, and bribing. All has failed. By the time that the family enters therapy, the parents and the anorectic may be struggling over the girl's refusal to eat, or the parents may have given up entirely. In either case, they expect the therapist to deal with the problem as it appears to them.

The family's denial of conflict feeds into their formulation. Family members often make a point of insisting that there is no reason for the child to act this way, though in some cases they may offer a variety of historical data indicating happenings external to the family which may possibly have precipitated the child's illness. They are a normal, happy family—or they were until this happened.

To the family therapist, however, an anorectic child is part of a psychosomatic system. The most effective way to change the symptoms is to change the patterns that maintain them. The goal of therapy is not only a changed individual, but a functional family system, one that can meet all of its members' needs for both autonomy and support. This goal can be achieved only by submitting the mutually restrictive involvement of family and child to the therapeutic process.

Short- and Long-Range Goals

The initial phases of therapy with an anorectic must focus on the life-threatening syndrome. A combination of behavioral interventions and family therapy techniques, specifically directed toward the presenting problem, can usually achieve symptom remission in a few weeks. With the use of such short-term strategies, the child begins to eat and to regain weight. But at this point, therapy has only begun. Now the therapist must address the transactional patterns that sparked and reinforced the anorexia syndrome. Unless change in the family system is achieved, the effects of the short-term strategies may, in the long run, be nil.

When we began working with anorectic families, we were not in the position of explorers charting an unmapped territory. Our research had already given us a blueprint of the psychosomatic family. The therapists were therefore able to use the model as a guide in zeroing in on the family characteristics that were closely associated with the anorexia syndrome.

The anorectic family is a system whose adaptive and coping mechanisms have become unavailable. Accustomed patterns, though ineffective, have become so rigid that no alternatives seem possible. The therapist's general, long-range goal is therefore to shake the family system and to facilitate the appearance of alternative modalities of transacting. The therapist enters the family by focusing on the immediate life-threatening symptoms of anorexia and moves toward the primary goal of helping the patient to relinquish these symptoms. Then he moves beyond the symptom bearer, zeroing in on the family interactions that supported the symptoms. In the process, a shift occurs in the therapeutic goal. Because the anorectic patient is freed to experience herself as only one part of a dysfunctional system, the family transactional patterns become the target of therapy. As the position of family members vis-à-vis each other changes, new modalities of transaction become possible. In time the exercise of these new patterns become self-reinforcing. The family members, experiencing a new freedom and effectiveness, finally learn to prefer the more adaptive patterns.

Forming the Therapeutic System

The treatment of an anorectic family starts with the meeting between the family and the therapist. The therapeutic system which represents the mutual accommodation of these two entities is formed. The family is incorporated in a larger system that becomes the context of therapy.

The therapist facilitates the formation of the therapeutic system by joining the family and by assuming the system's leadership. He joins the family by recognizing and supporting the family strength: respecting family hierarchies and values, supporting family subsystems, and confirming individual members in their sense of self. He assumes the leadership of the system by presenting himself as an expert, establishing the rules of the system, controlling the flow of transactions, organizing or unbalancing family dyads, supporting or stressing family members, and in general, exploring with family members their views of reality and offering alternatives which promise hope.

Interventions in a family cannot be made from "outside." The therapist has to join the field of stabilized family interactions in order to observe them. He must gain experiential knowledge of the controlling power that the system exerts. Only then can he challenge the family interactions with any knowledge of the range of thresholds that the system can tolerate.

At the same time, the therapist must maintain the authority and mobility of a leader. He will challenge and undermine the patterns that have become stereotyped, limiting the family members' experience. But his must be the planned flexibility of the explorer-participant. As a systems member, he is able to support the other members of the system through the sometimes painful processes of change. Inputs that go beyond the family's range of tolerance elicit responses that affect him, too, as a participant, warning him that he has reached the limits of acceptability.

Joining the family with an anorectic patient offers challenges to the most experienced therapist. Anorectic families have a deceptive capacity to accept without accepting. These enmeshed, conflict-avoiding people welcome the therapist warmly. He quickly experiences himself as a member of the extended kin group. The family members are friendly, cooperative, and obedient. The therapist positions himself as the leader of the therapeutic system without difficulty. The family members are eager to accept him. They are flatteringly attentive. They affirm that they will do everything in their power to help the anorectic patient.

But in this warm, comfortable proximity, the therapist finds that his power to demand change is radically undermined. The family cooperates enough to create the semblance of cooperation, but they maintain the system unchanged. The kind of gentle interventions that fit the anorectic family's conflict-avoiding style have little effect. Mild interventions are easily absorbed by the system with little effect on its homeostasis. The therapist must be able to execute therapeutic maneuvers of a high intensity in order to make any impact at all.

Anorectic families, then, require a therapist who is comfortable with proximity. But he must also be able to challenge, presenting his messages with the intensity necessary to have an impact on the enmeshed system and to push it beyond the usual homeostatic thresholds.

Challenging Realities

The patterns of interaction that the anorectic family now experience as real are only those that are most available to them. The therapist's challenge to the family members' experience of reality is the first step in the process of change. Challenging the way in which the family members punctuate the flow of their experiences offers hope of other solutions and other realities.

The first family transformation occurs as a result of the formation of the therapeutic system. In the process of therapy, the therapist joins, probes, clarifies, mystifies, and pushes, helping the family members to experiment with alternative interpersonal responses in the context of the therapeutic system. He assigns tasks to be carried out at home, where the family members will try out the new transactional patterns with the therapist symbolically present. When the process becomes self-reinforcing, the therapist has become unnecessary, and treatment is ended.

In the anorectic family's framing of reality, the daughter is sick, the parents are helpless, and the process is beyond their control. They come to an expert expecting that he will take charge of the situation. The expert challenges the family reality, declaring that the parents and daughter are not helpless, and recasts the problem. "This girl is sick; her parents have tried unsuccessfully to help her," becomes, "Both parents and daughter are involved in a fight for control." Clearly this new framing doesn't do justice to the complex humanity of the family members or to the many subtleties of family transactions, but as a scenario for therapy, it offers the advantages of allowing the fast mobilization of family members in unaccustomed transactions. This therapeutic framing activates conflicts around autonomy and control that transcend the area of eating; it also permits the actualization of different levels of intensity in therapy, depending on the therapist's style and the family's need.

In very rigid families with seriously ill anorectics, we have used this strategy of pitting the anorectic patient against the parent in a special way. By increasing the affective intensity of the family members' transaction around issues of control and disobedience, the family reaches a therapeutically induced crisis.

Achieving such a crisis is difficult, because rigid family systems utilize inappropriately swift homeostatic mechanisms. When interactions approach the permitted level of affective intensity, a family member acts to muffle the conflict. The affective component of the family members' interactions has to be pushed beyond the usual threshold.

To do so may require a number of interventions of high intensity. For example, the therapist may point out that the parents need to help their daughter eat because her survival depends on their help. But since the parents have already tried to help their daughter eat and have failed, this alone is inadequate to motivate them to try the process anew. The therapist then points out a variety of ways in which the girl is competent. He may state that her refusal to eat is an act of disobedience, not of illness. He thus reframes her not eating as a voluntary act, oriented toward defeating the parents, rather than being an involuntary symptom. The patient is declared the winner. This maneuver puts the spouses, who have been battling each other through the girl, together in defeat by her.

By this tactic of joining with the parents, challenging them, and then insisting on their power to save their seriously underweight daughter, the therapist mobilizes the parents to treat their daughter as a rebellious adolescent, not as an incompetent, ineffective invalid. The anorectic patient, who has expressed her own sense of powerlessness, is also challenged by the reframing of her symptoms as acts of power and manipulation.

What sparks change is the experience of alternative transactions that seem more hopeful. It may or may not be useful to help patients to understand how narrow their reality has become. But to provide the experience of an expanded reality creates the potential for change. It may or may not be useful to explore an individual's feelings. But to explore the system of mutual complementarity that elicits those feelings opens the pathway for change. The statement "You feel dependent on your mother" simply affirms the patient's feeling. To point out to her that she is dependent, angry, or depressed only reinforces the crystallized interactions that relate to those feelings. But the statement "Your mother keeps you from growing up; help her to let you grow up" suggests an avenue for change.

In other words, family therapy deals with a field that is larger than the individual symptom bearer. The process of change occurs through the activation of alternative modalities of interpersonal transaction in the family which creates the experience of new realities for all family members.

The whole process of therapy is like a play of lights and shadows, where what is not presently highlighted seems nonexistent. When an anorectic family comes for therapy, its members are in a tableau that highlights certain aspects of their transactions. This partial aspect of their present reality overshadows other aspects. Linear therapists, in their concern for cause and effect, address themselves to the highlighted areas, the symptoms and their underlying causes. Systems therapists, schooled in feedback circularity, look for ways to bring the submerged alternatives to the fore.

The psychosomatic model posits that five modalities of transaction are directly related to the appearance and maintenance of the anorectic symptom. For heuristic purposes, we presented these as distinct and separate variables, though in life they are intertwined in the fabric of family transactions. The same approach can be used in distinguishing the therapeutic strategies directed toward enmeshment, overprotection, conflict avoidance, rigidity, and the involvement of the symptomatic child in detouring conflict. Much of therapy with anorectics is concerned with challenging these characteristics and, in the process, with supporting the family's use of more functional alternatives.

Challenging Enmeshment

The operations that challenge enmeshment fall into three categories: supporting the individual's life space, supporting subsystem definition, and supporting the hierarchical organization of the family system. The quality of enmeshment is usually claimed with pride by anorectic families, since they see themselves as being loyal, protective, responsible, and responsive, which in effect they are. But when carried to the pathological extreme, their concern curtails autonomy, accommodation, and growth. The therapist must find ways to support individuation and challenge enmeshment, but it will help if he does so without challenging the value of family "togetherness," which can be a functional characteristic.

All operations that challenge enmeshment are also operations that increase the possibility of autonomy. The therapist therefore underlines the right of each individual, not only the anorectic child, to have and defend his own psychological space.

Accordingly, the therapist generally insists that all family members speak for themselves. He stops one family member from explaining how another thinks or feels, though he may encourage the first to ask the second how he feels. Two family members are not allowed to discuss a third member without that person's participation. Family members are discouraged from asking each other for data that they should know, or from verbally or nonverbally checking for approval.

Competent acts are spotlighted whenever they occur. This is particularly true for the anorectic child. The therapist pays particular attention to whatever the anorectic says and makes certain that she is heard and attended to. Often the simple operation of providing a forum has a powerful effect on the anorectic's sense of competence.

In some cases it is useful to develop a ritual after each family session. The therapist may take the anorectic away from the family to be weighed. This can be organized as a secret operation that establishes a boundary separating the therapist and child from the parents and siblings. During this ritual, the therapist can continue to discuss the need for operations of autonomy and differentiation.

The therapist's encouragement of each individual to talk and to give his point of view reinforces the right to individual operations and tends to increase differentiation. Conversely, the therapist may encourage a family member not to talk, on the grounds that any individual has a right to keep secrets. If a family member begins to cry, the therapist may encourage him to cry but block the attempts of other family members to become supportive or to explore the reasons for the crying. The family therapist's position is different from that of the dynamic therapist, who would encourage the ventilation of affect as therapeutic in itself. The family therapist in this case is not involved in the exploration of content or the ventilation of affect. He is interested in sending the message that the individual has a right not to explain his behavior.

The right to individuation can also be highlighted by nonverbal means, such as using space and pantomime. The therapist can create spatial changes, such as separating chairs, moving a family member so as to prevent him from catching paraverbal cues, or seating himself between two family members who habitually check with each other. The therapist can use his hands like a traffic cop to create a physical impression of separation.

It is essential that the therapist insist on communicating the message of separation continually and consistently. Anorectic families have a remarkable capacity for drawing others into family transactions. The unwary therapist may soon find himself a member of the family, sharing secrets and participating in transactions that undermine boundaries. He must avoid this pitfall, consistently reacting to enmeshed transactions by stressing the desirability of respect for a person's life space. His message can gain salience only by repetition.

These operations are necessary throughout therapy. The family members are consistently alerted to the fact that they cannot say "we" without first checking with each other, cannot talk for somebody else, tell someone else's story, finish someone else's phrase, request help in an area where they should be competent, or intrude on someone else's areas of competence. Often the therapist can track the content of the family's communications to find a metaphor that communicates their lack of differentiation. "This is a family which cannot close doors." "In this family, everybody watches everybody." "This is the family without traffic lights." If the therapist is consistent, the family members will become self-conscious about their intrusive maneuvers. Separation becomes labeled as an operation for health. The family's value of protectiveness is not challenged, but it is redefined to include protecting individuality.

Other operations that challenge enmeshment have to do with the protection of subsystem boundaries. It is characteristic of pathologically enmeshed families that dyads immediately attract other family members. If two people are talking, others join in, so that the two cannot finish their transaction. Often the intrusion is part of a conflict-defusing system: others join a dyad to save the dyad from a stressful situation.

The process is so automatic that family members rarely realize to what extent they both interfere and trigger interference. The therapist must find ways to block the intrusion and to underline the desirability of clear boundaries, but without getting involved in the content. The therapist may say to the intruder, "Did you ask them if they want your participation?" He may ask the dyad, "Did you ask for help?" Or he may be more specific. "This is an issue which concerns your parents, not you." "Let your children work this out by themselves." Sometimes the blocking can be done humorously, especially under the guise of protection: "Don't try to rescue your children all the time; that's why you get so tired."

It is also important to protect the generic subsystems. If the spouses elicit a child's participation when discussing a husband-wife issue, this must be blocked. Similarly, the sibling subsystem must be protected from parental intrusion.

The parents in an anorectic family typically intervene in arguments among the children, often to protect the anorectic child. Such intervention allies the anorectic inappropriately with her parents and robs her of the opportunity to participate in peer negotiations as an equal. The therapist must create a buffer zone, delineating the sibling subsystem. He may talk with the anorectic about the necessity of learning to fend for herself among her siblings. If the sibling subsystem operates in a protective fashion, he can assure the siblings that they do not have to worry so much about the anorectic. The child needs opportunities to learn how to accommodate to positions when she has less power and to act autonomously in situations of more power. Human social systems and life itself are organized hierarchically. It makes sense for the child to learn how to negotiate and to accommodate in hierarchical situations in the family.

Still other operations that challenge enmeshment have to do with supporting the hierarchical organization of the system. Difficulties in dealing with hierarchical organization are characteristic of anorectic families. It may be that the family's value system is inordinately child-centered. Or the family may function with the misguided notion that the democratic family does not have hierarchical organization, confusing authority with authoritarianism. It is therefore important to point out that the authority necessary for parenting is actually part of the responsibility that parents have for giving their children a sense of protection. The growing child needs to know that there are external controls which will provide protection and corrective feedback while she is learning.

The issues of hierarchy may be relatively clear when the children in the family are young. In the family with adolescent children, such issues are less defined. The therapist must make clear to them that there are still areas of parental power and responsibility, though there are also many other areas in which the parents and children can relate as equals. The anorectic child is frequently caught in transactions in which she is regulated to respond either like a very young child, or like an adult on a par with her parents. A therapist can say to an anorectic, "You sometimes act like a twelve-year-old, and sometimes you are forty-five, but very rarely do you act like a fifteen-year-old for any length of time." Then whenever the child acts in an age-appropriate manner, this behavior can be reinforced with the same metaphor, "I like you when you are fifteen." Using age as a metaphor for developmental level is invariably understood and accepted. Any fifteen-year-old feels insulted if a therapist calls her twelve. The statement "I like you when you are fifteen" carries a recognition of age-appropriate behavior in concrete, immediate fashion.

In supporting hierarchy, the therapist is seeking not to create an authoritarian *pater familias* structure but to reinforce a respect for idiosyncratic positions within the family. When parents feel effective in their executive functioning they will also be able to respect a child's need for growth and autonomy, even though this need brings conflict and change.

Hierarchical matters too can be supported humorously. The therapist may explain that he is agreeing with his grandmother. The support can also be given directly. The therapist can block a child from intruding in the parents' conversation or taking a protective position on behalf of one parent. He can chastise the child for intruding, or he can criticize the parents for allowing the child to do their job. When the child is supporting one parent, the therapist may criticize the spouse for not supporting his partner himself. In general, all therapeutic operations that challenge enmeshment are operations that support individuation.

Challenging Overprotection

Another characteristic of the families of anorectics that must be challenged is overprotection. The overprotective maneuvers in these families are an extension of the family members' intrusiveness. Many of the operations that are useful in challenging enmeshment also challenge overprotection.

As with enmeshment, there are many small operations which, repeated over a period of time, make the family self-conscious about its overprotectiveness. For instance, if a parent helps a child move a chair or take off her coat, the therapist can comment that the child is quite old enough to do that for herself. Such operations are small enough to be received by the family without defensiveness. But when they are repeated, together with the disenmeshment operations, they carry the vital message of protecting the individual member's right to try and fail, learning how to cope in the process.

It is important to signal overprotective operations in relation not only to the anorectic but also to other family members. This can be done by blocking the operation. When the therapist blocks unnecessary protection among family members, he can generalize by stating, "This is the style of the family X." Or he can say, "In this family, whenever somebody itches, everybody scratches." At times he may ask, "If there are so many people who support each other, how can anybody learn to fend for himself?"

In addition to challenging overprotection, the therapist supports coping behavior. Whenever the anorectic child operates in ways that display competence, the therapist frames that moment by responding to her with interest, asking questions that highlight her behavior and prolonging the moment of competence. By simply increasing the time span of the coping behavior, the therapist gives it salience to the anorectic as well as to her family.

Frequently both parents are extremely overprotective of the anorectic. Sometimes one parent may feel that the child should be treated more autonomously but is stymied by the "concern" which cloaks the other parent's intrusiveness. The parents cluster around the noneating syndrome reinforcing the symptoms in this area. And because the child is so visibly underweight, they fear to demand the same things that they demand of the other children. In such cases, the therapist can point out that they are putting the child in an impossible position, blocking her autonomy and exposing her to the resentment of the sibling group.

It is common to find that the anorectic child cooks for the rest of the family, even preparing gourmet meals. She may in general take a protective stance toward her siblings and even her parents. When the therapist finds the anorectic patient taking over the functions of the mother, he can challenge the behavior with humor, as in saying to the anorectic, "When you're your mother's mother, you must be your sister's grandmother." Or the therapist can challenge the father for allowing the daughter to protect his wife, which is the father's job. The therapist may state that the anorectic is intruding into the father's territory and taking over his tasks. In some cases, the therapist uses the value of protection to challenge the family members' misuse of protection.

A strategy that is sometimes useful to decentralize the anorectic is to direct the parents' concern toward another child. The therapist finds some area of concern and pays attention to that sibling's problem in such a way that the family's protective mode is channeled toward another member, freeing the anorectic a little from the intrusive concern of the family. The anorectic patient is specially positioned in the family as the center of overprotection. To generalize this pattern as belonging to the entire family also helps to decentralize the anorectic child as the sick person.

Overprotective operations spring from a natural warmth and concern. To challenge them, therefore, requires a therapist who is in some way comfortable with being unfair. The therapist's task is to encourage coping and individuation.

Challenging Conflict Avoidance

The avoidance of conflict in the anorectic family must not be confused with harmony. Clinicians have identified strife and conflict as pathological, so therapists are accustomed to recognizing their ill effects. Challenging the gentle facade of people who are seemingly not in conflict may seem destructive to the respectful therapist. However, the conflict-avoiding transactions of the anorectic family are part of the pathogenic pattern that maintains the symptom, and are among the most resistant dysfunctional characteristics of the family.

There are different forms of conflict avoidance. In some anorectic families one of the parents tries to confront the conflict avoider, but never succeeds. Or two family members, after entering a disagreement, signal the increase of stress so that other family members join in to diffuse the conflict.

In general, the therapist challenges conflict avoidance by creating boundaries that help the disagreeing family members to discuss and resolve their conflict. These operations can be relatively simple. When two family members express a difference of opinion, he may ask them to sit close to each other, using space to signal a boundary, and then insist that they discuss the matter. He blocks the attempts of other family members to help or intervene in any fashion. This operation challenges the family's tendency to form coalitions as a mechanism of conflict avoidance.

In anorectic families the therapist is often invited to take the position of referee, or judge, because the family members in conflict tend to use him in the same way that they use other family members, namely to diffuse conflict. It is important for the therapist to withstand such demands, participating only to increase or maintain the intensity of the conflict. He acts only as gatekeeper, preventing intrusion and escape, and maintaining the dialog longer than usual. He uses the boundaries of time to force the dyad to face conflicts by blocking escape.

In the families where one spouse is a conflict avoider, it may be necessary for the therapist to ally with the challenger. Such an alliance triangulates the therapist's ally, who must increase the intensity of his challenge if he wants to keep the powerful coalition. In other cases, the therapist uses the same strategy to ally with the conflict avoider. His ally can then keep the therapist's support only if he deals with his spouse. In such unbalancing operations, the therapist has to be unfair. He knows that the spouses are involved in complementary transactions in which each organizes the other, but he operates as though one spouse is to blame. Although the therapist's understanding is systemic, his intervention is linear. But sometimes an unfair operation is the only way to jolt the spouses from the transactional patterns in which they have been trapped.

Can a therapist, knowing that reality is more complex, operate with a partial reality, assisting one family member and blaming the other? This is a complex ethical issue. But we are always dealing with partial realities. When we say, "I see an apple," we are seeing part of the apple and assuming that the part we cannot see is there. Similarly in therapy, when the therapist joins with one family member against another, he is operating with a partial construct, but not a false one. The therapist knows that his intervention is partial, but he also knows that it is a transitional move. Later he will be able to support the attacked spouse. The therapist must be comfortable with the knowledge that this is a part of the healing process. At different points he supports different system members, with the purpose of helping the entire system out of a dysfunctional groove.

Besides supporting conflict and conflict escalation between the spouses, the therapist facilitates the development of conflict resolution between the parents and the anorectic patient. He focuses on areas outside the issue of eating, conflicts in the interpersonal arena related to the child's ability to do things on her own and the parents' ability to make proper demands on the child. Issues like the child's performance of household chores allow the increase of conflict between parents and child and the development of dialogs about alternative ways of resolving differences that are essential for the disappearance of the anorectic syndrome. The therapist supports the parents' right to establish rules in the house, and the child's right to command respect for age-appropriate autonomy.

Challenging Rigidity

The rigidity of the anorectic family is not the rigidity of the stone, but the ebb and flow of water. The difficulty faced by the therapist is that when he pushes, the family moves. He thus repeatedly has the illusion of making an imprint on the family structure, only to find that he has been sweeping back the sea. The therapist must therefore be wary of the family's seeming acceptance of his therapeutic interventions. He should be forewarned, so as not to feel betrayed and angry at the family. The family has the ability to convince the therapist that they are trying, but that change is impossible. This can result in the therapist's accepting the family image of their cooperativeness and helplessness, and taking over the responsibility for change. At this point the therapist will find himself utilizing the same mechanisms with the anorectic that the parents used before, and he will fail.

Because of the spongelike quality of the family, subtleties, light measures, or one-shot interpretations are no help. The problem of working with anorectic families is the problem of achieving intensity. The family blunts the intensity of the therapist's messages. He must increase his intensity until it makes an impact. The repetition of messages is one means to give intensity. Intensity can also be increased by lengthening the amount of time that family members are in a conflictual situation. The creation of no-exit boundaries and drama or affective ritual are equally related to the need for high intensity in rigid families. It is important for the therapist to realize that words convey only ephemeral messages to anorectic families. The enactment of issues and the development of concrete, clearly differentiated tasks are much more effective.

Challenging Conflict Detouring

The utilization of the anorectic child to diffuse stress in the family is part and parcel of the enmeshed characteristics of the family. Family members are continually utilizing each other to diffuse stress and to maintain their pseudoharmony. Furthermore, the anorectic child has been in a special position in the family since long before the development of the anorexia syndrome. The syndrome was incorporated into already existing transactional sets. But the child's role carries special privileges, which she does not want to give up. Therefore, the anorexia is supported by both parents' and the child's responses. It will be highly resistant to the therapist's attempts to create change.

The therapist uses two different modalities for increasing the strength of the boundaries between parents and child. Sometimes he uses his authority within the therapeutic system to block the intrusive maneuvers of parents and child. This requires a therapist who can function like a director, working at some distance from the family. At other times, the therapist uses himself in the close style that characterizes the family, affiliating and entering into coalitions against some members to unbalance the family system.

Challenging the structures that keep the child involved as a conflict-detouring pathway is perhaps the hardest of the therapeutic strategies to discuss in the abstract, requiring, as it does, an ability to run with the hares and to hunt with the hounds. In the process of protecting a triangulated family member, a therapist can affiliate with her too closely. The triangulators must be challenged, but they must also be supported. The therapist has to work both sides of the street, affiliating sequentially or simultaneously with all family members in such a way that they all feel respected, responded to, and affirmed.

To combat enmeshment, overprotection, conflict avoidance, and rigidity demands a therapist who is able to work in high affective moments, who can create and be comfortable with moments of dramatic intensity, and who can maintain their intensity without being drawn in to "help," thereby diffusing the intensity. The task requires a therapist who can feel comfortable allying with one family member against another, being ethically unfair but therapeutically correct. Issues of ethics and morality are important, but they must not undercut the healing process.

The Opening Moves

6 ———————————————————————————————————

The initial phase of family therapy with an anorectic focuses on the symptom and the symptom bearer. The goal is to help the patient relinquish her anorectic symptoms. This phase ends when the patient is eating and thus out of immediate danger. Then the therapist and the family can address themselves to the exploration of the family characteristics that are dysfunctional and the discovery of alternative transactional patterns that support system flexibility and individual growth.

It cannot be emphasized too strongly that improvement in the anorexia syndrome is only the beginning of the cure. Nevertheless, symptom remission in the early stages of treatment is essential for two reasons. First and foremost, anorexia nervosa is a life-threatening illness. The therapist therefore has a primary commitment to reversing the destructive process and helping the patient regain health. Second, the emotionally-charged salience of the symptom, which mobilizes the obsessional preoccupations of all family members around food and eating, restricts the exploration of other significant conflicts and dysfunctional behavior. As the symptom recedes in importance, alternative transactional patterns become available for exploration. Furthermore, the utilization of the anorectic as a conflict detourer is inhibited, forcing a search for new interactions.

The opening moves in the treatment of the anorectic follow different sequences if the patient is treated in the hospital or on an outpatient basis. The inpatient phase includes pediatric evaluation and management and a behavioral program with the anorectic, family meetings with the pediatric-psychotherapeutic team, and family interviews around lunch. In treatment on an outpatient basis, the

Note: Ronald Liebman, M.D., collaborated on this chapter.

pediatric evaluation of the child may be conducted by the child's pediatrician, and the first family interview can be a lunch session.

The Inpatient Phase

Whenever possible, we prefer not to hospitalize a child. Just as the conceptual framework of a problem dictates the way in which research questions are posed, the way in which health care is delivered is dictated by the conceptual framework. Thus in linear models, focused on the child as the site of pathology, hospitalization of the anorectic is logical and necessary. The anorectic child formerly remained in the hospital for eight to twelve months. Even with the recent emphasis on inpatient treatment with behavioral modification or drug therapy for anorexia nervosa, the mean hospitalization time in several large recent studies is on the order of three months.[1]

But since the conceptual model underlying the systems approach to anorexia nervosa sees the patient as the symptom bearer of pathology that is located in the family, hospitalization of the symptom bearer is not obligatory unless pediatric considerations dictate it. Treatment can take place entirely on an outpatient basis.

Several factors are involved in the decision for hospitalization. The primary decision as to whether a child requires an initial period of hospitalization is made by the pediatrician, who must respond to two medical issues. One is the desirability of performing a careful medical evaluation in order to rule out any organic cause for the anorexia; the other is the need to determine the degree of cachexia in the child, which may be so hazardous that it is unsafe to allow her to remain outside the hospital. In such a child with severe cachexia, an initial period of pediatric supportive therapy may be necessary.

Anorexia nervosa is also potentially lethal, with reported mortality rates of 5 to 15 percent.[2] The fact that these children have lost weight in a very gradual manner apparently gives their bodies a chance to adapt, and it is frequently difficult to tell how close to cardiovascular collapse they may be. To put the problem in perspective, an acute weight loss of 5–10 percent leads to severe dehydration and generally requires hospitalization for intravenous therapy; an acute weight loss of 15 percent may result in shock; and an acute weight loss beyond that figure is almost incompatible with life. All the patients in our studies had lost at least 20–25 percent of their body weight before referral, and weight losses of over 30 and 40 percent were not uncommon. The children had adapted to this chronic weight loss by developing a relative bradycardia or low pulse rate, and their blood pressures were usually low for their age, but not in the range where one could consider shock to be a serious threat to life. Postural hypotension could sometimes be demonstrated in these children with anorexia nervosa, but it was more frequent to have the incongruous situation of a cachectic child jogging beside the bed because she felt the need to exercise in order, as one patient expressed it, to "keep up muscle tone and not get fat." Because of the lack of specific guidelines as to how close to the edge any given patient may be, we adopted the conservative approach of hospitalizing any patient with anorexia nervosa who demonstrates serious postural hypotension or whose blood pressure raises serious concern as to what would happen if any intercurrent illness should afflict the child.

In addition to the medical issues that the pediatrician must address, hospitalization may be requested by the therapist for other reasons, usually involving strategic considerations. However, there has to be a clear separation of decision-making power between the two specialists in this process. The pediatrician must assess the need for further medical evaluation and the need for supportive therapy, and he must make these decisions independent of the therapist. But even if the pediatrician considers hospitalization unnecessary, the therapist retains the option of recommending that therapy start from an inpatient admission. Factors involved in the therapist's decision include the degree of willingness of the family to accept the family-oriented approach as a focus for therapy, and the possible effect of the treatment approaches prior to referral, which may have been so deleterious that hospitalization is helpful in order to sort out the disease process itself from the consequences of the previous therapy. In patients with severe problems who have failed in therapy elsewhere, there is often a very strong iatrogenic component to the continuation of the disease.

In practical terms, therefore, the pediatrician and the psychotherapist make independent judgments as to the necessity for hospitalization based on their specific areas of responsibility. The decision that is agreed upon is then presented to the family in a joint interview.

When hospitalization is judged necessary, children with anorexia nervosa are admitted to a pediatric rather than to a psychiatric unit. The pediatrician has charge of this portion of the treatment. There are three key periods during hospitalization: the evaluation, the institution of a behavioral program, and presentation to the family of the results of the diagnostic phase, at which time the formal family therapy begins and specific plans for the outpatient management are made. At this point the responsibility for the case is transferred from the pediatrician to the psychiatrist.

The Evaluation

The pediatrician meets with the family at the time of admission in order to explain that the diagnostic evaluation will proceed along two parallel tracks. On the one hand, a thorough screening will be performed to look for organic causes of anorexia. On the other hand, psychological evaluations of the family and the child will be performed in order to assess the phychosomatic components of family interaction.

The organic evaluation is thorough, but not extreme. Although a list several pages long could be made of the organic diseases that may present as anorexia, the three key ones of concern in the differential diagnosis are central nervous system tumors, gastrointestinal disease, and endocrine or metabolic abnormalities. A reasonable and appropriate screening program therefore includes at least two elements: careful physical examination with a meticulous neurological examination and laboratory tests.

Physical examination of the usual patient with anorexia nervosa is essentially unrevealing except for providing evidence of malnutrition and cachexia (cheilosis, desquamation, and generalized hirsutism), decreased vascular volume (low blood pressure and occasional postural hypotension), dehydration (poor skin turgor and fecal masses in the colon), hypothermia, bradycardia, and bradypnea. Any abnormal physical finding other than these demands investigation and further follow-through. Any neurological sign, no matter how minor, must also be further pursued.

The laboratory studies should include a complete blood count, urinalysis sedimentation rate, electrolytes, BUN, SGOT, SGPT, calcium, phosphorous, alkaphosphatase, plasma proteins, X rays of the skull, and EEG. These studies can be performed within the first day or two of hospitalization. Abnormalities such as leukopenia, an elevated BUN, and a metabolic alkalosis are not incompatible with the diagnosis of anorexia nervosa. Abnormalities other than these, however, should be investigated further. Extensive X rays of the gastrointestinal tract are usually deferred. If the sedimentation rate is normal, and if the child begins to eat and gain weight on the behavioral program without any manifestation of gastrointestinal symptoms, further studies of the gastrointestinal tract by X ray are considered superfluous.

Within the first day of hospitalization decisions must be made regarding supportive therapy. The pediatrician must make an initial judgment as to whether the patient presents a nutritional emergency. In such a case, vigorous supportive nutritive and caloric therapy will be necessary, possibly including nasogastric tube feedings. Any attempts at psychiatric therapy (including the behavior modification program) should be deferred until the patient is nutritionally reconstituted to the point where she is no longer in danger. Psychotherapy with a patient who is toxic is dangerous and ineffective.

In the difficult task of assessing how close to the edge of potential disaster any given anorectic patient may be, one possible clue is the presence or absence of urinary ketone bodies. The presence of ketones in the urine of a very cachetic patient indicates that peripheral fat stores are still being mobilized to provide fuel. The absence of urinary ketone bodies in a severely cachetic patient is an ominous sign, since it signifies the exhaustion of the fat stores upon which survival in long-term fasting is dependent. When this occurs, protein catabolism becomes more accelerated, and a point of no return may be quickly reached, leading to the death of the child.

Blood pressure measurements are also very important in assessing the need for supportive fluid therapy. If the child is not considered a nutritional emergency but postural hypotension or low blood pressure indicate the need for volume expansion, we give 20cc/kg physiologic saline on the first hospital day. This re-emphasizes to patient and family the serious threat to life that this disease poses, and it allows us to begin the behavioral program without fear that the patient will be thrown into cardiovascular collapse.

At the same time that the organic evaluation of the child is proceeding, psychological assessments of the child and the family are made. All families taking part in the research studies were asked to participate in both the family task and the family diagnostic interview. Otherwise the family task alone is used as an important part of the diagnostic protocol. The psychiatrist also sees the child and the family in relatively informal ways during the hospitalization, for the purposes of establishing a relationship and of gaining further information.

One of the advantages of the systems approach is that one can use information about the family in order to help make a specific diagnosis in the child. In the classic medical approach, the diagnosis of anorexia nervosa is always derived by the process of exclusion. In other words, one rules out endocrine or metabolic disease, one rules out bowel disorders, and so on; when all of these organic disorders have been excluded, one is left with the diagnosis of anorexia nervosa. The observations of family interaction are positive pieces of evidence that help to make a specific diagnosis. In one case, for example, a fifteen-year-old child with anorexia who had been treated for the condition by a psychiatrist for three months without significant improvement was referred to us. Her original screening studies were not markedly abnormal, and she started to eat and gain weight slowly when placed on the behavioral modification program. However, two discordant pieces of evidence prompted further investigation. In the family task session it was noted that the family did not display in excess the features associated with the psychosomatic family. This observation was reinforced by the nurses on duty with the patient, who reported that the family-child interactions which they had observed were not generally typical of what they had seen in other families of children with anorexia nervosa. This information prompted a re-evaluation of the borderline high potassium level, and the child ultimately proved to have hypoadrenalism or Addison's disease. Her anorexia responded dramatically to physiological replacement with cortisol.

The Behavioral Program

Since the report of B. J. Blinder and his colleagues, the use of behavioral modification has been adopted by many groups, with reported rates of success that are impressive.[3] Indeed, behavioral modification has become the major focus for the inpatient management of many patients. In our approach, however, the behavioral program is a small part of the whole approach to the patient. It is used during the inpatient stage, primarily to remove eating as an area of power struggle between the child on the one hand and the nursing and medical staffs on the other. Eating is an area in which the child has already demonstrated her power over her parents. We agree with the child that she is extremely powerful, but we define this power in a very narrow sense: she can exert this power only over herself.

The behavioral program is explained by the pediatrician to the family and the child. The analogy often used is that of a checking account: weight represents the balance of the energy deposits made by eating, minus the energy expenditures used in any activity, physical or mental. The patient will control her own eating, but the medical and nursing staff will control her energy expenditure, based on whether her weight balance indicates that she has sufficient energy to expend. If there are sufficient calories in the bank, the child can spend them; if not, like the hard-hearted banker, the staff will bounce her requests for expenditures, and the child will be forced to remain inactive.

In practice, the behavioral program is adapted to each patient. The age of the child and the areas of activity that are most pleasurable to her are important factors in designing the program. In the younger child, a sense of authority is established by setting up a yes-no behavioral situation. If the child gains 200gm per day, she is permitted full activity; if she fails to gain that amount, even if she has gained some weight, she is completely restricted to bed rest. In the older adolescent, strong guidelines are established, but room is left for negotiation and the exercise of some autonomy. These requirements often result in a more complicated program, in which activity and restrictions are related to amounts of weight gain or loss (table 1). The restriction of activity may be a powerful weapon for the classic hyperactive anorectic but of little consequence to a passive and submissive child. The restriction of mail, visitors, and even reading material may be necessary in order to motivate such a child.

The rules concerning eating are also kept simple: the child must order well-balanced meals, and she is allowed a set time in which to eat. These requirements avoid bizarre situations where the child orders an apple plus six packs of mustard and considers it a meal, or where the child develops a ritual that requires hours to eat the meal. The child meets with the dietitian in order to discuss her food preferences and calories. In actual fact, most anorectic children are more knowledgeable about calories than is the standard medical

Table 1. Behavior protocol during hospitalization of anorectic patients.

Weight gain of 200 gm or more—Up ad lib
1. May walk around unit, go out into hall to make phone calls, down to first floor with parents or nurse
2. May go out of the hospital for lunch only when weight gain is progressive and patient seems stable

Weight gain of 100 gm—Bed rest with bathroom privileges
1. May answer phone when someone calls but may not go out to make phone calls
2. May have visitors
3. May watch T.V., receive mail, bathe in bed

No weight gain or loss—Bed rest, no bathroom privileges
1. No phone calls, but may know who called
2. May have visitors
3. May watch T.V., receive mail, bathe in bed

Weight loss of 100 gm—Bed rest, no bathroom privileges
1. No phone calls, but may know who called
2. No visitors
3. May watch T.V., receive mail, bathe in bed

Weight loss of 200 gm—Bed rest, no bathroom privileges
1. No phone calls
2. No visitors
3. No T.V.
4. May receive mail, bathe in bed

Weight loss of 300 gm—Strict bed rest
1. No phone calls
2. No visitors
3. No T.V., mail, bathing
4. MAY ONLY EAT

---

student. The child orders the well-balanced meal, but it is left up to her whether she will eat the food on the tray. The tray, including any uneaten food, is removed after forty-five minutes. The child is given choices concerning the number of meals that she would like per day, the number of snacks, and whether she wants a running feedback concerning the calories ingested during the course of a given day.

In addition to being extremely powerful in the area of eating, these children are very manipulative. They try to divide the nursing and medical staffs by making them feel guilty and punitive. In particular, the nurses must be included as part of the therapeutic team, since they need to deal with the child's manipulations. It is imperative that the behavioral program not become the total focus of the inpatient stay. In particular, it is critical that the program not degenerate into yet another power struggle which will result in a "no-win" situation for both sides. This can be avoided if the rules are kept simple, the approach of the nurses and the medical staff are kept consistent, and the child is made responsible for her own condition. If the latter point is stressed, eating no longer becomes a power struggle between the child and opposing forces; rather, the child knows clearly that she can use her power only to influence her own situation and to control her own activities.

Most children begin to gain weight after five to seven days of such a program. Children who defy the orders to stay in bed are surprisingly rare. When this occurs, the acting-out behavior is regarded as a favorable sign. The parents are asked to come into the hospital to control the misbehavior that their child is demonstrating. In this way the family can be moved away from the eating issue and into dealing with the behavioral aspects of the problem.

All children with anorexia nervosa test the behavioral program and the strength of those administering it for the first several days. The ritual of the morning weigh-in, the results of which will determine the day's range of allowed activities, is often accompanied by plaintive pleas: "I tried to eat; I deserve some credit for that." Or, "If you let me out of bed so that I can eat my meals with the other children, I will eat more." The pediatrician and the nursing staff take a firm and inflexible stance: intentions and promises can be believed only if actual behavior results in a documented weight gain. They are not interested in motives; they are interested in the net balance in the energy bank. Although the behavioral program should be kept as simple and consistent as possible, it is frequently necessary to modify some of the rules, utilizing the information concerning the patient and the family as it becomes available under direct observation.

Our hospitalization program for anorexia nervosa has a number of significant differences from other inpatient programs, as shown by three major studies that have appeared. R. Galdston, reporting on fifty patients in a children's hospital, stated that their need for hospitalization derived "not only from the hazards of a medical sort, but also from the difficulties of defining the problem of learning to take care of the self in its broader dimensions."[4] The duration of hospitalization in this program ranged from one day to nine months, with an average stay of over three months. The inpatient program combined features of behavioral modification, such as activity privileges being contingent on weight gain, with intensive individual psychotherapy. No information was given, however, as to the outcome status of these patients.

A. R. Lucas and his co-workers studied thirty-two young patients with severe anorexia nervosa, whose hospitalization took place in the psychiatric unit for adolescents in a general hospital.[5] The hospitalization itself was dictated, according to the authors, not only by the need to treat malnutrition but also by the need to separate the child from the family in order to "interrupt the power struggle between child and parents, and to remove the child from an atmosphere emotionally charged on the issue of eating." The average hospital stay was between three and five months, with several hospital stays of eleven months. The main inpatient therapy consisted of individually planned psychotherapy, generally focusing upon a revision of body image and body concept with some milieu therapy. Each patient who remained with the program, three patients having left against medical advice, gained weight. There was also an improvement in such secondary symptoms as apathy, mental fatigue, and depression, and an increase of spontaneity in relationships with peers and adults. Although several of the patients were followed for as long as three years, the authors stated conservatively that it was "too early to draw definitive conclusions about the success or failure of treatment."

Joseph A. Silverman reported a successful hospitalization program for anorexia based on twenty-nine patients which was subsequently expanded to sixty-five children.[6] The hospitalization consisted of a mixture of behavioral modification (refusal to take fluids resulted in three makeup days of intravenous fluid therapy), "realistic regression" (all personal clothing was taken away, no decision-making was allowed, and limited contact was permitted with the parents, who visited briefly once a week), and intensive psychiatric treatment (four sessions per week). Hospitalization was required for an average of three months; no mention was made as to the actual range of hospitalization.

In our studies, however, only thirty of the fifty-three children with anorexia nervosa were hospitalized. The original patients were hospitalized because of the research aspects of the protocol. With other anorectic patients, for whom the decision concerning hospitalization rested completely on medical and psychological issues, the ratio of patients admitted to those started on an outpatient basis eventually dropped from three out of four to one in two. The median duration of the hospital stay was two weeks. The longest hospitalization recorded was one month. Rehospitalization was required for only two children, one of whom developed a pattern of weight gain at home that was bizarre and almost uninterpretable. When she was admitted for closer observation, she was found to be drinking excessive quantities of water in order to falsify her weight. Once this behavioral abnormality was documented, the child was discharged and the therapy focused on this and other aspects of misbehavior rather than on the specific issue of eating.

Our program is thus in contrast to the three others with regard to the actual therapy while in the hospital, the duration of hospitalization, and the need for rehospitalization. However, the critical difference was in the conceptual framework from which all these approaches emanated. When the child with anorexia nervosa is seen as the sole locus of pathology, hospitalization is mandatory, and it frequently is long in duration and intense in therapy. In contrast, when one starts from the premise that the child with anorexia is merely the symptom bearer, the flashing red light which brings attention to the problems of the entire family, then it is clear that the hospitalization of the individual child is not an absolute mandate but rather depends upon precise medical and psychological issues. It also follows that the duration of hospitalization, if required, can be short.

The Family Presentation

Presenting the results of the evaluative process to the family of the anorectic is one of the crucial phases of therapy. It generally takes place in session with the family. The family must experience the pediatrician and psychotherapist as one consistent team.

In the middle of the patient's second week in the hospital, a pattern has usually been established. The diagnostic portion of the hospitalization has been completed, and the results of the behavioral modification program can be evaluated. The meeting with the family is then arranged. At this meeting, attended by the family, the child, the pediatrician, and the psychiatrist, the results of the diagnostic evaluation are explained. The pediatrician and the psychiatrist jointly inform the family of their conclusion that a specific diagnosis of anorexia nervosa has been made in the child. They also present their recommendation for family therapy. The pediatrician indicates that he will continue to be in charge of the child while she is in the hospital but that increasing responsibility will be handled by the psychotherapist so that by the time of discharge the family and child will be completely under the psychiatrist's care.

The next meeting with the family constitutes the first formal family therapy session. This session is frequently organized around the serving of lunch. Such a setting is useful to intensify and highlight the problems that must then be dealt with throughout therapy.

Prior to discharge, another family therapy session may be held, usually three to five days following the luncheon meeting. At that time, the results in terms of the child's weight can be assessed, and plans for discharge and for outpatient management can be formulated. In our experience, the children gain weight rapidly following the luncheon therapy session. The goal is to have the child achieve a weight halfway between that with which she entered the hospital and the ideal weight for her height and age. However, when the child is gaining in a consistent manner, discharge can be considered. Further requirements for weight gain are set for the child after discharge. The specified weight, which is usually two pounds per week, can be monitored by the parents at home and documented by the psychiatrist in family visits.

By now, the pediatrician's role has become essentially that of consultant. From this point, the psychotherapist will carry the therapy into the whole-family context.

The Lunch Session

The family therapy usually begins with a lunch session, whether it takes place within or outside the hospital. The lunch session lasts two or more hours and is, in general, divided into two parts. In the first part the therapist joins the family and develops the therapeutic system: the therapist assumes therapeutic leadership, develops family trust, supports areas of competence of family members, and in general prepares the therapeutic system for the stress of the following sequence in the session. The second part of the session starts when the food that the family members have ordered is introduced in the session and the actual lunch starts.

The rationale for the technique is related to the generic advantage of enacting issues instead of talking about them. This technique facilitates the participation of the therapist in an area in which the family's description can only be partial, and is generally distorted.

When the therapist participates with the family members in the lunch session, he can observe the rigid family patterns that maintain the anorectic symptom and decide on the strategies to challenge the family system.

The goal of the session is to transform the issue of an anorectic patient into the drama of a dysfunctional family.

The lunch session can be organized to increase the focus on the eating problem. Or it can be organized to de-emphasize the focus on eating. The strategy adopted depends on the developmental stage of the child as well as on the other idiosyncratic characteristics of the case.

The strategy of overfocusing on food has been used successfully in families with young anorectics where the increase of parental control is frequently accompanied by a quick relinquishment of the anorectic symptom or in families with dangerously sick anorectics who are losing weight. This strategy is also used to create crises with older adolescents when the family is very rigid or the anorectic is in physical danger.

Overfocusing and Underfocusing

In a number of cases in our project the therapist overfocused on eating by framing the behavior of the anorectic as disobedient and challenging the parents to increase their effective control over that behavior by demanding that she eat. This had the effect of increasing the controlling contact between parents and child followed by increased conflict and distancing between them. By increasing the impermeability of boundaries between parent and child, it detri-angulated the anorectic.

A different overfocusing strategy was used with a male anorectic.[7] The therapist asked the family to agree on one diet that all family members would follow, and the family decided to follow the anorectic's diet. This situation lasted four days, in which the family members became increasingly stressed by their meager diet. It produced a family crisis, increasing the proximity between the spouses and highlighting the position of the identified patient as a controller of the other family members.

In another case the therapist used a strategy of overfocusing when he prescribed for a sixteen-year-old adolescent anorectic a week of limited eating and bed rest at home accompanied by daily phone consultations with the therapist around the acceptable kinds of and quantities of food.[8] This task was designed to keep the parents out of the initial transactions with the daughter around food and to increase the proximity between the therapist and the anorectic. In carrying out the task, the anorectic fought with the therapist for more food instead of fighting with the parents to eat less.

The overfocusing strategy is successful in starting the anorectic to eat. If it is continued beyond that period, the family homeostasis reasserts the old organization of parental control of the anorectic's body. The overfocusing strategy, therefore, needs to be short and should be followed by a period of therapy in which the focus moves away from food and eating.

In the opposite strategy the therapist de-emphasizes the concentration on the anorectic symptom and focuses on general family issues, specifically on the differentiation of family members. In one case the therapist applied this strategy by explaining that the patient would begin to eat when she attained her psychological age. In another case the therapist focused on the spouse transactions and ignored the anorectic patient, so that she could eat while her parents were "distracted."

In the case of the family that insisted on open doors, the therapist underfocused the eating problem in the lunch session by stating that the anorectic patient would not gain weight because the parents treated her as if she were the younger sibling. She would eat only when she became the older sibling. The focus was shifted to support adolescent autonomy and to challenge parental intrusion. The strategy of increasing the proximity between spouses is complementary to the process of separating the child from the parents.

In one case with an adult chronic anorectic the therapist attacked the patient for using anorexia as an "identity card." As soon as a minimal weight gain had been achieved, he stated that the anorexia had been cured but that the emptiness and thinness of the patient's world view remained. The family was discouraged from protecting their daughter's incompetence, and therapy, mostly on an individual basis, emphasized the increase of skills and competence in life. When the focus moved away from coping with the presenting problem to facing realistic problems in the daughter's life with increased competence, the anorexia gradually disappeared.

In another case of a sixteen-year-old anorectic whose symptoms were eating binges followed by vomitings, the family maintained the symptom by a continuous fight around control of the refrigerator, which even had a lock. The strategy of underfocusing was to allow the girl to eat whatever she wanted as long as she would vomit only in the bathroom, and unobtrusively. The disappearance of the usual transactions around food brought into focus the spouse conflict and facilitated a movement of the identified patient toward a world of her peers.

In still another case of underfocusing, the therapist turned to the problem of the anorectic's accommodation to the world of her siblings and emphasized her incompetence in such a world. As the girl's competence improved, her eating increased in the same measure. Lastly, in the case of eighteen-year-old twins of whom one was anorectic and the other had somatic complaints and phobias, the therapist challenged the family hypochondriac organization, which had been supported by more than ten years of individual psychotherapy for the twins, by using the family's sophisticated sense of humor to embarrass them and to satirize their imbedded style of paying attention to each other's bodily functioning. A follow-up a year later showed both twins to be functioning effectively in college with their sense of humor undented by psychotherapy.

These vignettes indicate that the strategies of overfocusing and underfocusing can take many shapes and utilize different family subsystems. The success of the strategies depends on the therapist's ability to accommodate to the family's idiosyncratic channels and to use his experience and imagination to activate the family's resources toward the therapeutic goal. If the therapist is clear about the goals, the end result will be favorable regardless of the road traveled to reach it.

Effectiveness of the Session

A frequent and surprising result of the first lunch session is that directly afterward, the anorectic begins to eat.[9] In our formal study of anorexia, from among the thirty cases that were hospitalized, eight cases had sufficient pre- and post-session weight data available to determine the effect of the lunch session on the weight

of the anorectic. The remaining cases were discharged for therapeutic reasons too soon after the lunch session to permit comparison, and there was insufficient data on the weight of the anorectics treated only on an outpatient basis.

The changes in weight for each of the eight patients during the
four days immediately preceding the lunch session differed sharply
from the changes in weight during the period from the lunch session until the hospital discharge (fig. 5). For ease of comparison,
all patients' weights on the day of the lunch session were assigned
the baseline value. Six of the cases had been declining in weight dur-

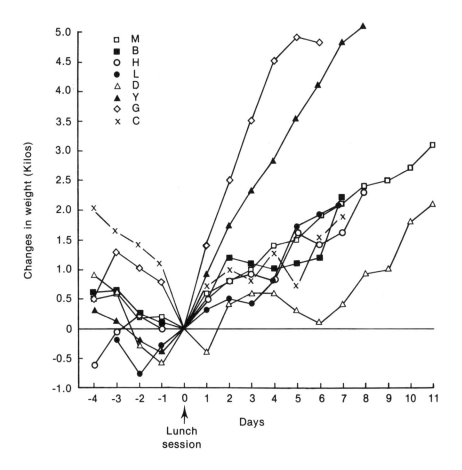

Figure 5. Individual weight changes of eight anorectic patients
before and after lunch session.

ing the week preceding the session but showed a marked reversal following the session and a fairly steady increase in weight thereafter. The other two cases had shown minor improvement prior to the lunch session, but the weight gain seems to have accelerated following the session. Both types of lunch session, overfocusing and underfocusing, were represented within this group, and both approaches appear to have been equally effective, as shown by a composite graph of the weight changes of the eight patients (fig. 6). The weight increased dramatically after the family lunch session.

The direction and magnitude of changes for the four days prior to the intervention were compared with a similar period immediately following the lunch session. The results were significant at the .02 level, using the McNemar test for the significance of changes as being 6.0 (table 2).

Despite the generally impressive rate of weight gain following the lunch session, the strategy is not regarded as a quick cure, be-

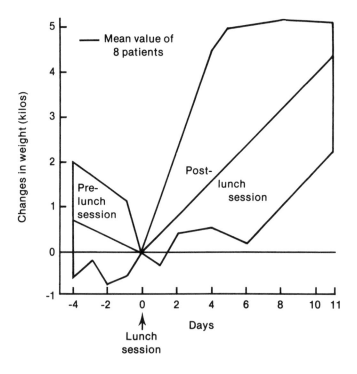

Figure 6. Composite weight changes of eight anorectic patients before and after lunch session.

Table 2. Weight changes of eight anorectic patients
four days before and after lunch session.

Patient no.	Weight change before session (kg)	Weight change after session (kg)
1	−2.0	1.3
2	−0.5	1.4
3	−0.3	2.8
4	−0.5	4.5
5	−0.6	1.0
6[a]	0.2	0.4
7	−0.9	0.6
8	0.6	0.8

a. Based on only three days before and three days after lunch session.

cause the results do not last unless treatment continues. The lunch session comes at the start of therapy simply because of the logic of this context for the therapy with anorectics; that is, if the patient does not eat, it makes sense to look at the field of family transactions around eating.

The efficacy of these strategies in producing a rapid challenge to the anorectic symptom is related to the transformation of the therapeutic system around the issues of eating. The therapy after symptom remission is similar to therapy with other enmeshed families and follows the same general rules.

The utilization of the lunch session in working with anorectics offers a significant example of the relationship between theoretical formulation and therapeutic implementation. In the linear epistemology a lunch session can be conceptualized only as a manipulation on the part of the therapist to increase the effectiveness of family control over the anorectic's body. In the systems model the lunch session offers the necessary context to explore and transform the dysfunctional processes of mutual regulation of a psychomatic family system. It is therefore an experimental field where the therapist can observe and intervene in family transactions around issues of individuation, autonomy and control, demands of loyalty and protection, the multiple maneuvers of conflict avoidance, and the ways in which the anorectic symptomotology is used by the family to maintain itself unchanged.

The Outcome

7

In the final analysis, the value of any rationale for psychiatric treatment can be established only on the grounds of efficacy. The approach to etiology and treatment may be clear, elegant, and logical. But did the patients get well? Elucidation is not enough. Scientists and healers must also evaluate their therapies. Yet too often, treatment is not evaluated. Established therapeutic procedures are adhered to as if they represented a moral code. To establish criteria for evaluation offers the challenge of defining goals and methods more clearly.

In anorexia nervosa, what does "getting well" mean? Sheer weight gain alone is of limited value as a criterion for treatment outcome, however desirable it may be as an initial step. Of much more importance are other questions. Has the weight gain been sustained? Has there been a personality change, enabling the patient to cope with the world outside the therapy room and the hospital? Have the processes of psychological and emotional development been reinstituted, so that new issues of growth can be met?

The issue of short-term weight gain as an outcome measure has been raised by Hilde Bruch, who criticized behavioral therapists for their unjustified optimism based solely on treatment success in the hospital.[1] While her critique was based only on the referral of "failed cases" to her, a more controlled study reported by M. J. Pertshuk did indeed indicate a high relapse rate of 45 percent for both weight and psychiatric problems in anorectics who had improved on a behavioral regime while still in the hospital.[2] The value of any short-term weight gain in anorexia is at best debatable.

A second issue encountered in outcome studies with anorexia is the comparability of the success rates reported. Can a study reporting on one group of patients be evaluated in the light of another study carried out with another group? Furthermore, can the therapy used be assumed to have been instrumental in the results attained? In a study of the field in general, Bruce Sloan reported that while patients being treated by behavioral or by psychoanalytic therapists improved significantly, so did patients on the waiting list.[3] The difficulties of evaluation are formidable. Some comparisons can be made by surveying the published literature, defining the range of recovery rates with and without treatment and placing one's rate of success with reference to these parameters.

An overview of the anorexia literature suggests that the poorest levels of outcome with any kind of treatment or no treatment at all are probably as follows: about one-third recover; about one-third remain at borderline levels, stabilized but with subnormal weight and constricted lives; and about one-third are chronically hospitalized for physical or psychiatric disorder. A. H. Crisp estimated that about 40–60 percent of anorectics make good recoveries.[4] However, K. Tolstrup emphasized that the removal of overt psychopathology is achieved by a lesser number of patients.[5] Finally, fatality rates approaching 10 percent have been reported, even in pediatric populations.[6]

Theoretically, controlled studies comparing different treatments with each other or with no treatment would be ideal. However, the vast majority of reports on the effectiveness of anorexia treatment describe programs like ours, conducted within clinical contexts. Thus, controlled comparisons of different treatments on matched populations are neither clinically nor ethically feasible. But within these limitations, we strove for accurate descriptions of the characteristics of the study group and clear definitions of the criteria used to assess outcome. Comparisons are made only with those studies that seem, to the best of our knowledge, to parallel our own conditions.

Assessment of the Study

Over a period of seven years we saw an increasing number of anorectic patients, all of whom were treated within a systems model. A detailed study was made of the first fifty-three cases treated, analyzing them according to the presenting characteristics of the patients, the course of treatment, and the follow-up data (tables 3–4).

Table 3. Characteristics of fifty-three anorectic patients prior to participation in family therapy research program.

Patient no.	Sex	Age at onset	Weight loss (%)	Onset-referral interval (mos)	Previous therapy
1	F	9	32	2	None
2	F	14	32	3	2 wks inpatient; 1 yr psychotherapy
3	F	9	26	2	None
4	F	12	30		None
5	F	15	42	2 9	1 yr inpatient; 2 yrs psychotherapy
6	F	13	26	18	6 mos psychotherapy
7	F	12	36	1½	None
8	F	14	23	12	None
9	F	15	56	27	2 mos inpatient; brief psychotherapy
10	F	14	30	6	None
11	F	14	42	15	None
12	F	9	22	3	None
13	F	13	35	5	2 mos psychotherapy
14	F	12	44	7	1 yr psychotherapy (for asthma)
15	F	15	29	5	3 mos family therapy
16	F	16	28	6	None
17	F	15	41	6	None
18	M	15	25	12	None
19	F	14	30	7	Brief psychotherapy
20	F	13	39	6	None
21	F	9	41	18	None
22	F	16	18	3	None
23	F	13	29	4	None
24	F	12	—[a]	6	None
25	F	15	21	3	Brief psychotherapy
26	M	12	26	3	2 wks Valium
27	F	15	36	9	1 mo inpatient
28	F	14	40	12	7 mos inpatient (tube-feeding)
29	M	15	22	6	None
30	F	14	36	6	None
31	F	15	35	36	Inpatient 2 times, 1 mo each, individual and family psychotherapy
32	F	11	27	6	Brief psychotherapy
33	M	12	35	15	4 mos psychotherapy
34	F	15	40	24	7 mos inpatient
35	F	10	20	6	None

Table 3 (continued)

Patient no.	Sex	Age at onset	Weight loss (%)	Onset-referral interval (mos)	Previous therapy
36	F	16	23	6	None
37	F	15	50	5	None
38	F	18	41	9	9 sessions individual and family psychotherapy
39	F	12	30	3	None
40	F	17	26	9	Brief psychotherapy
41	F	14	30	6–9	1 mo psychotherapy
42	F	14	23	4	Brief psychotherapy
43	F	18	30	6	6 wks inpatient with psychotherapy
44	F	17	32	7	2 mos psychotherapy
45	F	17	28	6	None
46	F	17	24	3	12 sessions family therapy (unrelated to anorexia)
47	F	15	27	6–8	2 visits psychiatric consultation
48	F	13	23	6–9	None
49	M	20	26	12	None
50	M	21	33	18	None
51	F	16	37	15	Brief psychotherapy
52	F	17	—	12	None
53	F	13	23	6	None

a. Unknown.

Table 4. Treatment and follow-up of fifty-three anorectic patients.

Patient no.	Treatment duration		Follow-up interval (yrs–mos)	Follow-up rating	
	Inpatient days	Family therapy (mos)		Medical	Psychosocial
1	11	12	2–9	Recovered	Good
2	21	12	2–6	Recovered	Good
3	8	4	4–0	Recovered	Good
4	13	6	2–6	Recovered	Good
5	16	4	2–5	Fair	Good
6	15	6	3–6	Fair	Fair
7	14	9	2–3	Recovered	Good
8	7	10	—	Unimproved	Treated elsewhere
9	13	3	2–0	Recovered	Good
10	13	7	3–4	Recovered	Good
11	15	Dropped	—a	—	—
12	20	7	2–0	Recovered	Good

Table 4 (continued)

| Patient no. | Treatment duration | | Follow-up interval (yrs–mos) | Follow-up rating | |
	Inpatient days	Family therapy (mos)		Medical	Psychosocial
13	22	7	2–6	Relapsed	Relapsed
14	24	7	4–2	Recovered	Good
15	25	6	2–9	Recovered	Good
16	14	6	2–8	Recovered	Good
17	14	6	2–11	Recovered	Good
18	0	12	7–0	Recovered	Good
19	0	6	3–9	Recovered	Good
20	0	12	3–9	Recovered	Good
21	0	2	2–3	Recovered	Good
22	0	4	5–0	Recovered	Good
23	0	3½	4–9	Recovered	Good
24	0	8	—	Unimproved	Treated elsewhere
25	0	12	Lost contact	Recovered	Good
26	23	6	2–8	Recovered	Good
27	9	12	2–6	Recovered	Good
28	23	12	2–5	Recovered	Good
29	14	7	1–6	Recovered	Good
30	29	3	2–5	Recovered	Good
31	29, 12	16	3–0	Recovered	Good
32	0	5	2–2	Recovered	Good
33	8	Dropped	—	—	—
34	0	8	2–2	Recovered	Good
35	14	3	2–5	Recovered	Good
36	8	7	2–0	Recovered	Good
37	14	Dropped	—	—	—
38	0	5	2–2	Recovered	Good
39	0	3	1–6	Recovered	Good
40	10, 10	6	2–3	Recovered	Good
41	0	3½	2–5	Recovered	Good
42	10	3½	2–4	Recovered	Good
43	21	5	2–11	Recovered	Good
44	0	4	2–4	Recovered	Good
45	0	8	2–11	Recovered	Good
46	0	7	2–7	Recovered	Good
47	0	9	1–8	Recovered	Fair
48	0	6	1–10	Recovered	Good
49	0	7	1–6	Recovered	Good
50	0	5	1–6	Recovered	Good
51	0	9	2–2	Relapsed	Relapsed
52	0	3	—	Unimproved	Treated elsewhere
53	0	6	1–8	Recovered	Good

a. Unknown.

Analysis of the data shows that the patient population was essentially adolescent, though including some preadolescents and young adults. Thirteen patients, a fourth of the group, were preadolescents, ranging in age from nine to twelve. The thirty-one adolescents, aged thirteen to sixteen, represented 60 percent of the patients seen, while the remaining nine patients, 15 percent of the group, fell in the age range of seventeen to twenty-one. The median age for the entire group was fourteen and one-half years. Six male patients, 11 percent of the group, were included. They were comparable to the females in diagnostic characteristics and course of treatment.

The weight loss at the time of admission ranged from 20 to 50 percent of body weight, with a median of 30 percent. In addition to weight loss, the patients exhibited the common signs of anorexia nervosa: amenorrhea, denial of hunger, hyperactivity, delusional body image, and fear of fatness.

Forty percent of the patients had been treated with individual methods prior to referral. About 20 percent had been previously hospitalized elsewhere. All cases diagnosed as anorectic at our own hospital within a three-year period were referred to us for treatment. About 20 percent of the cases were additional private referrals. The median interval between the onset of illness and the start of family treatment was six months, the range being one month to three years.

Slightly more than half of the patients were hospitalized at the beginning of treatment. They were admitted to a pediatric medical unit for a brief period of from one to four weeks, usually in order to make a medical evaluation, to restore the most debilitated patients, or in some cases to test the effects of disengagement of the patient from the family. None of the patients were tube-fed or received intravenous feeding. A higher proportion of the cases were hospitalized in the early years of the program than in the later, when we were more likely to begin treatment on an outpatient basis unless the need for medical care or for differential diagnosis required inpatient admission.

All of our patients were involved in family therapy, which typically was conducted at weekly intervals. Three families dropped the treatment after one to two sessions. For the fifty families who remained involved, the median course of treatment was six months, the range being two to sixteen months. The therapy was conducted by sixteen different therapists—senior staff psychiatrists, psychologists, social workers, and psychiatric residents—representing three "generations" of practitioners trained in the family approach.

Whereas all treatment was conducted within the broad systems framework, the formal characteristics and specific goals of treatment varied with the development status of the child in the family context. According to a survey conducted among the therapists, a different trend emerged in the treatment plan for each age group. For the preadolescent patients and their parents, the therapists almost universally stated as their primary goal "increasing parental effectiveness and parental control, and strengthening the parental coalition." When working with this age group, the therapists initially used conjoint or whole family sessions, shifting to spouse-couple sessions in the later phases. The preadolescent patients were not seen individually. For children in the adolescent age group, the therapists' goals were to develop autonomy, individuation, and independence. In working with this age group, the therapists occasionally saw the patient individually or in sessions with her siblings, in addition to seeing the entire family and the spouses alone. For the older adolescents and young adults, the therapists focused on issues involved in the separation from the family, which was impending or had been attempted and failed. The therapists worked in family sessions only at the beginning, moving quickly to separate the patient into individual sessions and the parents into marital sessions in order to foster disengagement.

The therapeutic outcome was evaluated in two areas: a medical assessment of the degree of remission of anorexia symptoms, and a clinical assessment of psychosocial functioning in relation to home, school, and peers. In the medical assessment the patients were scored as recovered from the anorexia when their eating patterns returned to normal and their body weight was stabilized within the normal limits for their height and age. If a patient improved, that is, gained weight but still showed some effects of the illness, such as a borderline body weight, obesity, problems around eating, and occasional vomiting, a score of fair was given. Patients who did not respond to treatment were rated as unimproved. When the anorexia symptomatology reappeared in patients after an apparently successful and completed course of treatment, they were scored as relapsed.

In the clinical assessment of psychosocial functioning, a patient's status was similarly scored as good if the adjustment in the family situation, the participation in academic and extracurricular activities at school or work, and the involvement with peers were all judged to be satisfactory. A rating of fair was given when the adjustment in one or another of these areas was unsatisfactory. Patients were judged unimproved if they were unable to function even at borderline levels and continued to show disturbances of behavior, thought, and affect.

These evaluations were based not only on the patient's condition at the termination of therapy but also on the information obtained through follow-up contacts with the patients, families, and pediatricians. The follow-up periods ranged from one and a half to seven years. Eighty percent of the sample was followed for two or more years. All of the follow-up times were dated from a point six months after the start of treatment, since this was the average duration of treatment.

The results from the two assessments (table 5) reveal that 86 percent of the cases were recovered from both the anorexia and its psychosocial components.[7] These results indicate that the vast majority of the cases seen had made complete recoveries, with respect to both the eating disorder and the psychiatric symptoms or other psychosocial dysfunctions, for substantial periods following the completion of treatment. Many of the children had become more independent and age-appropriate in their social relationships and activities than they had ever been prior to the illness.

Comparison with Other Studies

If we attempt to place our findings within the parameters of results reported by others, it is apparent that our results are dramatically successful. However, it has been suggested that this level of success may be accounted for by the young age and fairly recent onset of the illness of our patients.[8] Bruch in particular emphasized this point in evaluating our early reports of conjoint family therapy with anorectic patients.[9] For purposes of comparison, therefore, we examined accounts of other treatment programs for patients in the same age range as our own sample.

Bruch had carefully described the course and outcome of treatment for a sample of fifty anorectics treated by herself and other therapists. From the cases cited we selected for comparison all those involving patients from ten to seventeen years of age whose interval between onset and consultation did not exceed one and a half

Table 5. Medical and psychosocial assessment of fifty anorectic patients following family therapy.

Rating	Characteristics	Number of cases	Percentage of total
	Medical assessment		
Recovered	Eating patterns normal, body weight stabilized within normal limits for height and age	43	86
Fair	Weight gain but continuing effects of illness (borderline weight, obesity, occasional vomiting)	2	4
Unimproved	Little or no change	3	6
Relapsed	Reappearance of anorexia symptoms after apparently successful treatment	2	4
	Psychological assessment		
Good	Satisfactory adjustment in family, school or work, and social and peer relationships	43	86
Fair	Adjustment in one or another of these areas unsatisfactory	2	4
Unimproved	Inability to function even at borderline levels; disturbances of behavior, thought, and affect	3	6
Relapsed	Reappearance of anorexia symptoms after apparently successful treatment	2	4

years. Twenty-two of the cases, including males and females, fit these criteria. Of them, only 40 percent made complete recoveries. Two patients died. One of the fatalities, a fourteen-year-old boy, had been ill for four months when brought for consultation; the other, a fourteen-year-old girl, had been sick for six months. At the time of follow-up, two children were in state hospitals, and one other was still anorectic; the remainder were "restricted" in their functioning.

L. I. Lesser and his colleagues reported on a sample of fifteen anorectic children, ages ten to sixteen.[10] The treatment included pediatric hospitalization and psychiatric care. At the time of follow-up, which averaged five years later, all were described as in satisfactory physical health. These findings led the authors to conclude that the prognosis for this age group was better than for others. However, only seven of the fifteen were described as free from psychiatric disease, while six showed evidence of emotional malfunction and two suffered marked impairment resulting from psychiatric disturbance.

For an even younger group of fifteen children, ages seven to fourteen, with an onset-to-treatment interval of six months or less, J. R. Blitzer and his colleagues reported a 60 percent recovery rate.[11] The majority of the patients were hospitalized. Both patients and parents were seen in intensive psychotherapy for an average of one year, ranging from five months to four years. Nevertheless, four improved only slightly in the course of therapy, and one died. Similar results were reported for improvements in their personality problems.

The most gloomy report must be that by W. Warren, who described the treatment of twenty children, ages ten to fifteen, who were hospitalized from three to twenty-three months, averaging six months.[12] All patients were kept on bed rest. Other treatment included shock therapy, insulin treatment and tranquilizers. Sixteen of the twenty required subsequent hospitalization for anorexia or other psychiatric disturbances. Eighteen patients were contacted at the time of follow-up. It was found that eleven of the patients were recovered from anorexia but, of the recovered group, only two were considered psychiatrically normal. One patient had developed schizophrenia, another was leucotomized, two more were considered severe personality disorders, and five others showed "neurotic personality disturbance of varying importance." Two patients had died, while five had not yet recovered from the anorexia from two to six years after onset.

Several other studies have reported more optimistic results with a pediatric population. Although these studies present incomplete data on the outcome, making comparisons difficult, they have been considered to be examples of "successful treatment efforts."[13] R. Galdston, for example, reported on fifty children treated over a course of twelve years in a pediatric-psychiatric inpatient program.[14] The patients ranged in age from eight to sixteen years. The treatment program combined behavioral features, such as making

privileges and activities contingent on weight gain, with supernur-
turant care by the ward staff, who sometimes fed the patient or
more often sat with her during mealtimes, encouraging eating efforts. Patients were hospitalized for an average stay of about three
months, ranging from one day to nine months. While the authors
described at length the characteristics of these children, their psychodynamics, their families, and the rationale for both inpatient
care and individual psychotherapy, they gave little information
about the outcome and follow-up. The authors indicated that of the
patients fulfilling certain criteria at time of discharge, none had
required readmission. It is not clear how many fulfilled these criteria nor what the mental or physical outcomes were for any of
the patients.

A. R. Lucas and his colleagues reported on their treatment of
thirty-two hospitalized anorexia patients, aged ten to twenty-one.[15]
Their approach combined pediatric care, psychotherapy, and work
with the family. Whereas they claimed that the undescribed family
treatment was essential, it clearly took a back seat to the more detailed explication of individual psychotherapeutic goals and techniques, to which the medical regime and milieu therapy were also
subordinated. The hospital stay was usually between three and five
months but could last as long as eleven months. While data were
presented on the weight gain in the hospital, the report on the subsequent outcome was more impressionistic. Although "the great majority of patients" were described as doing well for periods of up to
three years after discharge, the authors felt that it was too early to
draw definite conclusions about the ultimate success of the program.

J. B. Reinhart and his colleagues reported on thirty-two anorectic patients who were treated on an outpatient plan.[16] They had individual psychotherapy with one therapist, while the family was
treated by a separate therapist. A brief pediatric hospitalization
was used only occasionally for medical reasons. Although reference
was made to a good outcome at follow-up, the results were not given
in any detail. A more recent report describing long term follow-up
on thirty of these cases indicated a very high rate of success with
the eating disorder as only a few cases showed residual effects. However, only 60 percent of the cases were described as having made a
good social adjustment. The remaining group gave evidence of
"emotional malfunction" or "morbid impairment resulting in psychiatric disturbance."[17]

A more optimistic view is reported by Joseph A. Silverman, who described sixty-five patients admitted to a pediatric unit especially devised for the treatment of anorectics.[18] The ages at onset ranged from nine to twenty; the ages at presentation ranged from ten to twenty-one. The pediatric hospitalization program was, on the average, of three months' duration. Psychoanalytic treatment commenced immediately and continued four times a week, with the parents seen separately once a week in therapy by the same therapist. This program was continued on an outpatient basis for two years on the average after discharge from the hospital. The intensive and prolonged treatment was reported as highly effective. Only nine cases were said to have relapsed, owing to "severe emotional disease on the part of the patient or to 'sabotage' . . . on the part of the parents, who, because of their own psychopathology undermined the therapeutic regimen." No follow-up data was presented on this large sample, however, nor was it stated what proportion were still in treatment. Also in question is the cost-effectiveness of the program, involving as it does both significant hospitalization time and prolonged psychoanalytic outpatient care, when less of each might be just as effective.

It is disappointing that some of the more positive studies of the treatment of young anorectics do not present sufficient data concerning outcome and follow-up. It is important in this area, where so much of the research occurs in clinical settings, that clear statements be made of the criteria used for medical and psychological outcome, the number of cases followed, the degree of success, and the follow-up time. Only in this way can an appropriate standard for comparability be developed.

Probably it is true that younger anorectic patients are more amenable to treatment. First, they are less likely to have been sick for a long time, to have developed chronic patterns of behavior to which they and their families have adapted, and to have lost important years of psychological and interpersonal development. Second, if a therapist is willing to intervene in the patient's context, the most immediate contextual field for the child, which is the family, is accessible and relatively malleable. However, to the extent that the condition is allowed to persist and the opportunities for altering the significant contingencies in the patient's environment that support the illness are not seized, then the outcome is bleak. Some of the studies revealed such poor outcomes, and suggested from whence come some of the older, chronic patients who present a formidable challenge to treatment.

In contrast, the results that we have achieved with our methods have been maintained consistently throughout subsequent follow-up and, further, at a psychological and financial cost to patients and families which is absolutely the most cost-effective of any yet reported. Specifically, the treatment approach has been effective in 86 percent of the cases. The program of family therapy lasts approximately six months, with brief periods of hospitalization employed only when necessary. And the anorectic symptomatology disappears two to eight weeks after the beginning of treatment.

These results are a challenge to the sense of hopelessness that has accompanied many follow-up studies on the anorectic patient. Without any doubt, when anorexia nervosa patients are treated within a year of the beginning of the illness with a systems approach in the context of their family, they can be cured in a short period of time.

The Kaplan Family

8

The cases appearing in this and the three following chapters provide actual models of therapeutic strategy as it is determined in the beginning phases of treatment. The content of these sessions, as in all case presentations, is idiosyncratic, representing a meshing of the family's style and the therapist's style. But at a more generic level, the interviews exemplify models of intervention.

The first two cases, the Kaplan and Gilbert families, are examples of crisis induction in a situation where the life of the identified patient is in danger. They reveal the strategies of treatment used until the symptoms of anorexia nervosa are alleviated and the patient is out of danger, which in each instance took about two weeks. The Kaplans highlight the difficulties and complexities of working with this type of family, for although Deborah relinquished her anorexia after two sessions, her psychological problems were more persistent, and she has continued treatment on an as-needed basis for four years. The response of the family of Judy Gilbert, who was the patient in our sample closest to death, and Judy's fast recovery clearly shows the effectiveness of this initial strategy with seriously ill patients.

The last two cases, the Priestman and Menotti families, present an initial approach that de-emphasizes the symptom. The Priestman case reveals a strategy of dealing with the anorexia nervosa by not looking at the eating. The therapist formed a therapeutic system in which he engaged the parents and focused on the spouse interactions, so that whenever the parents tried to triangulate the identified patient, the therapist offered himself as a substitute member of the triad. In the Menotti case, which involves an older adolescent, the approach emphasizes problems of negotiating adolescent privileges and parent rights. The therapist focused on issues of autonomy and control, dealing with the anorexia as an area in which these issues were transacted.

Individual data on the four identified patients are not emphasized, because the focus is on the development of strategy in the beginning phases of family therapy. All possible identifying characteristics have been changed. The transcript of each session appears in the left column, interspersed with analysis of the family transactions and the therapeutic techniques, presented in the form of an interview with the therapist. A more detailed analysis of specific family interactions and therapeutic interventions appears in the right column.

We met the Kaplan family briefly before. Now we will observe the complete lunch interview. Present in the session are the identified patient, Deborah (case no. 6 in the outcome tables in ch. 7), her seventeen-year-old brother, Simon, and her parents, both of whom are in their late forties.

About eighteen months prior to this interview Deborah, a normal, bright, and active child, weighed 115 pounds. Upon deciding to go to modeling school, she was told to lose some weight. She began a reasonable diet, then cut back more and more on her foods. Finally she adopted a vegetarian diet, which became increasingly restricted. Menarche had occurred just before her diet; after a few cycles, her menses ceased. A gynecological consultation indicated that there was no specific gynecological problem.

A year after the start of the diet, her family physician made the diagnosis of anorexia nervosa. The family sought a second opinion, which confirmed the diagnosis. Psychiatric treatment was recommended. In six months of individual psychotherapy her weight loss continued. Finally, at the age of fifteen years and four months, she was admitted to Children's Hospital of Philadelphia. At the time of admission she weighed 84 pounds, having sustained a weight loss of over 30 pounds.

On admission, her physical appearance was striking only in the degree of cachexia and wasting. The intern described her as "angry, but reluctantly cooperative." Her blood pressure was 110/50, her pulse 64 and regular. No specific abnormalities were detected. She was seen by various consultants. No evidences of either neurologic disease or specific endocrine disease were detected.

In the nurses' notes during the first days of hospitalization, Deborah was described as being depressed, tearful, and anxious. Deborah told the nurses that she wished her parents would die and that she herself had nothing to live for. She did exercises before going to bed. She insisted on wearing bulky street clothing even in bed, getting into hospital garb only for her morning weigh-in. She cooperated with the nurse when blood had to be drawn, but cried throughout the time. She asked if she could help with chores in the unit. She ate several packages of mustard but refused her meals when they were brought to her.

Deborah was placed on the behavior modification program. She tried to manipulate the nurses and argued with the physician, contending that bed rest would only cut down on her appetite, so that she would eat even less. During this time her family therapist, Salvador Minuchin, visited her daily for short social visits. He learned from her that she had been in Israel and was passionately invested in the future of that country, and he taught her a few words of Hebrew. They discussed science fiction, another common interest, and he gave her Isaac Asimov's *Foundation Trilogy*. He took every opportunity to commiserate with her about her need to be in the hospital. He made it clear that Dr. Baker was her pediatrician, but that Dr. Minuchin would be her family doctor once the sessions began, since her illness was related to the way in which she and her parents behaved with each other.

Just prior to the first lunch session, the pediatrician met with the family to review the findings of the physical workup. He told the family that there was no physical reason for Deborah's refusal to eat. He also told them that, in spite of the behavioral program, Deborah had lost four more pounds while in the hospital. Therefore, the first family session, scheduled to take place after five days of hospitalization, would seek to evaluate how the family handled Deborah's not eating.

Excerpts from the first two sessions are provided here. By the end of the third session, after roughly two weeks, Deborah was eating normally and regaining weight, and the focus of therapy was shifting to the family interactional patterns.

The lunch session, as in all cases where anoretics have not responded to the behavioral program, was organized to develop a crisis around eating. The whole session lasted over two hours. The first half of the session, before the food arrived, shows exploratory maneuvers. The second half builds to crisis intensity. For heuristic purposes, the interview is here divided into three parts around the key therapeutic maneuvers of joining, fostering dyads, and inducing crisis.

The processes of joining and fostering dyads occur in any first session, though they may not be clearly delineated. The third process is unique to sessions with anorectic patients. Therapeutically induced family crisis has been used for families with other psychosomatic presenting problems. But only with anorexia nervosa is it possible to induce a confrontation, in the present time and context, immediately and dramatically related to the presenting symptoms.

At the beginning of the interview, the family seated itself in a semi-circle, from left to right: Father, Simon, Mother, and Deborah.

FATHER: When you mention she has lost additional weight—she has been eating more than she did in the past. I wanted to know if medically she checked out okay. Tuberculosis? Something like that maybe?

MINUCHIN: She is okay. Deborah is involved in trying to gain weight, so she will. It is just a question that she needs to eat the proper food, and she's involved in negotiation. Deborah, you talked to the dietitian—what's her name?

DEBORAH: Mrs. Beasley. (*She begins to take off her scarf. Her father, sitting next to her, reaches out to help her.*)

MINUCHIN: She's fifteen, and she can do that.

FATHER: Okay.

MINUCHIN: Father is trying to help, but that's not so necessary when your daughter is fifteen. You talked with Mrs. Beasley?

DEBORAH: Yes.

MINUCHIN: And you talked with her about what kind of food you need to eat. So that today you ordered some food that has more protein.

DEBORAH: I don't want that hot dog, but

When contacting identified patient, therapist approaches her as a normal teenager, supporting her autonomy.

she said I had to take it. So I took cottage cheese also.

MINUCHIN: So you are involved with her in trying to change your diet so that your body responds to it. Mr. and Mrs. Kaplan, the fact that Deborah has lost four pounds is not important. She will gain it back because she is involved in doing it herself. It is important that she have control of the thing. Okay?

Therapist affiliates with daughter, supporting her autonomy.

———

INTERVIEWER: Why did you interrupt the flow of the session to highlight an event that is almost invisible, father's helping Deborah with her scarf?

MINUCHIN: This is the first example of organizing events that will frame the therapy—what Montalvo calls "creating a therapeutic reality." I take a small transaction and, by focusing on it, achieve a new dimension. Overprotection is highlighted by pointing out an automatic interaction between father and daughter. During the session there will be dozens of other situations that are dissimilar in content, but formally the same. I will focus on them. By highlighting these isomorphic operations, I will be chiseling away at the overprotective binds that immobilize family members.

Notice that the challenge is mild. I do not make an interpretation of overprotection or control. I say, "She is fifteen, she can do it." And as I block the father, my tone of voice becomes softer. Thus while I am blocking him, on the nonverbal level the gentleness of the intervention makes it a maneuver of joining the father. This is part of my style. I challenge frequently, but I tie challenges with joining maneuvers.

———

(*A secretary enters to take orders for lunch.*)

MINUCHIN: You can order some food from Children's Hospital.

FATHER: I just want a cup of coffee, that's all.

MINUCHIN: For lunch, a cup of coffee?

MOTHER: Abe, have a sandwich.

FATHER: All right. I'll have a sandwich also. Whatever kind of sandwich you have is okay. Just a regular sandwich—like a ham sandwich. Ham and cheese sandwich with mustard on it, and a cup of coffee.

> Enmeshment: mother orders for father.

MINUCHIN: Now you're swinging.

DEBORAH: You can have my hot dog.

> Daughter's enmeshment.

FATHER: Hot dog? I eat plenty of hot dogs.

DEBORAH: You used to tell me how much you liked them.

FATHER: I ate five hot dogs yesterday. Simon?

SIMON: I don't know what I want. I'm still trying to think.

MOTHER: Well, I'll have ham and cheese. Do they have Swiss cheese, perhaps? With mustard. And also coffee, please.

SIMON: Do they have any milkshakes? Okay. A strawberry milkshake.

MOTHER: What kind of sandwich do you want, Simon?

SIMON: Nothing.

MINUCHIN: Great. You know in this family, everybody orders for everybody else.

> Therapist challenges enmeshment, but simply by commenting on an event in which therapist and family are involved and which is in the present. However, the challenge is neutral, since it deals with a small, not very meaningful area. The repetition of mild challenging and blocking operations will give the therapist's input intensity.

SIMON: That's right. Exactly.

MINUCHIN: I want a shrimp salad and ginger ale. A double shrimp salad.

DEBORAH: If I didn't have to get the tray, I could order something.

MINUCHIN: You can order. What would you like to order?

DEBORAH: No, it's okay. They got me cottage cheese.

MINUCHIN: It's your decision, you know. So if you don't like this other thing and would prefer something else, order.

> Therapist supports anorectic's autonomy.

DEBORAH: No. It's just that I was never in the cafeteria.

MINUCHIN: Oh, you were never in the cafeteria?

INTERVIEWER: It seems unusual to have a therapeutic session around a lunch table. Is this part of your making events concrete?

MINUCHIN: It seems to me that if we ask the parents or the girl to talk about the problem, what we get is their selective perception of the issues. And since they have been trapped in an impossible situation for a year, what they will present is the stereotype of that year's transactions. As much as possible, I want to participate, to experience what the family experiences. It's like asking people to dance, instead of asking them to describe how they dance.

MINUCHIN: Simon, you said something that I liked, so we will continue with that. I said that in this family, everybody orders for everybody else, and you said, "That's right." Is that something that happens at home?

Therapist affiliates with son around issues of enmeshment.

SIMON: Well, not really. They might not order for me, but sometimes my mother might inch me onto something. Like, you know, like she might say—you know, she always bothers me about food. That's her only fault. (*The therapist gestures to Simon that he should speak directly to his mother.*) That's your only fault.

MINUCHIN: She's a Jewish mother.

SIMON: Yes, she's a Jewish mother. Right. And sometimes she just—she might take my voice, you know, in certain things. Not that she means it. She might just want to do what's best for me.

Therapist's nonverbal intervention is in the same formal category as his previous intervention to stop the father from helping Deborah. The rule is that family members shall not talk about other family members, but to them. The individuality of each family member is to be protected in therapy.

MINUCHIN: That's a nice expression. She takes your voice. That's a beautiful expression. That means she talks for you?

SIMON: Yeah, at times.

Therapist highlights competence. Son has provided a telling phrase, which therapist will use as a metaphor for family's style.

MINUCHIN: And she makes decisions for you?

SIMON: Not important decisions, but technical—just very small decisions. Like, I can do it on my own. I'm capable. But she likes to—

MINUCHIN: Be protective?

SIMON: Yeah. Protective, I would say.

MINUCHIN: But you feel a lump on your back.

SIMON: From time to time, you know. She is overprotective.

MINUCHIN: How do you shake her off your back? Do you have techniques of doing that?

SIMON: I wind up sometimes yelling at her. By saying, "Just stop, I can do it on my own. I'm a big boy." And sometimes it just doesn't work. She might do it without thinking that she's doing it, you know, for the love that she has for me. But she just keeps on doing it. Not that she means to, but, you know. I just try to shake it off inwardly. I just kind of forget about it because—it's not really a problem, but, I mean, I can control it inwardly. And if I can't, I normally yell at her.

MINUCHIN: What happens when he yells at you, Mrs. Kaplan?

Therapist challenges enmeshment and overprotection.

Therapist maneuvers to join with son. At the same time he deals with the enmeshing transactions, common in the family, which operate to maintain the anorexia syndrome.

INTERVIEWER: First you contacted father and daughter, then you had a long dialog with the son. Now you are moving to the mother. Do you always contact each family member individually?

MINUCHIN: Yes. In a first session, each family member should have the experience of having been touched and confirmed as a person. For instance, I really liked Simon's phrase, "She takes my voice," and I wove around it my appreciation for his intelligence and poetic imagery. In this very simple way I enhanced his self-esteem and became a significant person to him. His phrase is a very good metaphor of enmeshment. Furthermore, it is a metaphor that is clearly identified as having come from the family. They will be able to relate to it.

MOTHER: Nothing happens. It just ends right there.

MINUCHIN: Do you yell back?

MOTHER: No, I'm not a yeller.

MINUCHIN: I thought that you were not a yeller. I had a phone conversation with you, and I knew that you were not a yeller. It means that you are a retreater.

MOTHER: M-hm.

SIMON: She's very compassionate.

MINUCHIN: Wait a moment. Now you are taking her voice.

SIMON: All right. Yeah, you're right. I just wanted to tell you—

MINUCHIN: No, no, no. Do you have your own voice, Mrs. Kaplan, or do you need his? Because if you need his voice, he can talk for you. Okay?

MOTHER: I—I lost my thoughts.

MINUCHIN: We can wait. The idea was that when he yells at you, you retreat.

MOTHER: Well, that's right because it's not usually important things. If it were important, then I would keep at it. If it were an important matter, I would talk about it further. But if it's not important, I just let it drop, because I still want peace, and I feel that there are other important problems to discuss further. You don't have to argue about everything; give in a little bit. He's old enough for me to give in to.

MINUCHIN: You are a peacemaker.

MOTHER: M-hm.

MINUCHIN: Who else is a peacemaker in the family?

Therapist affiliates with mother. To refer to the phone call is a way of collapsing time. Therapist is already an old acquaintance. Quick involvement is characteristic of highly enmeshed families.

Therapist begins to use the descriptive metaphor to challenge. Pointing out that an individual boundary has been invaded is a disenmeshment operation. As the spotlight has focused on each family member, the identified patient has receded as the center of interest.

Because therapist's challenge to son has gone past mother's threshold of acceptance, she responds with a conflict-avoiding statement.

MOTHER: Well, Simon is also a peace-maker, really. Deborah is a peacemaker. She has never fought with any of us. She has never argued with any of us.

MINUCHIN: I would expect that.

MOTHER: My oldest daughter, who is married now—if she didn't like something, she let me know. We sort of rubbed each other the wrong way until she was married. No kitchen is big enough for two women, even though she's my daughter.

MINUCHIN: So you kicked her out?

MOTHER: She just left me willingly.

MINUCHIN: Well it's a pity that you didn't kick her out. That would have been good for you.

MOTHER: Well, I can't do that.

MINUCHIN: Yeah, you are the kind of person who loves things smooth. So who roughs it up in the family? (*The father laughs.*) Okay, let's go to you. Because I would be surprised if you can really make a lot of waves in a family where she always puts oil on the water. How do you do it?

———

INTERVIEWER: Are you now beginning to work with the spouse subsystem?

MINUCHIN: Well, as you can see, I am still taking part in each transaction. But I am building toward the experience of reciprocity and complementarity, which is essential for moving the individual from the experience of "I am" to the systemic experience of "I am affected by the re-sponses of the people I contact." Many of my comments highlight complementarity. For instance, to describe husband and wife as a yeller and a peacemaker describes a unit: roughing/smoothing. It is an "I/thou" Buberian unit: "I" exist as a part, and a complement.

———

FATHER: Well in business, many people say to me, "Wait a minute, stop yelling."

Conflict avoidance is a family pattern.

Therapist uses a bantering tone to soften his challenge of mother's pattern of avoidance.

Having contacted all family members, therapist begins to contact father as a member of spouse subsystem.

And the minute they say that, I honestly tell them, "Look, I'm not yelling." I talk in a loud tone of voice. I don't know how to talk low. I have certain feelings about the family and about what a household should be, and I probably am responsible for a lot of things that are carried out in the household. For example, I argue with my wife that she shouldn't ask the children what they want for dinner. She should put it on the table. And I get very angry when she says, "Simon, what would you like to eat?" He'd like lamb chops. What would she like to eat? She would like cottage cheese. What would I like to eat? I would like a steak. I was born and raised where whatever is put before me, I will eat, because when I was younger, I didn't—

MINUCHIN: Simon, change seats with your mother. Yes, continue.

FATHER: So one of the things that irritates me is when she asks them what they want. You know, if we all decide on having a baked ham, fine. It would be baked ham. But I don't think that she should cook different meals for every person.

Father describes eating as an arena of interspouse conflict. Mother had previously noted her conflicts with the older daughter in the kitchen. Conflicts around food are not the sole prerogative of identified patient.

INTERVIEWER: Why did you ask the son to change chairs?

MINUCHIN: This is an operation I do frequently, changing the family's space arrangement. It is one form of working with boundaries. As you saw, the boy was sitting between his parents. Husband and wife began an argument about food that moved in the direction of the therapeutic goal— to transfer the symptom from the girl alone to the family as a whole. Moving the boy signified that the argument was a spouse transaction that should not be blocked by a child. Creating geographic spaces to separate subsystems can be very effective.

FATHER: Now second of all, my wife and I have always had a very good rapport between one another. We love one another's company, we enjoy being with one another, and—I can speak for myself, I don't know about her, but I feel she feels that way. We've never had any problem, or very few arguments.

Having suggested an area of conflict, husband moves immediately to a statement of family harmony, diffusing possible stress.

MINUCHIN: Simon said that mother sometimes takes his voice. Now you are taking mother's voice. You are talking for yourself and for her. It would be nice if you talked just for yourself. So we will begin to change this—

Therapist challenges the conflict-avoiding operation, using family's description of enmeshment.

FATHER: Family structure.

MINUCHIN: My goodness, you have read my book. That's very good. Yes. I think we should change a little bit the way in which the family functions so that, for a moment, each one talks with his own voice.

———

INTERVIEWER: You are still quite central.

MINUCHIN: Yes. In this first part of the interview, I joined with each of the family members individually. I also began to challenge a major structural feature of the family—the tendency of each member to speak and act for another. The first stage of the session was characterized by one communication pattern: a very active therapist taking part in each new communication. This pattern is necessary early in a first interview. When family members meet with a therapist who is a stranger, they communicate only in their public voices. Not until the therapist has fostered trust can he move to create interpersonal scenarios in which he will be the observer.

At the end of this stage the family members are comfortable about transacting with each other. As a result, the next phase of the session will be under less control, and spontaneous material will begin to appear. The conversation will be casual, seemingly unrelated to the anorectic's symptoms. My therapeutic goals can best be perceived by ignoring the content and focusing on the way I align myself with the different individuals and groupings. One hallmark of the enmeshed family is the instability of dyads: a third party commonly intervenes in a dyadic interaction, deflecting the stress to maintain the surface harmony. In the second stage of the interview, therefore, I deliberately force the dyads to function as such. Different pairs are formed and protected from outside interruption. This experience of uninterrupted dyadic interaction extends the family's behavioral repertory.

FATHER: Well, I have certain opinions and impressions of how a family should be run. And I base these opinions upon other children that I have raised, that I haven't had too much of a problem with. I think that a family should sit down at a certain hour for dinner, and—

MINUCHIN: Talk to Candy. Candy, you listen to him.

FATHER: I feel that—

MOTHER: But we did, all the years. We always had—except when you worked late. Except when they had to go to Hebrew School, where they were away from 4 to 6:30. You see? I mean, there were times when you couldn't sit down as a unit.

FATHER: In other words, when I ran into all those problems—

MOTHER: Yes. When you were working late every night. I mean, you didn't come home any night for dinner.

FATHER: But you see, I have often said to you that anything good that I would do with the children would be undone by you because of your mild manner. And have I

Therapist insists that husband talk to wife. Often family members resist such instructions. Having come to an expert, they want him to exercise what they think is his function of giving advice. Therapist may have to insist a number of times before family responds to such instructions, leaving him free to observe.

Wife responds to husband with her own brand of soft criticism—a curve ball.

said hundreds of times, "Candy, you're so mild in manner that even the dog takes advantage of you"? In other words, I feel that there should be a certain discipline in the house. And if I set down a disciplinary action, I expect you to carry it out. I don't like the way Carol treated you. I never gave in to her, but she practically pushed you out of the kitchen. And she said to Deborah, "One of the reasons I eat up in my room is that Mother and Dad make me nervous." And several other things that she told Deborah. Now, you know, there are certain ways that I would want to run the household, but you see, Dr. Minuchin—I've got to stop talking to her and talk to you for a minute.

MINUCHIN: I am listening, so don't worry. I am listening.

FATHER: I have had certain ideas in my life about running a family today. I thought a family should have a lot of love. I don't remember ever hitting my wife and children, but I do remember being a discipline fellow if they did something wrong. Simon had a stage of playing hooky, and I was ready to kill him with my hands. I took him and practically threw him out. Didn't I, Simmie?

SIMON: Yes. But the—the thing is, I had you under my thumb, really.

FATHER: Did you?

SIMON: Yes. Because when I was away, I knew that I could come back. Because you loved me, and I knew you were going to give in.

FATHER: What did I tell you when I saw you coming back? I said you're coming back to this house because your mother is crying every day—

SIMON: You felt—Oh! I don't want to get into taking his voice.

Conflicts around food have now been expressed between spouses, mother and son, and parents and older daughter, as well as identified patient and parents. Eating is clearly an issue for the entire family. In the midst of a challenge to wife, husband suddenly tries to involve a third person, in this case the therapist. He has probably reached the acceptable limit of conflict.

Therapist responds, but refuses to participate in conflict-detouring pattern.

So father changes content, talking about harmony in the family.

Now father chooses to involve another third person: his son.

Son accepts the ploy and engages father. This transaction is less charged than husband-wife relationship.

Father calls mother into the dyad, both now and then.

Son accommodates to therapist. The small maneuvers challenging enmeshment have

FATHER: I did feel it, Simon. Because I love you.

SIMON: I knew that. Do you know what I mean, Dr. Minuchin?

FATHER: I did love you. However, you've got to admit that I gave all my—

MINUCHIN: Hold on a moment. If you two are going to talk—Candy, change seats. You're sitting between Simon and his father, and you are usually in the middle. I want you out. Continue talking with Simon, Mr. Kaplan. I think that's great.

SIMON: We'll have to change later, because—

MINUCHIN: That's fine. We'll change later.

FATHER: This is musical chairs.

MINUCHIN: Absolutely.

———

INTERVIEWER: Why did you let the son interrupt the transaction between Mr. and Mrs. Kaplan?

MINUCHIN: Mr. Kaplan and Simon colluded to avoid conflict. When the father put the mother down, an alarm signal went reverberating through the family. Both father and son responded to the signal, and in seconds the husband/wife conflict had become a father/son conflict. I had two options. I could have protected the husband/wife dialog instead of furthering the new father/son discussion. But I chose the second because I felt that it was impossible, at this point, to change the nature of the spouse transactions. The father/son discussion looked more promising.

———

FATHER: Yet when you felt that you wanted to go out on your own, I treated you like a seventeen-year-old boy. Because I remember when I was a kid at seventeen, I went to work and then enlisted in the army. So my thinking was that I know what

resulted in son's sensitivity to previously automatic transactions.

Again therapist uses spatial arrangement to reinforce the messages about boundaries.

Family members are beginning to recognize and accept rules of the therapy session.

What started as a dialog becomes a monolog. Father begins to speak faster and faster, and louder and louder.

you are going to face when you get out into the open world, and I said, "Go ahead, go away." Now you've got me very upset with this religious business. You're hanging around with these "Hare Krishna" types, and that's a conflict between you and me. I remember when I was a kid, I broke a lady's window because she said something against my religion. Now I don't know much about religion, but your arguments irritate me, and—

Now father is almost shouting. But as the intensity reaches the acceptable limit, he moves to a childhood reminiscence that diffuses present conflict.

MINUCHIN: Hold on. Simon wants to say something.

FATHER: Go ahead, say it.

SIMON: No. I just wanted to say, it has nothing to do with religion—that little mess-up you had with that lady. She was jealous of you because you were Jewish.

Obedient to family rules, son accommodates to father.

FATHER: All right. Now you're a Jew. You have a Jewish heritage—

SIMON: Of course I'm a Jew.

FATHER: And there are very few of us in this world that are left. And as far as I'm concerned—I can't speak religion to you because I don't know that much about religion—but I know that it's proper for my son to keep whatever religion he was born into! And to give the Jewish rabbi as much of a chance as you've given the other people you listen to. Simon, I love you. I think you're the greatest guy in the world. You're a good son. And the little problems that you're giving me now, I think you're going to come out of.

Just as in the sequence with his wife, father stops himself at the threshold of conflict and moves toward avoidance.

MINUCHIN: Hold on a moment. I just want to ask you one question. Simon, how easy is it to interrupt Father? Just now he was supposed to be in a dialog with you. Could you interrupt him to make your point?

Therapist supports the boy in order to maintain conflictual transaction past the point where father began to diffuse it.

SIMON: Well, yes—

FATHER: Do I listen to you when you talk?

SIMON: Yes, you listen to me. I know how

you are with other people. Sometimes people try to say something and, you know, you want to finish with what you're saying. But I'm like you. And when I want to get in a point, I'll say it. And then, you know, sometimes it's very favorable because—

FATHER: Would you say I try to run the house in a democratic manner?

SIMON: Yes.

FATHER: In a very democratic manner?

SIMON: Yeah. Sure.

FATHER: Do you really, sincerely mean that?

SIMON: Yes, I do. You misunderstand some things, but so does everybody else.

FATHER: Yes. Maybe I don't agree with you all the time, but I think I try to be as democratic as possible.

SIMON: Definitely. I don't think "democratic" is the word. I think—more than fair, you know. Understanding.

FATHER: I try to bend over backwards. But I blow my top once in a while. I'll take your damn pamphlets and throw them against the wall if I see them in your room, or something like that. I lose control. I'm too domineering.

MINUCHIN: Candy, what were you thinking? (*He signals to Deborah to move her chair near her mother's.*)

In response to therapist's support of conflict between them, father and son begin to demonstrate their harmony. They will continue to do so until their facade of nonconflict is acknowledged by therapist.

INTERVIEWER: Why did you interrupt the discussion between father and son to ask the girl to sit near her mother?

MINUCHIN: While the father and son were working toward a conflict-avoidance plateau, I was triggered by the two women's silence. Asking the girl to move her chair was in preparation for activating the female dyad. Again, I am challenging the organization of the family, this time around gender subsystems.

MOTHER: Just—I don't know.

FATHER: She might be afraid to talk, Doctor. I—

MINUCHIN: Are you going to take her voice?

FATHER: No.

MOTHER: I'm not afraid to talk. Not at a time like this, I'm not.

MINUCHIN: Very good. You know, I was thinking. With two guys that are as talkative as Simon and—what is your first name?

FATHER: Abe.

MINUCHIN: As Simon and Abe—do you have any space?

MOTHER: When I have something to say, my son will listen to me. My husband will listen to me.

MINUCHIN: Really?

MOTHER: I have a chance to talk.

MINUCHIN: Deborah, you know I have a feeling that the men in this house take all the space, and that the women are kind of quiet and demure, and not talkative. You are the listeners in the family, and they are the talkers in the family. Do you have space to talk?

DEBORAH: They are—

SIMON: Domineering. (*Laughs.*)

MINUCHIN (*getting up and walking toward Simon, gesturing*): Look at that. Look at that!

DEBORAH: I couldn't think of the word.

MINUCHIN: Oh, but he went into your mouth and he said the word. That's exactly what you said your mother does to you, Simon. That's exactly what your father did to your mother. And now you do that to Deborah.

SIMON: The whole family does it.

MINUCHIN: Okay. But please, you know, let people have a little bit of freedom.

DEBORAH: They have my voice. I don't have one.

Father's enmeshment.

Therapist challenges enmeshment.

Therapist frames an automatic act, making the transaction visible.

By noting the repetition of the operation, therapist makes the jump from individual to family dynamics.

Identified patient uses the family metaphor to explain her own circumstances.

MINUCHIN: They have your voice, yes. What do you do when you want to say something? When you have something to say?

DEBORAH: I don't say it.

MINUCHIN: Is your mother like you?

DEBORAH: To my father, yes.

MINUCHIN: That means she's a quiet one.

DEBORAH: Yes. Yes.

MINUCHIN: What about your older sister? Was she also like you two?

DEBORAH: Well, she would talk to me.

MINUCHIN: She would talk to you. Would she answer back, and fight, and disagree with Father?

DEBORAH: Um—very much.

MINUCHIN: So, she was different. And you and Mother are the quiet ones in the family?

DEBORAH: What did you say? Yes.

Therapist joins her, supporting individuation.

INTERVIEWER: Now you are again acting as a member of a dyad. Have you finished fostering the family subsystem transactions?

MINUCHIN: No. A therapist has to operate according to long-range goals. At the same time, however, the separate steps of the session are determined by the immediate pulls and pushes within the therapeutic system. It is also necessary for the therapist to accommodate to family members while pushing them to change. The mother and daughter required my support if they were to become active, so I changed strategies.

Furthermore, I have been working here with different family subsystems. I started first with the family as a system, then I made contact with each family member as an individual. Then I began working with dyads (husband/wife, father/son, and now mother/daughter). Each individual has been seen as belonging to a variety of subsystems, which highlights each individual as a subsystem. This type of maneuver—supporting individuals and separate subsystems—is essential in enmeshed families, where all individual and subsystem boundaries tend to be weak, individual differences are blurred, and there is far too much emphasis on family identity at the expense of individual acknowledgement.

———

MOTHER: I feel that Deborah is a quiet child. Yet she has as much to say as she wants to. She was never as quiet as she has been recently. She hasn't had friends to the house—

MINUCHIN: Let me make a little bit of a rule. When you talk about Deborah and you say that Deborah was a quiet person, you are describing something that you know—that she is quiet. When you said that she had as much space as she wanted, that is something you cannot know. Only Deborah knows what she wants or not. So that part you cannot do. That's entering into her—

MOTHER: Well, the reason I said that was because she used to talk more than she does now.

MINUCHIN: Then you can ask her if she talked as much as she wanted to. Because that thing, you do not know.

MOTHER: Do you talk as much as you'd like to—speak in the house, you know?

DEBORAH: Now?

MOTHER: Well, how about now and before.

DEBORAH: Before, I was much younger. And there was a different environment.

MOTHER: Why was it different, Deborah?

DEBORAH: You weren't as loud as you are now. You are changed, now that Carol is married.

MOTHER: Do you mean because of change in the family?

Therapist again challenges enmeshment, this time by a rule defining communication content. Formally, this intervention is isomorphic with changing chairs and pointing out that father does not have to help Deborah with her scarf.

Therapist fosters mother/daughter dyad.

DEBORAH: You've gotten much older.

MOTHER: And now you feel that your older brothers and sisters are out of the house, it's different—it is a quieter house? I grant you that. And you became more quiet. Is that what you mean? Well, don't you feel that you can talk as much as you want? (*Deborah does not reply.*) It's a quiet house now, I grant you that, compared to—two children compared to six is a third the noise.

MINUCHIN: Deborah, in a way, by being silent, you make Mother a talkative person. Just as Father, by his tremendous amount of talking, makes Mother a rather quiet person. You know, you don't have any space at all. Do you know that? They don't give you any space, and you don't take any space. When Mother asked you something, you didn't answer. So you took even less space than she allowed.

Therapist's affiliation with daughter supports her right to more space in the family. It is also a move to draw the girl closer to the therapist, in preparation for the lunch part of the session, when he will have to challenge her.

DEBORAH: But I don't know how to express myself.

MINUCHIN: You do. I disagree with you. I talked with you a couple of times in the hospital. And you know how to express yourself. It's not true, what you said.

(*Lunch is now served, and over the next fifteen minutes everyone but Deborah finishes. The therapist has directed the parents to make Deborah eat, but without success.*)

MINUCHIN: I'll move out and leave you together. I want you to negotiate this lunch and see if you can finish it. (*He starts toward the door.*)

INTERVIEWER: Why did you give them a task and then leave the room?

MINUCHIN: I had directed the parents to make their daughter eat, but the family's homeostatic patterns only continued, with someone intervening whenever the interaction reached the acceptable limits. Furthermore, the family was using me to maintain the family homeostasis. They asked me to intervene whenever there was conflict, and I found myself unwittingly responding to their cues by acting as a conflict diffuser. I therefore determined at this point to induce crisis by leaving the parents alone with Deborah with the assigned task of getting her to eat.

MOTHER: Doctor—the thing is, I would like to wait to see how much she does finish.

MINUCHIN: I will be watching through the one-way mirror. I will come back shortly. I want you to negotiate with her. Otherwise she is going to die, the way she is eating. She is starving herself to death. I don't want that to happen. And she is your daughter. (*He exits.*)

FATHER: Okay. Candy, you want to start negotiating with her, or do you want me to?

MOTHER: Well, she is still eating. I would like to see her finish it. Deborah, do you want to finish this half of my sandwich? It is very good.

DEBORAH: Dad, I told you last night that I didn't like it, but I tried it.

FATHER: Are you talking to me? Okay now. I told you that you are going to have to eat everything. And when you get up to a certain weight, you can pick your own shots, but right now, we are negotiating for your survival, like Dr. Minuchin said. Your life. And it is important that you eat whatever—not only here, but you said to me last night that you wanted to get out of the hospital. Now one of the things that I was going to ask Dr. Minuchin was: what happens if you eat everything here, gain weight, go home, and start the same nonsense again?

The following sequences show how the family members maintain the anorectic system without change.

Mother challenges husband and supports daughter, then asks for her cooperation.

Daughter gives the appearance of cooperation.

Father's monolog is a diffuse sequence of requests and demands:
1. "You are going to have to eat everything"—an authoritarian threat.
2. "When you get up to a certain weight . . . pick your own shots"—negotiation, suggesting a conditional reward.
3. "You wanted to get out of the hospital"—request for future compliance.
4. "What happens if you eat everything . . . same nonsense again"—a "no-win" premise.
5. "If my child is going to

Now as far as I am concerned, if my child is going to starve herself to death, and I know she has to eat, I am going to open your mouth and make you eat the goddamned food. But I would like to see what you eat by yourself.

DEBORAH: The dietitian was up here, and she asked me what I wanted to eat.

MOTHER: You are old enough to understand. Dr. Minuchin was just in here. And before you came to the hospital, I told you that you were going to die. Do you know what that means, Deborah? You are going to *die!* You have a beautiful life ahead of you—you are only fifteen! Deborah, this contains protein. This—

FATHER: Deborah, how many doctors have told you that you are *not* a dietitian? Dr. Bryan, Dr. Cole, Dr. Minuchin. Now wipe out of your mind what these things contain, and just eat them.

MOTHER: Let her finish eating. I think she is going to try to eat.

DEBORAH: I was talking to a real dietitian here. And she told me to order what *I* wanted. And she said that cottage cheese is a very good source of protein, and I don't have to eat all that—

MOTHER: You have been losing weight ever since you went on cottage cheese and apples. Doesn't that mean anything? You have to start to gain. Do you understand what that means? You have to order milk shakes, cakes, pies—

DEBORAH (*her voice rising to a whine*): I don't like that stuff. I don't want it.

FATHER: Your life is involved, and you have to eat. Listen, Deb, don't be one to grasp onto what a dietitian says or what a doctor says and use that as an excuse. To

starve herself . . . eat the goddamned food"—mixture of protection and threat.

6. "But I would like to see what you eat by yourself"—request for cooperation. These demands annul each other; their algebraic addition yields only inaction.

Daughter's mild challenge has the effect of postponing necessity to respond to father.

Mother joins in, disqualifying father's demand. She requests daughter's understanding, thereby increasing the intensity of affect and concern. She pleads with daughter, then immediately switches to rational explanation.

Father's interruption nullifies any effect from mother's pleading and explaining.

Mother challenges father on grounds of concern and protection for daughter.

Daughter brings an expert opinion into the discussion in order to disqualify both parents and again postpone the necessity for action.

Daughter's response to mother's escalated pleading is negative and childlike.

Father's demand for action is immediately followed by a plea that annuls the demand.

me, cottage cheese is a side order. Just a dish—

DEBORAH: Look at you.

FATHER: What's wrong with me? I weigh just what I should weigh. I wish to hell you looked like me.

MINUCHIN (*re-entering*): You are not doing well at all.

FATHER: I am sorry.

MINUCHIN: You have to think of how you can do this so that it works. As you are going, you are yelling, and she is resisting. But she has to eat. There is no way out of it.

FATHER: Okay, Doctor.

Daughter challenges father, making him the target.

Her gambit works: father's self-defense and attack carry no request for action.

INTERVIEWER: I was wondering why you broke in at that point.

MINUCHIN: Well, from behind the mirror I was observing a very delicate organization. Each of the three family members was controlling the others. In response to my demand, the father took a stern attitude: "You will eat." The daughter responded with an oblique complaint about her parents' overcontrol. This triggered mother to say to father, "Don't be so harsh." The mother took over, pleading, and the girl responded by rejecting the request. This activated father to take another stern position. The girl became pathetic, and the mother then interfered in her behalf, again intimating that the father was too stern. There was an escalation of tension which reached a plateau faster with each new repetition. I thought that my verbal intervention might change the sequence and give the girl the freedom of eating on her own terms.

INTERVIEWER: In other words, you were hoping that you could get the parents to pull together instead of cutting each other off.

MINUCHIN: Yes. That is why I said, "You'll have to think of how you can do this so that it works." But as you will see, the maneuver was unsuccessful, and the process continued. This system is regulated by all three members. Deborah can make the father become reasonable by turning pitiful. The mother is activated when the girl counterattacks or the father becomes demanding. But when the mother intensifies her demands, the father again turns reasonable in a way that keeps the girl in the same position. All three change according to circumstance, but the system remains unchanged.

FATHER: Deb, eat what's on your tray.

DEBORAH: I don't like this!

FATHER: But eat it.

DEBORAH (*shrieking*): No! No! I don't care! You can shove it down my throat! I'll get sick, and I *will* die!

Daughter's outburst expresses her perception of life in this family, and her only solution. Her only power is passive resistance; her only effective challenge is to threaten her own death.

MOTHER (*calmly*): Well, why don't you order something else then? Another piece of meat? Another kind of food?

DEBORAH: Because I ordered cottage cheese! And they said they would give me meat three times a day, if I wanted it.

FATHER: You *have* to eat meat three times a day, if they say so.

DEBORAH: No, no, no! You know a growing girl eats what she wants. Oh golly, you *make* me eat it!

Daughter's request for recognition of her autonomy is immediately linked with her feeling of helplessness against external power.

MOTHER: A normal growing girl can eat what she—a growing girl eats certain nourishing foods, and then she eats other things that she likes as well. You are starving your body.

DEBORAH: I am *not* starving it! My pulse went up. Everything is going up.

In response to mother's calm, daughter becomes reasonable. But she still rejects the request.

MOTHER: Then why are you losing weight? Over two pounds since yesterday, a

The intensity of mother's plea increases, particularly as father tries to get in a word.

half-pound the day before that. And you are eating. A pound a day before that. You have got to eat more. You have got to start to gain, because you are going to die, Deborah!

FATHER: You—

MOTHER: You won't have another chance. You only have one chance, right now.

FATHER: Deb—

DEBORAH: I won't die.

MOTHER: You will.

FATHER: First of all, you are acting just like a two-year-old baby. Now look Deborah, let me speak to you. And let's not cry, because that is no way to express yourself. Understand? I told you that last night. I told you that you can get your point across without crying. You are acting like a two-year-old child, honey. Now let me ask you a question, okay? I asked you a question, like are you going to eat any more food that is on your tray, and you said no. But I would like you to. Now, you said to me last night you want to get out of this hospital—you can't stand it in this hospital. And I told you that the only way you can get out of this hospital is to go up to 120 pounds. You said that you will *never* weigh 120 pounds. Now Dr. Minuchin said today you can get out of here at 88 pounds. I am not worried about that. I know that you are going to eat, and you are going to eat well, because if you want to get out of this hospital, you are going to eat. And you are going to put plenty of weight on. But the thing is this, Deborah. You are starting out on the wrong foot, and you are acting wrong. I cannot understand the difference in you between last night and this afternoon. Last night you told me, "Dad, I am going to *try*. I am going to eat."

DEBORAH: Dad!

But while the affective intensity is high, there is still no demand for change. Mother's plea is only for understanding.

Father responds to increase in mother's affective intensity by becoming reasonable.

During his long speech, father shifts between an authoritarian position and a request for cooperation.

MOTHER (*calmly*): Wait a minute, Abe.

DEBORAH: I ate the peas instead of apples. And this morning I asked them to bring me tea instead of milk.

FATHER: But I told you last night that *whatever* anybody gives you is not poison. It is food. It is not going to hurt you.

DEBORAH: I can't eat that much! You have to remember that I am—

MOTHER: Deborah, you don't have to eat that much. But eat food that will help to put weight on you. You don't even have to eat that much of that, but certain types of food are necessary.

MINUCHIN (*entering indignantly*): The problem here is you two! You say, "You should eat." And Mother says, "You shouldn't eat." Just now, Mother said that Deborah should not eat!

MOTHER: No!

MINUCHIN: No? No? Don't tell me no, because I am telling you yes! The problem is that you are supporting her not eating. You are supporting her starving, as an attack on your husband.

FATHER (*loudly*): I had that child on—

MINUCHIN (*silencing father with a gesture*): No, no, no. Why are you attacking your husband in such a way?

MOTHER: Because I feel that he is just upsetting her, and that she is going to rebel all the more.

MINUCHIN: You are attacking your husband. And you are killing your daughter.

INTERVIEWER: Why did you attack the mother?

MINUCHIN: The only way to separate the daughter from the parents is to break the sequences that maintain the homeostasis. One way the therapist can do so is to position himself in the system in such a way

Daughter's cry activates mother, who interferes on daughter's behalf, challenging husband.

Father identifies food as the vehicle for transacting cooperation and autonomy.

Mother is activated by intensity of husband and daughter, who are nearly screaming. She tries to diffuse the conflict, but her intervention, as usual, will only reinitiate the cycle.

that the cycle cannot repeat itself. At this point I am allying myself with the father in a way that will make the mother's soft protests ineffective. This alliance will prevent the father from responding to the mother's homeostatic signal. In effect, the father will be triangulated by my coalition with him: in order to maintain my support, he will have to change his responses to his wife. One of the family mechanisms for diffusing conflict will thus become unusable.

INTERVIEWER: You could have allied with the mother. Why did you choose the father?

MINUCHIN: Theoretically, it would be possible to ally with either of them. Probably something in the session—perhaps the way the father accepted an earlier intervention—organized me to ally with him.

INTERVIEWER: The intensity of the Kaplans' reactions at this point is shocking. Why did you elicit such a response? How will you develop it in a way that is therapeutic rather than destructive? And what happens to you when you see these people hurting each other? What do you do when they become psychologically exhausted?

MINUCHIN: First, when I have a conflict-avoiding family with a seriously ill member, organized in rigid patterns, I find the development of high-intensity interpersonal conflict a good strategy. It quickly moves the identified patient away from her morbid intrapsychic obsessions. At the same time, the therapist must always be aware that there are dangerous elements in a crisis induction, as shown by the Chinese character for crisis, which is formed by two other characters—opportunity and danger. In this case, the crisis is created by a rather economical therapeutic maneuver. I organize a dyad—mother/father, mother/daughter, later father/daughter—around a task: that the girl should eat. Then I prolong the time of the transaction, maintaining each dyadic transaction way beyond what would have been possible without my intervention. The intensity increases with each repetition of the nonresolution cycles. The family is caught in a "no-exit" situation.

Second, however, I join with each of the family members, as occurred during the previous hour. I support subsystem autonomy. I also learn to accommodate to the family and experience their stress signals. Such measures foster an atmosphere of respect and trust, and suggest that there *is* a way out of the private hell they have created. It is hope and trust, just as much as dependency, that will mobilize these family members to follow my lead in developing alternative ways of relating.

And third, the crisis is induced by allowing a pattern that has been repeated often at home to play itself out in the concentrated time of the therapeutic session. I know that the family members will respond to each other's signals, regulating their sequences. Therefore I can detach myself, becoming available to intervene when necessary in order to increase the intensity or, conversely, to support a member who is psychologically exhausted. You will see how this is done in the next segments.

MINUCHIN: Is attacking your husband so important that you want your daughter to starve?

MOTHER: No! No, I—

MINUCHIN: So why do you do that to him? Why do you attack him so heavily?

MOTHER: Well, as I said, I feel that he is getting her upset. And she should—

MINUCHIN: You are attacking him, and you are making her starve. If you want to kick him in the shins, kick him in the shins.

But don't handicap your daughter. And you, Deborah. You are obeying your mother in her fight with her husband, and there you are, in the middle. Your eating or not eating is part of this struggle. Can you succeed in making her eat, Mrs. Kaplan?

MOTHER: Well, I thought I could try to get her to.

MINUCHIN: Well, make her eat. Mr. Kaplan, you and Simon come with me. (*They leave to go behind the one-way mirror. After a few minutes the three men return because the sound system in the observation room has failed, but they remain silent during the entire sequence that follows.*)

MOTHER: Deborah, I want you to eat. Because it is going to be pretty bad. I want you to eat. After you get your certain weight back, you can eat anything you want. Deborah. Deborah!

DEBORAH: Why doesn't Dad get a sandwich? Why don't you get one?

Daughter uses a variety of postponement strategies in this segment. Whereas they all give the impression of cooperation, they serve merely to deflect conflict without complying with mother's pleas and demands. In this instance daughter's ploy is extraordinary: in the highly enmeshed system, where her eating is subject to parental control, she claims the right to control her parents' eating.

MOTHER: Because Dad has enough meat on him, and he is not in the hospital like you are. You are in the hospital, Deborah. You are here for a reason. You are here because you have to eat. You have to eat. There is no way out. You are an intelligent girl. You have to eat while you are in the hospital. You have got to eat. You have got to eat!

The ploy works, and mother cedes to daughter the right to control parental eating. In response to daughter's use of concrete thinking typical of much younger children, mother also talks to her as though she were younger. Then mother returns to pleading and demanding.

DEBORAH: I swear to you I won't die.

Another distracting maneuver: daughter reassures mother like a little girl.

MOTHER: You have to eat in order to start gaining. Deborah! You have got to eat because you are losing. You are staying the same weight. (*Her voice rises to a scream.*) You are going to die! Do you want to die when you have so much to look forward to in your life? Don't you understand? Can't you get that into your head? There's no way out! You have to start eating! (*She deliberately calms herself.*) Deborah, could you live if you stopped breathing?

DEBORAH: Did I stop breathing?

Mother has escalated the issue of eating or leaving the hot dog to a question of survival. In daughter's present physical condition, this is not unrealistic. But the repetition reflects the mother's helplessness: all she can do is to increase intensity.

Again daughter uses literalness as a way to deflect parents without open defiance.

MOTHER: No, but you had better start eating. It is the same thing as breathing. I eat enough all day.

DEBORAH: You don't eat the right foods!

MOTHER: No, but I eat enough—I don't have to eat the right foods! I am fully grown. I never left a piece of food. How could I eat and watch you starve? Hold your breath. See how long you can hold your breath. Food is like air! You didn't touch your milk or your beef.

DEBORAH: Okay, I will finish the beef. But I'll get sick and vomit all over.

MOTHER: I promise you, you won't get sick.

Mother offers her own eating as a model, just as father did a few minutes ago. Eating is a family affair, as though they all shared one body.

Mother accepts daughter's challenge and begins to explain her own pattern of eating. Then she returns to the issue, but her statements still carry no clear demand for change.

Mother and daughter talk as if both of them controlled daughter's physiological functioning: "If I eat and vomit, it will be your fault." "I promise you I won't let that happen." This is reminiscent of Bruch's comments on mother/infant transactions.

DEBORAH: I don't want it! You force everyon me. Everything I ever did! You have always forced me!

MOTHER: I have never forced you. After you decided to go on your diet, I talked to you like a person.

DEBORAH: You didn't talk to me at all.

Daughter breaks through to the issue of autonomy.

But after mother suggests that she respects daughter's autonomy, daughter labels this as rejection. Daughter participates actively in maintaining her own powerlessness.

MOTHER: I talked to you and told you that you would pay for it. And you are paying for it now. You need food, Deborah. You need it like the air you breathe. It's not much further that you won't have any flesh at all. And you said that you wanted to gain weight. You have enough time later on in life to eat the way I eat and be well nourished. Right now you're still growing. Right now you must be fed back to good health. And you have to eat everything. Everything! Your milk is very important. You are going to lose your teeth—

DEBORAH: I'm going to—I'm going to this, I'm going to that all the time—

MOTHER (*more calmly*): Deborah, from day to day we don't know whether you are going to survive. We don't know what is going to be tomorrow. You are losing weight so rapidly. I mean, you are an intelligent girl. I don't see why you can't reason this thing out. The only way to go home is to eat. Let me see you start eating again, and see how far you go. Then we'll discuss it further.

DEBORAH: No, no, no! I'll be defeated!

MOTHER: Well then, be defeated. And I lost my appetite! Because you have never known me to leave anything. Start eating the hot dog now. You said you were going to. Go ahead.

DEBORAH: No, no, no! After I finish that, you will start all over again. I am not going to eat this tray! You can shove it down my throat, and I will vomit it up like I did before. I said you're going to make me die!

MOTHER: You have got to eat to survive. Here. You have to eat to survive until tomorrow. Don't you understand? Don't you

Mother never issues a command; she reasons, or pleads, or threatens a bleak future. She may control daughter, but she does not "force" her.

Daughter's refusal to accept responsibility for her own actions makes it impossible for her to negotiate or compromise. Any concession becomes total defeat.

Again mother equates daughter's not eating with her own lack of appetite. In this overinvolved dyad, daughter controls mother's eating, as well as vice versa.

Giving in once means total surrender, total annihilation. Clearly daughter is talking not of food but of self.

understand that, Deborah? You have two doctors watching over you. Now why don't you start to eat? You don't have very much there. You don't even have enough to fill anyone up.

DEBORAH: I don't want to finish it—the whole thing. I don't want to eat any of it! What did you eat before you came up here?

Daughter condenses her thoughts, which in full might be, "If I could start to eat something and stop when I am satisfied, I would. But I know that you won't let me stop. Therefore, I will not start." Total refusal is necessary. Daughter does not have the power to negotiate. In her final question she again blurs the boundaries between daughter and mother.

MOTHER: I eat all day long, Deborah. I eat a tremendous meal at dinner.

Mother accepts daughter's control.

DEBORAH: Coffee! Mints!

MOTHER: I eat a tremendous meal! I'm not in the hospital. You are. Am I underweight, or are you? Yes, I should be in a hospital—a mental institute, that's where I should be. Because that's where you are going to put me! Now go ahead and eat. I said, go ahead and eat! Start wherever you want, and—

Angered by daughter's intrusion on herself, mother goes beyond her usual pattern and makes a demand. This sequence would have been of short duration at home, but in the session the therapist's insistence on continuing conflictual transactions has extended the interchange beyond its usual point of deflection.

DEBORAH: I am not going to finish it!

MOTHER: Let's see how far you go. You know, Deborah, I am desperate. Do you know what being desperate is?

As usual, daughter answers tangentially. Though she does not eat, she avoids a direct challenge. Her verbal statements are "almost" an acceptance.

DEBORAH: Yes, I do know.

MOTHER: Suppose you were me, and I were you. Would you let your little girl starve to death? Would you?

DEBORAH: I wouldn't force her.

MOTHER: If she were going to die, you wouldn't force her? If she were going to die?

Because of the extension of the transaction beyond its natural end point, the pattern of nonresolution becomes absurd and illogical. But mother and daughter have no other way available to deal with each other.

DEBORAH: I—no! She wasn't going to die.

MOTHER: Oh no, honey. You know she's going to die because she's not eating. You know she's going to die. Now what would you do in that case? Would you feed her, or let her do what she wants?

DEBORAH: I would let her eat vegetables and protein. This isn't going to kill me.

MOTHER: What kind of nonsense is that? You can't even differentiate between foods at this point. You have to eat what is given to you. You had no right to order cottage cheese instead of meat. The dietitian intends to give you a well-balanced meal. You start to eat! Last year you were eating every kind of food. You enjoyed everything.

DEBORAH: I was not! You never once gave me hot dogs.

MOTHER: That's a downright lie!

DEBORAH: Do you ever make them?

MOTHER: No, I don't any more. When you were kids—all kids love hot dogs. But I don't make them any more because there are other foods that are just as nutritious. Now start to eat, because we may not be sitting here tomorrow. Start to eat!

DEBORAH: I don't want it!

MINUCHIN: Do you think you will succeed?

MOTHER: Well, evidently I am on the wrong track.

MINUCHIN: Whenever you feel that you have been defeated, your husband will take over. At any point that you feel that you are beaten, call him in.

MOTHER: Deborah, please start to eat now. You know that you may not live.

DEBORAH: Be quiet!

MOTHER: Look. You can start with one slice of beef.

DEBORAH: I am not going to eat it. Because I know I'll have to eat the hot dog.

MOTHER: Well, when I was a little girl and I had to eat something I didn't like, we would always eat that first to get it over with.

The intensity fades, and a new cycle begins, maintaining the accustomed pattern. Once again, mother will beg, and daughter will maintain the semblance of cooperation by continuing to discuss the issue—ad infinitum.

Therapist's intervention underlines the power element of the struggle, moving daughter's starting to eat into the background.

DEBORAH: Well, I am not going to have all this. I'm not starving.

MOTHER: You are starving! You are starving to death! Why do you think we are all here? This is no picnic. Your father can't do any business. Your father is losing the business! Do you understand that? Now start to eat, because we may not be sitting here tomorrow, because you'll be dead. Start to eat!

DEBORAH: I don't want it!

MOTHER: Start to eat now! Start to eat right now! (*She is screaming.*) Right now! Because every minute means something to you. To all of us. Start to eat, Deborah!

DEBORAH (*crying*): I don't want it.

MOTHER (*screaming*): You've got to!

DEBORAH: But if I don't want it—(*She sobs hysterically.*)

MOTHER: I said you've got to! Now! (*She bursts into tears.*)

DEBORAH: Mother, I'm not—

MINUCHIN: Sit down, Mrs. Kaplan, and let your husband try. You have done the best that you could. (*He takes her arm and gently pushes her toward a chair.*)

> Therapist experiences mother's desperation and intervenes to protect her.

FATHER: All right, Deborah. Now I'm not going to play any games with you. And I'm not going to leave this room unless they carry me out bodily unless you finish everything that's on that tray. Now, you want my love. You want to walk the dog with me. You're going—

> To father, eating is a way of negotiating love as well as power.

DEBORAH: I don't want your love! I don't want anything.

FATHER: All right! Fine! You don't have to have my love.

DEBORAH (*crying*): I don't want to eat! I don't want this hot dog! I don't!

FATHER: Deborah, you can throw that hot dog on the floor, but by the time I leave this room, you're going to eat that hot dog.

> As before, father's language is loaded with the threat of immediacy.

DEBORAH: You can try, but I don't want it!

FATHER: Deborah, you can talk all you want, but—

DEBORAH: I don't want to talk. Now leave me alone! (*She begins to cry again.*) You are always making me do things that I don't want to do.

FATHER (*threateningly*): Deborah!

DEBORAH: You always force me!

FATHER: Deborah, listen to me. You say that I yell loud? You yell louder than I do. Now listen to me.

DEBORAH: This is not going to get me anyplace.

FATHER: This is going to get you plenty of places. But you're not going to be able to do things you want to in life unless you feel a little better. I don't want to talk about the rest of your life. Right now you'll finish what's on that tray. And I mean every morsel! You understand? Because if you had a little more flesh on you, I'd beat the shit out of you! Do you understand what you've done to this family? Now you eat every goddamn thing that's on that tray! And if you don't, you're not going to leave this room until you do. Now start eating! I'm going to give you three minutes to eat it, and if you don't start, you're going to find it in your ears and your eyes and down your mouth and everywhere else! Now you start eating! I'm not playing any games with you. Because we're past the game-playing stage. I lost my goddamn business and everything else. I lost my wife, and I lost my family because of you. And goddamn it, I'm not going to play any more games with you! Now you eat! Now come on. That's not poison.

DEBORAH: It is! Did you try it?

FATHER: All right. I'll eat a little of it. (*He takes a bite of the hot dog.*) Now, is this poison?

Daughter's answer is cry of the powerless and the subjugated.

The cycle ends without resolution, then begins again.

Father's monolog has a mounting intensity. It starts with reasoning, then goes into an all-or-nothing demand for immediate action.

Father's demand for compliance is softened by a three-minute reprieve, which turns into bluster, and then into a detour into the father's life circumstances that also delays action.

DEBORAH: I tried it! (*She sobs hysterically.*)

FATHER: This is good food, and you eat it. Deborah don't pull that shit on me. Now eat it! If I thought it would kill you, I wouldn't let you eat it. Don't you tell me about cottage cheese and protein. You're no goddamn doctor. Now you eat it! Or you'll find milk all over your hair and your body and on your— (*Still sobbing, Deborah takes the hot dog and crushes it.*) Now I told you I'm going to give you a couple of minutes, and then I'm going to feed you myself. Because eventually you're going to get fed with a tube down your stomach anyway. Look at your body, and look at your arms. Now come on, start to eat it. Start to eat it! And don't be like a two-year-old baby and make a big fuss out of eating a stupid hot dog. A lot of kids wish to hell they had a hot dog for lunch.

Father's pattern of transacting with daughter, like mother's, follows a cycle of escalation, then deflection, then escalation again.

DEBORAH: Well, give it to them!

FATHER: I'm not going to give it to them, I'm giving it to you! And I'm not wasting any food, either. Now Deborah, don't put me in a position where I'm going to get violent, goddam it. You eat the food, or you're not going to see me in this goddamn hospital again. I don't care if they carry you out of here on a stretcher. Now you eat it. Come on, eat the goddamn hot dog! Deborah, if you don't eat this hot dog, you're going to be sorry.

Father's responses to daughter are more directly negativistic, but the plateauing of his threats seems to be triggered by his wish to be seen as a good father. "Don't force me to get violent" seems to equal, "Don't force me to be a bad parent."

DEBORAH: I don't want it! (*She crumbles the mush in her hands.*)

FATHER: You eat it! Don't you destroy it, or I'll get you ten more. Now you eat it!

Daughter's visible challenge angers father into escalating his threat.

DEBORAH: I don't want it! Look at it. It's ugly!

FATHER: Eat that hot dog! I'm not leaving this place, I swear to God, until you eat it. Eat it! And drink this milk. And eat the peas. I don't mean leave it. Eat that hot dog! God damn you! You son of a bitch! You eat the goddamn hot dog! I told you to eat it! (*He takes the crushed hot dog and shoves it into Deborah's mouth. She resists, and is smeared with food.*)

MINUCHIN: Mr. Kaplan. (*He gets up, touches the father on the shoulder, and indicates his chair.*)

Here again therapist feels the need to intervene to protect both daughter and father.

FATHER: I'm sorry. (*He sits down, visibly exhausted.*)

MINUCHIN: I think that you have done your best. You have done your best.

FATHER: I'd like to bust her in her goddamn mouth! You little son of a bitch!

MINUCHIN: She has defeated both of you.

FATHER: I'm sorry I don't know how to make her eat.

MINUCHIN: Both of you did your best.

FATHER: I'd like to kill her!

MINUCHIN: Because she has defeated you.

FATHER: She's sick!

MINUCHIN: No, she has defeated both of you. Because she is stronger than both of you.

INTERVIEWER: What is the purpose of dividing the parents and having them deal with Deborah separately?

MINUCHIN: In this family, the spouse subsystem operates in such a way that whenever the husband says to the daughter, "Eat," the wife says to the husband, "You are too harsh." Whenever the wife says to the daughter, "Please eat," the husband says, "You are too soft." The parents operate as though Deborah would eat if one of the spouses changed. This leaves Deborah triangulated. Any action she takes regulates and is regulated by the spouse subsystem. If she eats, it will be experienced as a coalition with one parent against the other. That is one systemic reason why she experiences herself as "defeated" regardless of what she does. Eating has become a symbol of all the activities in which she experiences herself as controlled.

Dividing the parents is part of a strategy to break this system. The overall technique is to change a detouring protective organization into a detouring attacking organization. First, I asked the parents together to make the girl eat. They failed, but each felt that this was because the other was doing the wrong thing. By separating the parents and having them try individually, I made each of them experience failure in a power operation with Deborah. Now I will try to make the parents join in defeat and unite against the girl. This is the detouring attacking position. It increases the distance between parents and daughter, and is a first step in the process of detriangulation.

INTERVIEWER: Doesn't Deborah have a function in the symptom maintenance?

MINUCHIN: Of course. At this point, however, the possibility that the girl owns her own actions is not considered in this family. That will have to come later. Deborah is saying, "By not eating, I am maintaining my only way of functioning autonomously." This is a way of stating her individuality while preserving her position within the system rules, which require close proximity. That position in the system was being challenged when I told Deborah, "You are defeating your parents." This is a relabeling operation. Instead of being a sick, crazy girl, she is made a strong, rebellious adolescent. I will support her need to rebel and separate, but it will have to be pushed outside the eating area. She will have to learn to rebel in other ways.

MINUCHIN: She has defeated both of you

because she is stronger than both of you.

SIMON: Doctor, I think I can defeat her. I know if there was a hot dog and she had to eat it, I could defeat her. I think I could make her eat it.

Son, who was excluded from struggle between parents and sister, now wants to join the executive subsystem.

MINUCHIN: No, I really don't think so. (*To parents.*) At this point, Deborah has shown who has the muscles. You two have to really be together in this, because Deborah is involved in a struggle. It has nothing to do with food. It has to do with a struggle that she has with both of you, in which she is saying she will win. And she does.

Therapist blocks son because he plans to involve him later as sister's ally.

FATHER: She might win this time, but she's not going to win any more, I'll assure you.

MINUCHIN: She's concerned with this one. She defeated you, Candy. You tried your best, and you were defeated. And you, Abe, tried your best, and you were defeated.

Therapist insists on discussing the present, and ties parents together in defeat.

FATHER: That's right.

MINUCHIN: She is really involved in a fight with both of you, in which she wins. And that is all that is important to her.

FATHER: Her mother cried every day and night in front of me, and in front of her, and she didn't even care about it. My mother is dying, and she didn't even care about that. The only thing she cared about was herself. I started to think she was spoiled. I never thought she was spoiled before. I tried to give her love and affection and everything she wanted.

Father begins one of his long speeches that deflects action and diffuses conflict.

MINUCHIN: She's not sick; she's involved in a struggle.

Therapist insists on actualizing conflict.

MOTHER: I don't understand.

MINUCHIN: Ask your husband. He will explain it to you.

Therapist delineates spouse subsystem, separate from daughter.

MOTHER: I don't think he knows either.

MINUCHIN: About the fight? She's involved in a fight with you.

MOTHER: But why?

MINUCHIN: That's not important.

MOTHER: But she, of all six children—

> Mother begins her cycle of diffusing conflict.

MINUCHIN: Don't. It's not important.

> Therapist blocks it.

FATHER: She is rebelling against you and me for some reason.

MOTHER: You know, we've been very good to her.

FATHER: Maybe we've been too good to her, I think. Maybe. Maybe I should have disciplined her and not given her everything she wanted. I don't know. But she was really—she didn't deserve—

MOTHER: She's a good child.

FATHER: She's a good child. I don't understand this.

> Parents begin the old repair pattern.

MOTHER: We gave her these things because she was good.

FATHER: I got her a sewing machine. She wanted a sewing machine, I got her a sewing machine. She brought home good grades from school. I never tried to bribe her to bring home good grades. She's a reader. I love her, and everything else. But I can't love somebody that shows—I can't love somebody that shows—that tears me and my wife apart.

MINUCHIN: She has the pleasure now of having won that battle. I think you were very successful, Deborah. Very good. You don't have to hold your victory in your hand. Leave the hot dog on the tray. You can throw it on the floor. Here, throw it on the floor.

> Therapist highlights the struggle again.

DEBORAH: Why?

MINUCHIN: Because it's a symbol of your victory. When a fight has been as bloody as this one has, it's nice to have all the signs. Why do you want to defeat them? You feel that you have been so controlled that this is one of the ways in which you will express your autonomy? (*To parents.*) Well, you know you are on a really difficult boat. You will get out of this boat only by pulling together.

FATHER: What should we do?

MINUCHIN: We will help you. We will help you.

(*The therapist sends Deborah back to the ward then talks with parents for a few more minutes and sets next appointment.*)

INTERVIEWER: What were you after in this last part?

MINUCHIN: The goal was to delineate the spouse subsystem—two united parents, with Deborah excluded. I wanted them to leave the session feeling the continued seriousness of the situation, but also with a feeling of something accomplished, and of hope. It was an extremely intense session, but at the end the problem was relabeled. They now felt that they were dealing with a conflict between an adolescent girl and her parents, rather than with a mysterious individual disease. In effect, I declared this to be a normal situation.

INTERVIEWER: A behavior problem is more normal than a psychosomatic disorder.

MINUCHIN: Well, yes. The relabeling is not absolutely correct, but it is one of the steps in changing the family system. The therapist has to have a certain license in such matters.

INTERVIEWER: Why did you ask the girl to throw the remains of the hot dog on the floor?

MINUCHIN: People do not always experience the reality of their own actions. They see themselves as manipulated and controlled—as chess pieces being moved by the players. This feeling is one of the classic components of anorexia nervosa. In such situations, it can be helpful to frame their actions with a concrete literalness, so that

they experience, "I did it." The hot dog on
the floor became a dramatic result of Deborah's actions and symbolized her capacity
to act.

When Deborah returned to the ward after this lunch session, she
ordered a voluminous meal and ate every scrap. By the time of the
next family session, which follows, she was eating a normal diet
and gaining satisfactorily. She was still in the hospital and still on
the behavioral program, but eating was no longer a life-and-death
issue. Consequently, the therapist decided to make the second session a regular family session, not a lunch interview.

During the interval the therapist had visited her almost every
day. The pediatrician monitored her weight gain, administering the
behavioral paradigm. The therapist's interventions were again more
social, made with the goal of joining this patient to further the relationship that would be necessary to help her individuate.

MINUCHIN: Did she tell you that she has
decided to leave the hospital very, very
soon?

FATHER: I was very happy last night. I
went to visit her and found that she was
eating well.

DEBORAH: When you left, I still was eating. And I got such a stomach-ache!

FATHER: Well, when I left, she sent my son
down for a steak sandwich, and she ate the
steak out of the sandwich. And she had sent
me down and I got her two hamburgers.
Did you eat the hamburgers? I didn't see
you when I left.

DEBORAH: Then I had an orange and two
hamburgers.

MINUCHIN: She is on a campaign to leave
the hospital. She wanted to put on three
kilos in one day, and I thought that it was
too much. But you really did very well.

FATHER: Did she put on weight?

MINUCHIN: She put on two pounds.

MOTHER: Do you weigh eighty-five now?

FATHER: Well, there is more to it than just

Therapist emphasizes identified patient's capacity for
decision making.

leaving the hospital, you know. When you get home, you have to continue.

MINUCHIN: What prompted you to the decision of trying to get out of the hospital —to start eating?

DEBORAH: I can't stand doing nothing all day. It's horrible. And I'm not sick. I'm not as sick as the other kids. Somebody else could use my bed.

Therapist emphasizes daughter's decision making.

INTERVIEWER: I see that she has started eating, but I don't understand why.

MINUCHIN: First, it is interesting that Deborah herself does not know why; she offers not a psychological insight but a common sense explanation drawn from the logic of her present circumstances. Nor am I certain about the reason. Probably her response is multideterminant. The family went through an ordeal during the previous session, and I think that the idea of going through such an experience again must be considered as part of the pressure for a search for alternatives. My position in the therapeutic system blocked the homeostatic mechanism that kept the parents triangulating the daughter. Deborah found herself relabeled a strong, rebellious adolescent and was offered support for her struggle with her parents in another transactional field. During the previous session, at a point of heightened emotional intensity and in a "dead end" position, I offered them a different view of their dilemma and the possibility of solutions. By reframing their reality, I offer hope and promise a leader out of the labyrinth. I think that this is the mechanism for transformation in many healing rituals.

MINUCHIN: I told Deborah that I cannot begin to treat her until she's at home because the problem is the way in which you

Therapist continues to emphasize anorexia as a family illness, framing hospitalization as a short, if necessary, postponement of treatment.

two and Deborah work together and has nothing to do with eating. So, she's wasting time being in the hospital. I am pleased that you have decided to leave the hospital, Deborah.

FATHER: I think I know why she wants to leave the hospital. I have tickets for the ballet for New Year's Eve and she wants to go to the ballet.

MINUCHIN: That's your assumption.

FATHER: That's my assumption, that's right.

MINUCHIN: But she said something different.

FATHER: That's right.

DEBORAH: But, I want to go to that, too, and I want to go back to school. To get out of here.

MINUCHIN: Okay. I think that, you know, once Deborah is at home with you, the problem is: will you be able to let her grow up and will she grow up, or will you and your wife keep her as a little girl?

MOTHER: I've already made up my mind. The only thing is, I have to know from you where I can put my foot down. Do you know what I mean? I don't know.

MINUCHIN: You have a husband. Deborah, it is wrong for you to sit there between Father and Mother. I know that this is the only chair they left you—

MOTHER: It didn't happen intentionally. Now, where do we sit? Do I sit next to him?

DEBORAH: I'll sit here.

MINUCHIN: She is not supposed to be in between both of you.

DEBORAH: I know, but—

MINUCHIN: Your parents organized you that way. You didn't have any other chair. They left this empty chair that was set so that you would be caught between both of them, you know, and that is what's happen-

Therapist emphasizes separation, supporting daughter as different and challenging father's enmeshed view that he knows what daughter is thinking.

Therapist uses a strategy of isomorphic fields: instead of dealing with eating as the arena of power operations and individuation, he carries the problem to other arenas.

Mother's attempt to make therapist an expert on parental behavior is challenged, and mother is referred to father. Therapist is affiliating with identified patient, continuing to frame her behavior as organized by parents. This strategy supports her rebellion against parents and encourages conflict.

Position of daughter's chair in the middle is seen as a spatial metaphor of her triangulation by parents in other transactions. Therapist joins with daughter in challenge to parents, as in the previous session he joined with parents against daughter.

ing to you. You get caught between Daddy and Mommy.

FATHER: Well, you know, a lot of things that have happened I've analyzed when I got home. And I learned a lesson from the last time we were together. I'm very hard to teach a lesson, but I did learn a lot from you, Doctor, and I have changed. I feel, and probably I was wrong in my feeling, that we had a loving house. And I didn't think Deborah would rebel the way she has rebelled with the food or whatever it is. I run my house in a certain way. If I had to change that way, I would change the way I run my household, but I sort of felt that it was right.

MINUCHIN: Do you run the household alone?

FATHER: My wife and I run it, but I think that I dominate it most of the time. I set the pattern and my wife sort of carries through, and I'm probably at fault there. We probably should run it together, but—

MINUCHIN: You know, she's here. (*He signals that husband should talk with wife.*)

FATHER: All right. What do you feel about me running the household? Tell me the truth, Candy. You don't have to be afraid.

MOTHER: Well, I always thought that if a child came to us and he asked whether he could do something, I'd say, "No, but you can ask your father, and if your father says yes, it will be all right with me." Isn't that so? You always had the upper hand; even though I didn't agree with you, I'd always say to the child, "Ask your father, and whatever your father's decision is, it is also my decision." Well, I thought that was right. Doctor, isn't that right?

MINUCHIN: No, no. You continue talking together. Don't bring me into it.

MOTHER: Like I say, I mean, several times

Again therapist emphasizes need for mutuality in spouse subsystem while emphasizing separateness of subsystems.

The following sequences show how family members, on reaching a degree of conflict, activate a cycle of attracting or triangulating another member to diffuse stress.

Wife transforms husband/wife issue into father/mother issue.

Parents have tried to use therapist as third person in their conflicts, which is the position in which daughter

I would think you were wrong in your decision, but I always stuck by you.

FATHER: That's right.

MOTHER: Because I feel that the father is the man of the house and he has the say.

FATHER: Well, that's true. You have always stuck by me when I made a decision. And I have tried to make proper decisions, let me say. But Deborah, do you think I made the proper decisions?

MINUCHIN: No, no, no! That's exactly where you get caught, Deborah! Your father was trying to resolve a problem which is between Mother and him by bringing you in the middle. And that's crazy! You should not be in the middle.

DEBORAH: I guess he values my opinion of things.

MINUCHIN: Yes, but they should value your opinion on *your* things. They should not bring you in the middle, because you get caught. Continue.

FATHER: But I think the decisions that I make—Candy, can you give me an example of some of the decisions that I made that were wrong?

MOTHER: Well, I don't know if your decisions were wrong. Like, we would disagree on different things—for example, Deborah going to modeling school last year. She wasn't even fourteen. I didn't approve of her going to modeling school at that age. And yet, you said you would send her, you would do your best to send her because she wanted it and she was good and she was entitled to some good things because she was a good child.

FATHER: All right, now, do you know why I actually sent her to modeling school? Since that child has been born, I have tried to keep her out of your hair during the summer. You have always said she was an active

---

frequently finds herself. Therapist's strategy of blocking daughter's triangulation activates him as a possible pawn in their transactions. His participation would support system homeostasis; his refusal strengthens the boundaries around spouse subsystem and maintains conflict.

Father attempts to triangulate daughter.

Therapist blocks triangulation.

Daughter attempts to keep her position in triangle, for she will lose proximity and power with individuation.

Therapist blocks daughter's wish to be involved.

Wife again avoids direct conflict by bringing marital disagreement into the arena of parenting.

Father changes conflict between spouses into a situation in which he protects wife in her conflict with daughter.

child. She has to be kept active. Whether I could afford it or not. If she were around the house, you would say, "She is driving me crazy. She has to go here; she has to go there." Now, I tried to see to it that every summer she either went to camp or she went somewhere so you wouldn't have to be concerned about her. Now, my thinking— being very honest about it—is not so much for her. It was for you. To get her off your back.

Father's actions are for somebody else, which is his pattern of avoiding "I" position.

MOTHER: But I still felt modeling school was not the right thing. And then, the second thing is that I didn't approve of her going to Israel. And you felt that she was entitled to it, and she had saved toward it, worked hard and everything, so we sent her. That was another thing where I disagreed, but since I feel that you should make the final decision, you did.

Wife's marital pattern: feeling that she should obey husband, wife doesn't defend her position and acts as if accepting husband's. As a result she maintains a grudge against him. In this submerged spouse conflict, daughter is triangulated.

MINUCHIN: Wait a moment, I want to talk to Deborah about it. See, you have been in the middle between Father and Mother for a long, long part of your life. They have disagreements about you, but they did not resolve them. In the end, the problem was not resolved and you were in the middle. Now, I don't want you there, because that keeps you very helpless, and a loser. One of the things that I talked with you about is how you can begin to be a winner. You see, Simon, I think, fought his battles, and he has gained his right to go away, to move out of the family, to have a life of his own. So, move a little bit nearer to Simon. I want you there near him, because he is learning how to be independent and you need to learn from him. Simon, you will be a teacher. Talk with Deborah about how you gained your role outside of the family.

Therapist creates a sibling subsystem that can support daughter in her move away from the spouse subsystem.

INTERVIEWER: Do you frequently work with the sibling subsystem as a therapeutic tool?

MINUCHIN: Yes. It is unfortunate that for so long the only thing we observed in sibling transactions was "sibling rivalry." The position of a child in the sibling subsystem can be as important in the process of identity formation as are his relations with parents. In therapy, the siblings are always important elements in the therapeutic process. Sometimes, as in this situation, they can be part of the process of detriangulating from parents. At other times, the transformation of the structure of the sibling subsystem alone facilitates the experience of alternative ways of transacting.

SIMON: Well, I guess it was time for me to grow up and not be spoiled any more. And I think I gained the respect of Mommy and Daddy. And it's not over a small period of time; it's over years.

DEBORAH: Well, I know that all these things are true, but that doesn't really answer anything.

MINUCHIN: Okay, good. So push him to answer differently.

SIMON: Well, I—I'd like to get off the point for just one second. I think Daddy made a mistake by letting you go to Israel because you weren't ready for it. I'm not a doctor, but now I'm supposed to be your teacher. You didn't mature, you didn't get to that point where you finally showed them that you were ready, because it takes years of maturity—

Whereas therapist asked brother to become sister's teacher in gaining individuation from parents, brother takes the position of forming a coalition with parents.

DEBORAH: I think you're wrong. I think I was ready. Now I know what Israel is like and I want to go back. And I'm glad I went, because I don't think I would ever have a better opportunity to see. I appreciated it more than anyone I know who went.

SIMON: Yes, I'm sure you did, but, you see, I am the teacher now—

MINUCHIN: No, don't let him go on if you have a different point of view.

Therapist supports daughter in challenging brother, who is parents' ally. This operation

DEBORAH: You're the teacher now, but you're not going to change my past, are you?

SIMON: Yes, I know—

DEBORAH: And you are wrong. Because if I had stayed home that summer, I could have done something worse. You could have blamed the point on if I had gone to camp and come home crying. You could have said I wasn't ready to go to camp. But I didn't come home crying and I wrote letters and I don't think it was a mistake. I am very happy that I went, and if I go again, I'll go to the same places. I think you wanted to go. I think you really wanted to go also, and you didn't have the opportunity to go. Did you want to go?

SIMON: I didn't want to go because—because I know that I'm going to be there, in Israel. (*To mother.*) Do you have a Kleenex?

FATHER: Here, Simon, use my handkerchief. Here. It's a clean handkerchief. Spread it apart. Take it apart.

MINUCHIN: He's seventeen.

MOTHER: Here, give him this. (*She hands father a Kleenex.*)

FATHER: All right.

MINUCHIN: My goodness! Look how this family gets activated! You wanted a handkerchief, so Father moved and gave Deborah his handkerchief to pass to you, Mother gave Kleenex to Father—

MOTHER: We have togetherness.

MINUCHIN: Togetherness, but—

FATHER: I don't know. You'll have to show me if it's wrong.

MINUCHIN: You just don't seem to know when one finishes and the other begins. You know, you wanted to wipe your mouth. Is that what you wanted?

SIMON: Yes.

MINUCHIN: You activated your whole family. How old are you?

SIMON: Seventeen.

is isomorphic to challenging parents.

With therapist's support, daughter answers at greater length, becomes surer in logic, and is able to stand up to brother. It may be that she needs to practice disagreement with brother before she dares individuate from parents. But when daughter's increased disagreement with brother reaches the accepted threshold of conflict, it is diffused by her last question.

Brother accepts sister's signal and asks for care, which activates the cycle of conflict-avoidance in which the total family participates.

Therapist uses the opportunity to point out that the enmeshed approach to daughter is only one instance of a pattern that goes on in the whole family. This therapeutic operation moves patient out of the main focus and puts her into family context.

Therapist challenges enmeshment.

FATHER: Well, we try to please one another.

MOTHER: Yes, we try to please each other. I do want to tell you, Doctor, and you may not believe this, but Deborah has always had a say in the family. She is not as quiet as you think she is. She's the one that wanted to do different things and brought it to our attention and insisted on it in her own little way. She's always had a voice in the family.

Mother responds to therapist's challenge by giving a sample of "good parenting." In the following sequence the "nondecision-making" patterns are similar to the patterns around eating observed in the previous session.

DEBORAH: Did I insist on going to modeling school, or did I ask you?

MOTHER: Yes, you did, honey. You wanted to go desperately.

DEBORAH: Yes, but I didn't keep insisting and asking.

MOTHER: Well, you wanted to go very badly.

DEBORAH: I wanted to go very badly, but I didn't insist. I never did that. I didn't say, "I'm going."

MOTHER: No, you have to get permission. You can't insist on something at your age.

DEBORAH: Well, I did. That's exactly what I did, and you said I asked—

MOTHER: But you had me on that phone calling the different places and getting interviews set up.

DEBORAH: But I didn't insist.

MOTHER: It was almost like insisting.

DEBORAH: But it wasn't insisting.

MINUCHIN: Candy, you didn't agree with Deborah, did you?

Therapist frames conflict in a small area, in the process of training family members to negotiate disagreements and deal with conflicts in the session.

MOTHER: About going to modeling school? No, I did not agree.

MINUCHIN: Do you know that she did not agree, Deborah?

DEBORAH: I knew you didn't want me to go as much. But you wanted me to go for my own sake. You wanted me to have a good time.

Daughter signals the possibility of conflict—a yellow light—then backtracks.

MOTHER: Yes, I wanted you to have a good time for the summer. But, there were two reasons why I didn't want you to go actually.

DEBORAH: Why not?

MOTHER: One was financial reasons and, secondly, was because I just didn't feel it was for you. I wasn't objecting to your becoming a model later on in life, but I just felt that at age fourteen, I just couldn't see it.

MINUCHIN: You did not agree, then.

MOTHER: I did not agree.

MINUCHIN: Deborah had an opinion; Candy did not agree. Deborah, you said that you did not insist. Nonetheless, you went. Deborah doesn't know that you really did not want her to go, Candy.

MOTHER: Well, at the time she did, because I told her.

MINUCHIN: When you disagree, how strong is your voice?

MOTHER: Well, as I said before, not too strong, because I always leave it open for the child to ask the father. Now if the father disagrees with me—gives a different answer —the child knows that I will go along with the father. They can always go to him.

MINUCHIN: Even if you disagree?

MOTHER: Yes, even if I disagree.

MINUCHIN: That leaves you very powerless.

MOTHER: But I don't object to that. I can live with that.

MINUCHIN: No, no. You do object in very subtle ways. You don't object openly, but these things, in some way, work on you.

MOTHER: It doesn't bother me. Maybe another person with a stronger personality would feel it, but it doesn't—it bothers me —I keep it inwardly until it wears itself out, and then I am like it never happened. But even when I grew up in a family of four

---

Mother, trying to maintain affiliation with daughter, agrees with her and then, trying to maintain alliance with therapist, advances in spite of daughter's signal.

Therapist supports conflict.

Again mother enacts pattern of diffusing conflict by activating a third member. Now mother/daughter conflict is transformed into parental conflict with triangulated daughter.

Therapist focuses on mother's helplessness, trying to activate conflict between spouses.

Mother offers a model of womanhood to daughter that comes straight from the *shtetl*. This model, which was accepted in her own family and which both parents seem to support, provides Deborah as well as

children, I always felt that the father was the head of the family, and if my mother didn't agree with him, she would say, "Go to your father." And if he agreed, she would go along with it.

MINUCHIN: That puts you in a strange position, Candy.

MOTHER: Yes, but I always felt that a house should be full of harmony. And where there is harmony, then the children grow up in harmony, not yelling and screaming at each other all day long.

MINUCHIN: How old are you now?

MOTHER: Forty-eight.

MINUCHIN: And you still feel comfortable with being powerless?

MOTHER: That doesn't bother me. I myself like to depend upon my husband.

MINUCHIN: Do you like that, Abe? Because what she's saying is that everything falls on your shoulders.

FATHER: We have been married for twenty-seven years without too many arguments and very much love between us. And I can see where I have been responsible for all the problems in the family. I know the responsibility lies in me because I have been too soft with the children. I have some sort of phobia. I was just sitting here thinking, while we were talking, that if Simon had asked me to go to Boston today and I said you can't go, and if Deborah said, "I want to go to modeling school," and I said, "Deborah, I don't have the money. I can't send you to modeling school"—what would have happened? Would they rebel against me and say to me, "Well, I'm going to go out and commit suicide" or "I'm going to go out and do this," because I said no? I don't think I have the strength to say no to my children. I honestly don't. I never remember saying no, and I've been afraid of my children. I can see that.

Simon with an anachronistic view of woman that will handicap them in the extra-familial world.

Therapist moves the focus of concentration to flush out hidden conflicts, making mother uncomfortable with her position in husband/wife subsystem.

Father moves from implicit husband/wife conflict to conflict around parenting. Therapist's reference to wife's demands on husband to be decision maker flushes out a father caught in his own pattern of conflict avoidance when the family system allocates to him that function.

MINUCHIN: That's interesting. Because
Candy feels that you are full of strength.
But you cannot say no to your children.

FATHER: I can't say no to her.

MOTHER: I don't ask you for anything.

FATHER: Well, she likes to feel that she
doesn't ask for very much, but I have never
said no to anybody. Can I say no? To anything? If you ask me in the middle of the
night to walk somewhere, will I go for my
children and my wife? Do you ever remember me saying no to you in any way? In your
lifetime, Simon?

SIMON: You've always said yes.

FATHER: That's my problem.

MINUCHIN: Do you know something? It
seems to me, then, that you must feel very
exploited.

FATHER: I think I'm responsible for everything. I guess I'm sick in a certain way. I've
been working seven days and nights a week
since September and getting nowhere, and
I could tell you certain things that have happened, and I just can't say no. That's just it
where the family is concerned. Because I
have some idea that someday we are all
going to be together, and that is what I want
in life. I should have been more stern and
said, "Deborah, you can't go to Israel this
summer. You go get yourself a job." And
she would have been a better person for it,
maybe.

MINUCHIN: But, we are looking now at
your inability to—

FATHER: Say no.

MINUCHIN: To say when your needs start.
You really need Candy's help in many ways.
Candy is insisting that you are strong,
when, in effect, you are saying that you need
help.

*Father transforms a possible
conflict between spouses into
a triangle in which he asks
for son's affiliation.*

*Therapist's support of father
brings him to challenge his
own pattern of conflict avoidance in his relationship with
children.*

*Therapist moves away from
individual focus to frame
complementarity in spouse
subsystem.*

———

INTERVIEWER: I am confused. In the previous session, you seemed to have a clear map
that you were following. Now I see you

tracking the family and accepting their shift in dyads and in content. Do you have a rationale for this strategy?

MINUCHIN: The first session seemed clearer because I framed their transactions in terms of a definite goal: the girl should begin to eat. My strategy highlighted certain patterns of the family and elicited certain information at the expense of other patterns and other content. Having achieved the first goal in therapy, I feel free to relax, decentralize the patient, and begin to know the family. Still, while I encourage different family members to bring themselves into focus and to tell their stories, my interventions continue to focus on dysfunctional patterns, particularly enmeshment, conflict avoidance, and overprotection, challenging the triangulation of the identified patient and other family members. These elements of family transaction are the ones that have been identified as supporting the psychosomatic symptoms.

Now that the eating problem has lost salience, the focus can be on the family as a whole. The therapist has a clear idea of his therapeutic goals, but he functions like a sculptor who, depending on the material that the family brings him, uses a hammer and chisel, a spatula, sandpaper, and so on. Because the same formal transactions among family members occur and recur in different contexts and among different family members, they are available for therapeutic intervention in a variety of shapes. The therapist selects the transactions in the session that are most readily available and most suitable to his style in order to move the family in the direction of the therapeutic goal.

MOTHER: Well, I tried to take over some jobs, but he doesn't permit it. (*Therapist directs her to husband.*) You don't permit it. Well, first of all, getting back to the children, I am more strict with them than you would be. I would say no to something, and there would be reason for it, but then you would come along and say it was okay. I am a stricter person with the children than you would be, and I always felt that the children spend more time with me than with you, and I run the house, and I should really say yes or no to these things. But then your good nature comes up and spoils them, or whatever it is.

MINUCHIN: Do you disagree with him?

MOTHER: He always knows when I disagree.

MINUCHIN: But you could not help him to change his view.

MOTHER: No, no.

MINUCHIN: Then you are not helping him. He says he needs your help to draw boundaries sometimes.

MOTHER: It's true, but he has a very strong personality, and I—

Mother tries to maintain myth of husband's strength.

MINUCHIN: But you didn't hear him. Say again what you said just now. Say it to Candy so that she can hear you. Because I don't think she hears you.

FATHER: I don't know how to say no. And I guess it's been that way with all of them. But I'm going to change in that respect. I'm going to try to give you the responsibility—

MINUCHIN: The issue here is how can your wife help you to draw the boundaries. Apparently she can, a little bit more than you, but apparently she doesn't feel that she has that right.

FATHER: You've come to me, and you've said, "Abe, I don't know what to do. I don't know what to do with the children; I don't know what to do with so-and-so; I don't know what to do with Simon." I have always feared that when I would go away to work, the children would be able to run

Wife's dependence on husband has kept father in need of maintaining a facade of strength. Mother's value that husband should be boss has handicapped her possibility of using her competence in rearing the children. Father maintains the myth of the in-

rings around you. I have been easy with them as far as money is concerned, let's say, and trying to do for them, but I haven't been easy as far as keeping them on the right path. In other words, our kids have been in the right direction. As far as Simon is concerned, I think he's about the best, and Deborah has always been a model child in my opinion and we have never had any trouble with her. She would be the last one I would ever expect to go on a starvation thing like she went on. The one thing I always feared with Deborah is that she is the type of child that takes things too seriously, Doctor. I worry about the kids. I'm not going to do that, though, any more, I'm sure.

MINUCHIN: No, no. You will. You will continue. You cannot change a lot. See, in that thing, you need tremendous help from Candy. And you have organized a contract in which Candy cannot help you.

FATHER: Oh, I can change if I set my mind to it. I'll change

MINUCHIN: No, you cannot, you cannot change alone. I know enough about people like you to know that they don't change alone. Candy, he needs your help, but he cannot accept it either. How can you help him when he feels that you cannot help him? He thinks that he is a big macho and that he needs to do everything alone. And his spine is aching because he carries everybody on his shoulders. Now, when will you take some of this job?

MOTHER: Well, as soon as he—as soon as you will let me make a few decisions and make life easier for you.

MINUCHIN: How will you help your loving husband, here, who doesn't know how to let other people help him? How will you help?

MOTHER: Well, you see, that's a hard question because—well, like I say, we some-

---

Marginal notes:

competent mother that supports the myth of the strong father.

Cycle of husband/wife conflict finishes with a statement of harmony and a movement toward the ideal.

Father moves conflict between spouses to father's concern about children.

Therapist presents a paradox: husband cannot change alone, but wife could help him. But for wife to help, she would need to change, and husband would need to change to accept her change.

Wife resists therapist's push to change, reactivating myth of the powerful husband.

times differ in opinion on big problems. Now, I'm not brilliant. I don't know who's right. I mean, I can be wrong the way I think. And I don't want to go ahead with my decision for fear that I'm wrong. It's just the way I feel. And since Abe is more experienced—he's more in the open world. I'm always inside my little world.

MINUCHIN: This man, here, your husband, he needs your help. He needs to be able to say no when the demands of other people take away his needs. And he doesn't know how to do that.

Therapist persists in challenge to wife.

MOTHER: Well, I could say no for him. Many times I would say no. I've tried to inject my thoughts on a particular subject. Like if he—

MINUCHIN: Can you do that? Can you shake a little bit the peace in this family?

MOTHER: Well, I try to. Like the night she took him for one of those late walks. I said to Abe—well, I don't want to rehash it— but he had no right to leave at that hour. He should have gone earlier with her and not waited until she was ready. He was exhausted by that time, and I kept telling him, "Don't go, don't go," but it didn't matter. I tried to get it through to him.

Mother moves spouse conflict to parental conflict with triangulated child.

MINUCHIN: You will need to be stronger. Because you were right.

MOTHER: Well, I felt I was right. I kept telling him no while he was getting dressed.

Therapist encourages interspouse conflict which would detriangulate identified patient.

FATHER: I don't agree with you, Doctor, or Candy. At that stage of the game, Deborah was practically on the verge of God knows what. And the only time I could get to talk to Deborah was when we had these walks.

Father moves from relationship with wife to affiliation with daughter.

MINUCHIN: At what time was it?

FATHER: Twelve o'clock at night, or one o'clock.

MOTHER: But I feel that if you had gone two or three hours earlier, the same effect—

FATHER: You're right, in that respect.

MINUCHIN: But, you see, she was right. I think that in your family Candy is accustomed to say, "Okay, your ideas are correct ideas." But the truth is that many, many times Candy is right.

FATHER: See, we were going through a period in which Deborah was walking up and down the steps. Deborah correct me. Hundreds and hundreds of times. Walking around the kitchen table with Simon doing his homework, so that Simon couldn't do his homework. Bringing the garbage up and into the room. And I sat down, and I got through to Deborah. I stopped that. I saw a little progress. I was trying to play the part of a doctor or psychiatrist because we had nowhere to turn and nowhere to go to.

MINUCHIN (*to wife*): I still feel that you need to help your husband. To say to him, "Simon will survive without your help; Deborah will survive without your help. I want your help." You need to say to him, "I need you," and begin to work on stopping him from doing all these crazy, generous things that he does. He will not be able to do it by himself. I know that he will fight you. Can you keep the line if he fights you?

MOTHER: I will if I yell louder. He doesn't like anyone to yell.

MINUCHIN: But, can you?

MOTHER: Well, if I know it's going to help, I will.

MINUCHIN: Yes, it will help. It will help. You need to help him.

MOTHER: And you know, also, Doctor, I fall into the same category, though, because when he's not home and they ask me to do something for them, I drop everything and do it, too.

MINUCHIN: You cannot say, "I am busy"? Deborah, can you disagree with your parents besides in food? Do you disagree with them?

Therapist uses the value of protection to challenge enmeshment and to encourage conflict: wife needs to protect husband against his need to protect daughter.

Pushed by therapist to act in conflict, wife moves toward pattern of conflict avoidance.

Therapist tries to continue the issue of conflict with daughter, but in this maneuver unwittingly uses the

DEBORAH: Yes.

MINUCHIN: Openly?

DEBORAH: Not openly.

MINUCHIN: Why not?

FATHER: I don't agree with her. I think we have a democratic household. I'll always ask you, Debbie, "Do you agree with this? Do you agree with me?" and if you don't, we will always discuss it. I think that—in other words, when you say no, can you give me an example of what you mean? Or don't you understand the question? The doctor said, "Can you disagree with your parents openly," and you said, "Not openly." And when you do disagree, what happens when you disagree? You know, tell it like it is.

DEBORAH: Could you give me an example? Because I don't remember.

FATHER: I don't think we've had any disagreements.

DEBORAH: Yeah, I guess you're right.

FATHER: I really don't remember any disagreements.

MINUCHIN: So I will need to teach you to disagree. I saw what happened last week when you needed to negotiate something. Mother yelled at you, and Father yelled at you, and you held fast. In the end, in this disagreement, neither of you knew how to resolve anything. When you have a disagreement, you don't know how to resolve it.

FATHER: You see, Doctor, you're hitting the nail on the head. I am very worried, and although I know what I have to do to change and I think my wife knows what I have to do to change, I am very worried about getting Deborah home. I know she's going to eventually come home.

MINUCHIN: It can be tomorrow if she makes 88 pounds.

FATHER: I don't want her to just eat to get out of here and then when she gets home

family pattern of triangulating daughter.

Therapist has clearly gone beyond the accepted threshold of family conflict and activated father to initiate a cycle of conflict avoidance.

to do the very same thing and come back in the hospital again or come back somewhere again six months later. I am worried about getting you home because I know the type of personality you are and I know the type of personality I am.

MINUCHIN: How about Candy?

FATHER: And the type Mommy is and what's going to happen. Let's say you don't eat breakfast, lunch, or dinner, or you say to me, "Daddy, I want to eat at two o'clock in the afternoon; I don't want to sit down with the family." And I say, "Deborah, you've got to sit down with me at five o'clock to eat dinner." Now, what's your reaction going to be? I'd like you to tell me now.

DEBORAH: I will, but I don't want you to plan to have me around after dinner and before dinner. You see, you want me to always stay home. And I want to go out.

Daughter moves conflict away from eating and toward issues of autonomy involved in family's dining together.

FATHER: All right. Suppose you want to do something, and I say no, you can't do it.

DEBORAH: What?

FATHER: Suppose I say you're not supposed to go out tonight. I don't want you to go out tonight for some reason.

DEBORAH: What's the reason?

FATHER: Whatever it is. I don't feel that you should go out at night for some reason. And you want to go out, and I say no. Now, what is your reaction going to be? (*The therapist nods encouragingly to Deborah.*)

Father continues to deal with issues of autonomy and conflict around areas of separation and proximity.

DEBORAH: Well, it depends on what kind of —if you say I don't want you to go out, but everyone else is out with somebody, I'll question it and I'll be very upset about it, because unless you have a good enough reason—because I like to have my own life. If I eat with you and I talk with you, that's fine, but I still want to go out, and I want to have a good time.

With therapist's support, daughter begins to assert herself in an area of autonomy that is not related to eating.

FATHER: Suppose, as a parent, I don't think it is proper for you to go out. Let's say that I have to discipline you. I see that your weight—I want you to get on the scale and weigh yourself, and I want to have control of your weight—

MINUCHIN: No, that you cannot do.

FATHER: I cannot do that?

MINUCHIN: You cannot control her body. Deborah, that's one of the areas that will be between you and me. After you go home, I will weigh you at Children's Hospital when you come to the session.

(*The session continues for another ten minutes with a discussion of the possibility of Deborah's going back home in the near future and the need to negotiate the rights of both parents and children. The therapist promises to help them.*)

INTERVIEWER: Do you always take control of the weight gain when the child goes home? Doesn't this strategy carry the danger of putting you in the place where the parents were and giving the identified patient the power to defeat your therapeutic goals?

MINUCHIN: I use a variety of different techniques in my work with anorectics, whether they are at home or in the hospital, but the differences are superficial. The basic structure of all these strategies is the same. They represent variations on the theme of detriangulation. My strategy here is based on the idea of facilitating the Kaplans' use of other areas of transaction, so as to bring about therapeutic transformation in those areas. I want first to move their conflicts away from Deborah's eating. This strategy, which started in the first session where conflicts about Deborah's eating were transformed into conflicts about discipline around the table, will be the essence of the

---

Father brings issues of obedience and loyalty to the arena of eating.

Therapist blocks eating as an area of parent/child transaction.

therapy for the coming months. The iso-
morphism of many transactional patterns
in rigid families supports the notion that
the focus of therapeutic scrutiny and
change can be their conflicts in a variety of
safe areas.

Deborah was discharged from the hospital after five days. At home she continued to eat and to gain weight.

The treatment of the Kaplan family lasted for six more months. The majority of sessions included the total family, although a number of sessions were conducted with the parents alone or the child alone. Near the end of the treatment, the therapist divided the sessions into two stages, meeting first with the parents and Deborah together and then having an individual interview with Deborah. When the anorectic symptomatology subsided, Deborah refused to eat with her parents; at another point, she refused to talk with them. There was an increase of acting-out behavior on Deborah's part. Her demands on the parents also increased, but simultaneously, the parents' ability to resist her improved. Deborah's school performance remained satisfactory. She expanded her social activities and took a job after school for three hours a day and Saturdays, saving the money that she earned to pay for college. The work with the parents included sex therapy and encouragement for them to concentrate on issues relating to couples instead of concerning themselves continuously with parental issues. Treatment terminated with an indication to the family that if at any point in the future a problem arose, any family member could contact the therapist.

A year later Deborah called Dr. Minuchin to request an individual session. She arranged to pay for it with her own money and asked to maintain this contact separate from the family. At this point Deborah was concerned over her relationship with boys. She was seen individually for ten sessions. Two years later she was seen twice, at her request, to discuss issues related to her college life. The issues of anorexia did not recur in any of these interviews.

Four years after the termination of treatment, Deborah made a suicidal gesture by swallowing an overdose of tranquilizers. She was hospitalized for a week. Upon discharge she resumed treatment again. The precipitating event of her suicidal gesture was a frustrated love affair. In college, Deborah had maintained a B average, been very active socially, and made many close friends. Her relations with men, however, followed a destructive pattern. Deborah was an attractive person who started friendships with boys easily, but these relationships became conflictual when they reached a certain level of intensity. At this point she became anxious and afraid that she would not be liked if discovered in her full incompetence. She then started to eat compulsively, broke dates, and the relationship ended. Her binges were episodic, related to external stress.

Deborah was seen in individual treatment for four months, traveling from college for the sessions. At different times she invited a close friend to share a session with her. Her two closest friends were bright, introspective, articulate, and loyal. Deborah's training in her family had clearly been an asset in her adult life. The individual therapy focused on her expectations of fast success without effort and on the dynamics of avoiding stress by utilizing escape routes. The therapist encouraged Deborah to continue temporarily with the binges since they provided her with a release from stressful situations. He suggested that the binges would disappear when she changed her avoidance patterns. The binges subsided after six or seven sessions. Therapy has again ended, but the subsequent time has been too short to allow a real follow-up.

This is a complex case. It raises questions about the relationship of therapy to the continuing course of human development. Development always involves new challenges, new contexts, and inevitable periods of disequilibrium while individuals and social systems find new patterns of adaptation. For all our anorectic families as well as each of their individual members, it was a generic task after the official termination of treatment to meet the changing demands of new circumstances in their life. Like all of us, they needed to explore alternatives, to accommodate, to increase their repertoire of adaptive mechanisms—in sum, to cope and change. Most have been able to do so out of some mixture of competence in their own makeup, paralearning from the therapy, and fortunate circumstances in their outside life that support the transition. Some people like Deborah, however, almost predictably need intermittent help as they move into new circumstances, away from the family, at least until viable mechanisms for negotiating change in new contexts are learned.

Deborah moved out of her family into a college environment where demands and constraints are different and into the complexities of male-female relationships that characterize young adulthood. But her ways of coping relied too frequently on inappropriate patterns that had been viable in her family. The earlier therapy could not preview the issues since it concentrated on Deborah's psychological survival as an individuated member of a family system that was learning, with difficulty, to let go of its members. It was necessary for Deborah to move out and to face the new circumstances alone without the buffer of her protective family. In her attempts to cope, she developed new skills, but she also relied on old dysfunctional patterns that were now experienced as belonging to her. At this point it was essential that the therapist be available for the continuation of treatment. This model of continued treatment is analogous to the practice of the family practitioner, who is available as issues arise. In the long run, it seems an economic approach to therapy.

The Gilbert Family

9 —————————————————————————————

Judy Gilbert (case no. 28 in outcome tables, ch. 7) was fourteen years and one month old when she was referred to Children's Hospital of Philadelphia by the southern hospital where she had already been hospitalized three times for anorexia nervosa. She had been regarded as an active, normal child, with adequate weight and appetite, until the time she was thirteen. During that summer she began to diet. Thereafter, she completely lost her appetite and became moody and withdrawn. Her peer activities decreased. No specific precipitating episodes could be found.

Within four months of the start of the diet her weight dropped from 93 to 56 pounds. She was hospitalized for four months. An extensive medical workup failed to reveal any organic cause for the anorexia. The psychiatrist at the hospital described her as a rigid personality, suffering sexual conflicts. He reported that she drew pictures without hands, which was considered significant in the light of her extreme passivity. He also noted: "At the beginning of her stay in the hospital she would stand as opposed to sit, would rock back and forth in a very infantile manner and would never stop moving. Gradually she was tried on various medications and when she was placed on Thorazine, this seemed to help control this rather autistic-like rocking behavior."

She was placed on a behavior modification program, which was unsuccessful. When her weight continued to decrease, feedings via naso-gastric tube were instituted. With the forced tube feeding, it was possible to increase her weight to 70 pounds. Upon discharge from the hospital, however, her refusal to eat and her hyperkinetic behavior caused a weight loss drastic enough to necessitate readmission to the hospital for another program of forced tube feeding.

She was again discharged and readmitted, and at that point was referred to Children's Hospital of Philadelphia. Her father changed jobs, and after selling their home, the entire family moved halfway across the country to be with Judy.

Upon her arrival at the hospital, Judy appeared extremely thin and withdrawn, though she seemed to be in no distress. Her weight was 56 pounds, height 4 feet, 9 inches, blood pressure 92/54, and pulse 56. Other than the severe degree of cachexia, no obvious physical abnormalities were detected.

Because of Judy's extensive previous workup, only minimal screening studies were ordered. All of these proved to be negative. She was placed on a behavioral program. When the regimen was explained to her, the nurse noted that the patient "did not seem impressed. She stated that she would refuse to use a bedpan if confined to bed, and could hold her urine for three days."

True to her word, the behavioral program in this instance was not very effective. Because of her elevated BUN (54) and her low blood pressure, intravenous saline was used to expand her plasma volume. Though confined to absolute bed rest, Judy still persisted in eating only minimal amounts. She did not gain weight, but neither did she lose excessive amounts of weight. It was at this point in her therapy that the lunch interview was held.

The first stage of the interview was, as always, a time of joining and exploration. It is vital for the therapist to establish a supportive relationship with the family before entering crisis induction. In the following transcript, however, this first stage, which lasted nearly an hour, has been drastically cut.

MINUCHIN: Before we begin to have lunch, could I know a little bit about how the family works?

FATHER: The way the family works. You know, there is a uniqueness about a seaman's family.

MINUCHIN: I said that to Judy. "I don't know any ship's captains. Is your father a very strong, authoritarian person?" Because that's my stereotype.

FATHER (*laughing*): I'm not. I think that I'm probably very emphatic in many ways. I try to understand, at home and at work.

And "my word is law" is not necessarily the way it is. On the job, I'm the boss.

MINUCHIN: Yes?

FATHER: The ship has to have a captain. It has to have someone running the show. That's when the decisions are being made by one person. But when I am away—quite frequently my wife has a dual role as parent. Father parent and mother parent. She's got to be both.

MINUCHIN: A single parent family.

FATHER: Yeah, and this becomes a problem when I come home. You know, "Here I am again."

MINUCHIN: I think I see.

FATHER: Having been away awhile, you know? It's hard for her because she's got to play two roles, then go back to the one role again.

MINUCHIN: M-hm.

FATHER: Maybe she wants to expand on that a little bit. She said that was a problem.

MOTHER: No, I never considered that to be a difficulty. We have always made our decisions together.

FATHER: Yeah.

MOTHER: And I pretty much know what Gregory would like to have done in certain situations.

MINUCHIN: I am thinking about what your husband is saying. It seems a very sensitive way of looking at the family. This is a family that expands and contracts.

MOTHER: That's right.

Therapist joins with father, confirming him as a sensitive, articulate person.

INTERVIEWER: Is the way in which you started the session an example of your way of joining the system?

MINUCHIN: Yes. I begin supporting the father, who is an authority aboard ship and peripheral at home, by asking him for a description of family functions, which makes him an authority at home as well.

In this strategy I contact the identified patient only superficially and move the focus of the session toward generic family issues.

MINUCHIN: How is life when your husband is at sea?

MOTHER: It has varied. He used to be away for longer periods. When Judy was from seven to ten, he would be gone for three months, and then he would be home for about six months, and then he would go for three more months. But all the time he was gone—Gregory is very conscientious about keeping good contact with the family. He writes regularly and he calls occasionally. We never felt that he was gone, you know, for long periods of time without interaction.

Mother, having been directed by father to continue, takes over description of the early period of family life.

MINUCHIN: Is the life—

MOTHER: The everyday life of the children is certainly and was then, more controlled by me than by Gregory. But I don't think that changes much whether he's home or whether he's gone. I think children's daily lives are pretty much governed by mothers anyway.

Therapist directs his attention to wife, facilitating her involvement.

MINUCHIN: Oh, today there are all kinds of models, you know. But probably the tendency to centralize you as a parent is part of the way in which your family was organized.

FATHER: I think so.

MOTHER: M-hm.

MINUCHIN: This is what you were saying about the families of seamen.

MOTHER: M-hm.

FATHER: Yeah.

MINUCHIN: How was it, Judy? Do you remember these periods before? Can you describe what happened when Father went away? When Father came home? This accordion kind of family—what was the im-

Having contacted both parents and confirmed both as competent individuals, therapist moves to join with identified patient.

pact of Father coming and of Father leaving?

JUDY: Oh, it would be exciting when he'd be coming back—watching for the ship. When he was on the ship, I remember going down to the piers and watching for him. And going on the ship and getting to go on —and do stuff. And, you know, he'd bring back stuff. So it was always, "Oh, boy," you know. (*Everyone laughs.*)

MINUCHIN: What would you bring back, Gregory?

Therapist encourages the pleasant atmosphere.

FATHER: This was a period, Judy, in which your younger brother was a baby, or even before—

JUDY: Before he was there.

MINUCHIN: Not there. So, Judy, you stayed with Mother alone. And probably there must have developed a very close relationship between you and your only daughter. Is that true, Maureen?

MOTHER: I think so, yes.

MINUCHIN: Judy, did you talk a lot with Mother?

JUDY (*in a sharp tone of voice, indicating challenge and rejection*): I don't know!

MINUCHIN: I am not talking about now.

JUDY (*same tone of voice*): I don't know!

MINUCHIN: What do you think, Maureen? What are your memories? Can you remind her?

INTERVIEWER: What happened there?

MINUCHIN: Suddenly, I was powerless. I tried to involve the girl and was rebuffed. I tried again, and was rejected even more sharply. At this point, five minutes into the session, I could not afford to become involved in a power operation with Judy. So I brought the mother into the transaction.

INTERVIEWER: That sounds like the way these families detour conflict.

MINUCHIN: Yes, it is an indication of my

accommodation to the system that I unwittingly utilize now the same maneuvers
that the other family members use to detour
conflict. In terms of restructuring the system, the therapist has control over who
participates. In some cases he may find it
useful to keep other family members from
joining a dyad, thus forcing the pair to interact longer than they naturally would.
But at other times he may encourage a third
member to join in, as here, where the technique works both to deflect confrontation
and to gather different information.

———

MOTHER: Well, you have to look back, I
guess, to the time Dad was on the ship. You
know, Judy, we would do things together.
When Dad was gone, we would sometimes
go over to Gram's house—

JUDY: I really don't remember.

MOTHER: You don't remember any of
this?

JUDY: Nope!

MOTHER: And we'd sometimes invite the
cousins over to come and visit and stay with
us for a week or two. We had lots of relatives in the immediate area. When Gregory
was gone—

FATHER: This was when we were in Virginia. She's talking about when I was a
ship's officer.

Implementation of mother/
daughter dyad and development of stress between them
activates one of the mechanisms that family uses for
diffusing conflict: creation of
a triad, or a shift of dyads.

MOTHER: Yes. That's what she was referring to when she was talking about going to
meet the ship.

MINUCHIN: Gregory, I think you sent a
rescue mission to your wife because she felt
uncomfortable when Judy refused to remember. (*Everyone laughs.*)

By accommodating to father's
naval language, therapist
frames the transaction underlying a family pattern.

FATHER: Well, maybe I did. And what
you're saying is, "Don't send in a rescue
mission."

MINUCHIN: Well—did you need it,
Maureen?

Therapist challenges unnecessary protection between
spouses.

MOTHER: No. No, I don't think I needed your rescue.

MINUCHIN: This is how family members do trigger each other. It's kind of fun when you see how synchronized spouses are.

Therapist underlines the idea of family as a functioning system, phrasing his input supportively ("It's fun to see").

FATHER (*laughing*): What you're really saying is, I interfere in a way.

Father accommodates to therapist.

MINUCHIN: Maureen, did you feel that you made a movement toward Judy, and she cut you off?

MOTHER: Right.

MINUCHIN: Judy, did you notice that you slapped your mother? You know that you did slap her wrist?

Therapist challenges Judy in an area not related to food, preparing for further interventions that will transform the problem of not eating into a problem of behaving badly.

JUDY: No.

MINUCHIN: Yes you did.

MOTHER: Not physically, but he means by what you said. (*There is a pause.*)

MINUCHIN (*to father*): Maureen seems to be a very sensitive kind of person who can be bruised easily.

FATHER: Ah, probably so. I think we're both that way, frankly.

MINUCHIN: And you have a young girl that is extremely stubborn. That sometimes looks like strength.

Therapist begins to reframe daughter's position in family.

FATHER: Yes. You know, I don't think we've ever recognized that until recently. Maybe I'm stubborn as well, but I don't know it. I feel like I've got flexibility, but yet, at the same time, I know that I like to do things and that maybe other people don't necessarily—my wife may want to expand on that.

MOTHER: I smile because we always say that I'm very determined and Gregory's a perfectionist and so that makes Judy a determined perfectionist.

MINUCHIN: And how have you dealt with the problem of your determinist perfectionist daughter? I will use your terms. I think they fit like a glove for you, Judy. You have

Therapist uses family language to reframe family's view of daughter.

Therapist contacts daughter.

apparently been in a hell of a mess for what? Six months?

FATHER: We were apologetic about the situation, trying to say, "Hey, you know, please do this because this is the way we'd like you to do it," but never, "Do it or be damned." Simply because I'd never experienced such a turn-down.

MINUCHIN: Before, Judy was a nice, polite—?

FATHER: Yeah, Judy was always a great kid. Still is. You know, just a super kid. And did things—we did a lot of things together and enjoyed them. Camping, hiking, you know.

Father gives relatively common description of the anorectic child before the beginning of illness.

MINUCHIN: How did Judy express disagreement before expressing it so violently now?

Therapist continues to frame behavior of the anorectic in terms of voluntary expression of disagreement.

MOTHER: I don't think Judy did. That's what I think is part of the problem.

MINUCHIN: She never expressed disagreement?

MOTHER: Not really, no. She would glare at us occasionally.

FATHER: Yeah.

MOTHER: That was the only sign, I think, that we got that she was really unhappy with something that, you know, that we had decided or had done.

(*Lunch is brought in.*)

INTERVIEWER: That was a relaxed first stage.

MINUCHIN: Yes. I focused away from the anorectic, dealing with generic family issues. I joined with the family members, experiencing some of their strengths, the avenues that they either closed or facilitated, the range of their patterns, their thresholds of conflict, and some of their strategies for coping. At the same time, I learned something about their past life and present context.

While transacting with the family, I worked to strengthen my leadership by such simple maneuvers as directing the communication flow, requesting information, blocking family patterns, and supporting family members. By the time that the food arrives, the family members have learned to rely on and trust the therapist as the leader of the therapeutic system. This is essential, since the second stage of the session will involve the enactment of a family crisis. Family members will have to be motivated to go beyond their usual thresholds of conflict and to explore alternative ways of behaving.

(*Lunch is served. The mother, father, and therapist are given the sandwiches they ordered. Judy is given the tray she ordered earlier on the ward. Everyone begins to eat except Judy. The therapist gestures to Judy that she, too, should start eating.*)

JUDY: I don't want it now, Dr. Minuchin.

MINUCHIN: Gregory and Maureen, this is something that we will need to discuss.

JUDY: I am not going to eat it. I'm not going to eat it now.

FATHER: What?

MINUCHIN: Judy, this is something that you will not deal with me. You will deal with your parents. We have a very significant issue that we will resolve today. Let me be blunt. We all are afraid that Judy will die.

FATHER: Yes.

MOTHER: That's right.

MINUCHIN: I think that the treatment procedure in the previous hospital was worse than the illness itself. Not only doesn't Judy eat, she doesn't chew. She doesn't swallow. She learned there to be fed through a tube and now she's being fed here through the veins. She is your daughter and she needs to begin to eat.

Daughter's shift from postponement to refusal and back to postponement is characteristic of the evasive way in which all family members deal with confrontations.

JUDY: I am.

MINUCHIN: You are?

JUDY: Yes.

MINUCHIN: That's not the information that I have. This is something that I want to continue talking about with your parents. I want you two to deal with her at this point. She has to eat.

JUDY: I know.

MINUCHIN: I'm not interested in talking with Judy because she's childish—

FATHER: Yes.

MINUCHIN: —and infantile. And when fourteen-year-old people deal with me like a three-year-old, I get tired and just don't respond to them. There must be some way in which you two people who have lived with her for fourteen years, love her, and are concerned for her, have some keys to her survival. It depends on your ability to make her stop her hunger strike. So I will leave, and you can talk with her. You can talk as long as you want. You can command; you can insist; you can cry; you can plead; you can cajole; you can seduce. Do whatever you want, but she has to begin to eat something. (*He leaves the room.*)

Therapist contacts Judy, challenges her, avoids the power struggle, and puts her in a powerless position. He models for parents and puts them in charge.

INTERVIEWER: Why do you think that you will succeed in activating them since they have tried before and failed, have taken their daughter to the hospital, and the hospital has failed as well?

MINUCHIN: I have indicated that the daughter is in danger of death and that they could save her. These are very powerful ingredients to activate people. The stage for crisis induction is now set: Judy has been cast as an irresponsible, powerless child; her parents have been assigned the responsibility for saving her life; and food has been introduced as the issue.

INTERVIEWER: Do you always leave the room at this point?

MINUCHIN: No. It depends on the family. This family is very good at drawing a therapist in to help maintain their conflict-detouring patterns. From behind the one-way mirror I can easily avoid the system's demands for accommodation and intervene only at the times I must in order to redirect their transactions.

INTERVIEWER: What if a therapist doesn't have an observation room?

MINUCHIN: Then he has to develop techniques for becoming invisible, such as studying the floor or the ceiling, contemplating his navel—whatever fits his own style.

———

JUDY: I told you, I'll eat when I go back.

FATHER: Judy, you're going to eat now.

JUDY: No, I won't.

MOTHER: Why won't you eat now?

JUDY: 'Cuz I don't want to.

MOTHER: For any particular reason?

JUDY: Yeah.

MOTHER: What?

JUDY: 'Cuz I don't want to.

FATHER: That's the only reason?

JUDY: Yeah.

FATHER: Just because Judy doesn't want to eat now?

JUDY: Right.

MOTHER: Well, we would like you to eat now, honey.

JUDY (*nastily*): I don't care to, thank you.

MOTHER: You're starving to death, dear. You've got to eat. Please!

JUDY: I will when I get back, I said!

Daughter avoids challenge, this time by postponement.

Father makes a demand.

Daughter rejects it.

Mother enters, moving backward and using reasoning to avoid confrontation.

Daughter's confrontation with father stresses family system beyond its threshold, activating mother/daughter dyad.

Daughter responds to mother's signal to avoid conflict by returning to postponement ploy.

FATHER: We're not going to wait.

Father makes a forceful "we" statement.

JUDY: Well, I am.

Daughter challenges father and activates conflict.

FATHER: We've been waiting for a long time, Judy. If you really were sincere in what you're saying, you would eat now.

Father avoids conflict, then shifts ground to family values, revealing one of the family's inaction patterns.

JUDY: I don't want to. And I'm not going to.

Daughter rejects father and amplifies conflict.

FATHER: But you're not sincere. You're not sincere. You're telling us a fib.

Father keeps action in the field of values and emphasizes family loyalty ("You're telling us a fib").

JUDY: So what?

FATHER: Well, not so what. You're being deceitful.

JUDY (*mockingly*): Deceitful.

MOTHER(*pleading*): Is that what you want to be? I mean, what is it you do want, Judy?

Increased intensity of conflict causes mother to reactivate mother/daughter dyad.

FATHER: What is it you want? Do you want to be deceitful?

MOTHER: Do you want to be thin and starving? What is it you do want? That's what we don't know. If we knew what it is that you wanted, perhaps we could solve the problem, if you would talk to us about it. We don't know.

Mother pleads for the return of the good daughter to the fold of the harmonious conflict-free family.

FATHER: You don't talk to us.

MOTHER: You don't eat, but you don't say why. You just don't eat. Honey, we don't know what to do. We have pleaded with you, and we have promised you, and we have begged, we have cried, and we have been angry with you, and you still have not eaten. And until you decide that you want to eat, there really isn't much we can do. So, come and sit with us and eat. Just pull a chair up and eat something.

Mother's placating tone is a signal for avoiding conflict. Mother, like father, is unable to demand change and at the same time maintain family harmony.

JUDY: I don't want to.

MOTHER: Eat something, honey.

FATHER: Applesauce looks good, honey.

JUDY: You can have it.

FATHER: No, honey.

JUDY: I'm not eating it.

FATHER: Eat it!

Daughter refuses to accommodate.

JUDY: No.

FATHER: Judy, it's good food.

JUDY: Crap.

FATHER: It's not crap.

MOTHER: You know there's nothing wrong with the food, Judy.

JUDY: I'm not eating it now.

MOTHER: Why not?

JUDY: 'Cuz I don't want to.

MOTHER: You didn't give us a reason.

As daughter escalates conflict, parents alternate their requests to daughter, unable to go beyond their ineffective range of coping mechanisms.

INTERVIEWER: The family members seemed much more flexible at the beginning of the session and appear extremely rigid in their transactions now. Is that the effect of the task, or were they masking their real patterns before?

MINUCHIN: This family is not totally dysfunctional. In certain transactional arenas its members, like members of normal families, enjoy alternatives, and the homeostasis of the system endures wide deviations from the system's rules. When these family members transact in dysfunctional areas, however, the permitted deviations from the usual patterns are drastically narrowed. In the lunch session I created a task in a dysfunctional field which required a transformation of family patterns for its successful implementation. Faced with the need to enter into conflict in order to implement the task, the family members responded in their usual conflict-avoidance pattern, relapsing continuously into narrowed, emotion-centered transactions.

JUDY: So what?

MOTHER: Just not wanting to is not enough. I want more reason than that. Honey, we care about you. We care whether you live or not. Maybe you don't care, but we do. (*She cries.*)

FATHER: Judy, what is it that you want?

Parents try to mobilize daughter by eliciting guilt. They are, in effect, using a technique employed by some parents of much younger children when they ask the child to eat one spoonful for mother, another for father, and so on: "Eat

Do you want your mother to just keep tearing her heart out, waiting for you to eat, for some master thing that is so important to you that you won't eat over it?

JUDY: I don't want to eat now.

Daughter responds to this old conflict-avoidance signal not with rejection but with postponement.

FATHER: Why, honey?

JUDY (*exploding*): I already said I don't want to eat now! Tough it!

Father insists softly.

Daughter rejects him and elicits conflict.

FATHER: "Tough it, I don't want to eat now"?

JUDY: Right.

FATHER: You don't love your mother? You don't love your brother? You don't love your dad? You don't love us? Is that it?

MOTHER: Worse yet, worse yet, she doesn't care about herself.

FATHER: You just don't care about Judy. You don't care about your family. You don't care. You just don't care.

JUDY: That's all you ever say. "You don't care. You don't care."

FATHER: You do care?

JUDY: Shut up, Dad.

FATHER: All right, I will shut up when you stop your hunger strike.

MOTHER: Does it make you feel good to talk like that to Dad?

JUDY: No.

Father avoids conflict and elicits loyalty. To daughter's statement of affirmation ("I don't want to eat now"), both parents respond with a request for love and family allegiance.

Mother comes to father's defense. The issue of daughter's starvation is lost in the labyrinth of attempts to regain family harmony.

for us, because if not, we suffer."

INTERVIEWER: Is this last set of transactions an example of the narrowed pattern?

MINUCHIN: Very much so. The struggle between parents and daughter is related to the acceptance or rejection of input (eating, acceptance of rules, taking orders). The daughter increases the stress by challenging the parents when she feels trapped into accepting. The family members then move into emotion-directed transactions, and the stress diminishes.

MOTHER: You like to say, "The food is crap," and tell him to shut up and things like that?

JUDY: No.

MOTHER: Does that make you feel big and important?

JUDY: No.

FATHER: It's more important to say that, though, than to eat.

JUDY: Yeah.

FATHER: You're saying that you'd rather stay in the hospital than come home. Is that what you're saying to us?

Parents continue to empha-size family loyalty.

JUDY: NO!

MOTHER: You're saying that by not eating.

FATHER: Yeah, that's what you're telling us. Exactly.

JUDY: I don't want to eat now.

Daughter reverts to postpone-ment instead of rejection.

MOTHER: You know, by not eating, you're saying, "I don't want to come home. I'm not ready to come home and face you yet. I don't want to be part of the family."

Parents function in tandem, emphasizing love and har-mony as a motivation for change.

JUDY: I don't—can't eat it now, sorry.

MINUCHIN (*re-entering*): I don't think it will work like that.

FATHER: No.

JUDY: *You're* not going to get anywhere, Doctor.

Daughter first persists in her challenge, then hesitates and postpones. Daughter's shifts and postponements are an expression of the narrowed transactional range. Post-ponement is a pseudo-accept-ance of the parental order to "eat now."

MINUCHIN: What has happened is that you have allowed your fourteen-year-old daughter to be extremely disrespectful with you, to crap on you and on your food. And you accept that. She has the ridiculous idea that she is able to do whatever she wants to you: to walk on your dignity, to step on you, to make you feel impotent, helpless—

Therapist shames parents for being helpless. He as-sumes that in this family the language of dignity and pride will serve as a lever to make parents move away from their conflict-avoidance position.

FATHER: It seems so.

MOTHER: It's true.

MINUCHIN: I am coming in because the way in which you are going, your daughter will not eat. Because she feels stronger than her father and she certainly feels stronger than her mother. And when you try to say to her that she should eat, you get a little bit concerned about your strength. She has trampled on your dignity. On both of you!

FATHER: Right.

MINUCHIN: There's something very wrong. So I want you to try something different. (*To mother.*) Can you change seats?

MOTHER: M-hm.

MINUCHIN (*to father*): I want you to sit next to her. And I want you to make her eat.

FATHER: I feel like my—I—I'm physically too powerful to do what I really want to do.

MINUCHIN (*leaving*): You talk with your wife.

FATHER: Are you ready, Judy?

JUDY: No.

FATHER: It's so unlike you, Judy.

JUDY: I don't like to be rude to you.

MOTHER: I know you don't like to be. Then why are you?

FATHER: Honey, I know you don't.

MOTHER: Why are you being rude to us? Why are you not eating? Why don't you sit up and eat?

JUDY: 'Cuz I'm not hungry.

MOTHER: Sometimes you have to eat when you're not hungry though, right?

FATHER (*giving Judy a piece of bread, which she throws to the floor*): Judy, goddamn it, give me that bread back here. Now put that in your mouth and eat it. (*He gets the bread from the floor and gives it to Judy.*)

JUDY: No.

FATHER: You ready? (*He takes another piece of bread and shoves it into her mouth.*)

JUDY (*spitting it out*): No!

FATHER: Here, you're so disgusting. You're a mess. And I am really upset with you. What am I going to do? What is it you want? Forcing food into your mouth like an infant? That's what we do to infants. Hold

Therapist tries tactic of having father work alone with daughter. As with Kaplan family, the strategy at this stage of the session has four steps: first, both parents together were asked to help the girl to eat; now each in turn will be asked to try separately; and finally both parents will be asked to join in opposition to daughter.

The level of activity in the room changes as father, in coalition with the "ghost" of therapist, goes beyond his usual range of responses.

But faced with daughter's confrontation, father moves back to reasoning and pleading.

you, brace your mouth open, and push the food in. Like a three-year-old. That's what we do. That's Judy, the three-year-old, right here.

JUDY (*mimicking an infant's voice*): Mama.

FATHER: Yeah, okay, "Mama."

JUDY (*infant's voice*): Papa.

FATHER: Here, open your mouth. (*He gives her more bread.*)

JUDY (*infant's voice*): No, Daddy.

FATHER: Open your mouth.

JUDY: No, Daddy. (*Father feeds a spoonful of applesauce to Judy, who spits it out. Father pushes it back, and Judy bites his finger.*)

FATHER: Ouch!

MOTHER: Judy, I'm going to give you a good slap. Knock it off.

JUDY: I'm not eating applesauce. Gross.

FATHER: Stop slopping that all over the place. And I mean it. And you're gonna eat before you leave here this afternoon.

JUDY: I'm not eating it.

FATHER: Yes, you are.

JUDY: No, I'm not.

FATHER: Yes, you are. There's chicken there that you like, bread that you like, and applesauce that you like.

JUDY: No, it's not.

FATHER: It is, and I know it is.

JUDY: I'm not eating it.

FATHER: Yes, you are.

JUDY: You're a pig.

FATHER: Oh, I'm a pig! Well, you are full of fancy words today, aren't you?

JUDY: Yep.

FATHER: You got some more?

JUDY: Yep.

FATHER: Let's hear them.

Mother's intervention supports father but interferes with development of intensity between father and daughter.

Daughter responds with selective rather than total rejection.

Father's threat is reminiscent of Mr. Kaplan's delaying techniques.

Daughter's confrontation is followed by father's conflict avoidance.

JUDY: Pig, pig, pig.

FATHER: That's upsetting to me. You've never been like this before, and it really upsets me.

> Symmetrical interaction between father and daughter escalates to daughter's last provocation.
>
> Father moves conflict to a personal statement that signals a warning.

JUDY: Me, too.

> Daughter responds, acknowledging warning.

FATHER: Well, if it upsets you, Judy, why don't you stop it? Honey, change, Judy! Change back to the Judy that was so much a part of the Gilbert family. Is it that hard? Judy, I love you. You don't think I love you, do you?

> Father returns to a request for family loyalty and family harmony.

MOTHER: Answer him, Judy.

JUDY: I'd rather not.

MOTHER: It's rude not to answer.

> Mother intervenes to protect father.

FATHER: Yeah, well, that's what you just told me. You don't love me. Now I'm perplexed over that.

> Father moves to issues of interpersonal acceptance and hurt.

JUDY: I didn't say that.

FATHER: Yes you did, honey.

JUDY: No, I didn't.

FATHER: You said, "Hum."

> Daughter responds with a literalness that avoids conflict without giving in, as did Deborah Kaplan.

MOTHER: The question was, you asked her if she thought that you loved her, not whether she loved you.

> Mother intervenes to diffuse conflict. Wife's joining with husband frequently includes a disqualifying element.

JUDY: Uh-huh.

FATHER: I love you, Judy.

JUDY (*in a mocking voice*): Thank you. I love you, too.

MOTHER: Do you care about Dad?

JUDY: Yeah.

MOTHER: You do really?

JUDY: Yeah.

> Mother moves to protect father, bringing mutual care and concern into focus again.

MOTHER: Why don't you show him that you do then. Why don't you sit up and eat? Here, have some chicken.

> Mother's push for change conforms to family's values of harmony and love.

JUDY: No, why don't you? I don't want it.

> Daughter's request that mother eat is similar to Deborah Kaplan's.

MOTHER: Why don't you really show him that you care, Judy, by sitting up and eating something?

> Mother takes over in the name of father, avoiding his defeat. As before, she asks daughter to eat *for* father.

JUDY: I don't want any of it.

MOTHER: All right, this is one of the things you have to do that you don't want to do. Sit up and eat.

JUDY: I don't want to sit here and eat now, with you.

To mother's reasonable approach, daughter answers not with rejection but with two postponements (not "with you" and not "now").

MOTHER: But we're saying that you must sit up and eat with us whether you want to or not. We're not giving you a choice, honey.

Now mother makes a demand.

JUDY: I don't want to.

Daughter rejects it.

MOTHER: We're telling you that you must do it. Now do you want to do it yourself or do you want Dad to end up throwing it all over the room here?

Mother assumes the forceful "we" stance to make her demand, then shifts to father as disciplinarian.

JUDY: He can throw it all over the room.

MOTHER: Well, he's going to aim for you, though, so you know, if you don't want to cooperate, that's what's going to happen. He's going to force it into you. Now, would you like to sit up and try so that won't happen? Because Dad is going to have to feed it to you.

Despite the lack of power in father's demand, mother maintains the myth of male strength. This statement also carries a disqualification.

JUDY: I'll have my napkin, thank you.

MOTHER: I'm going to come and slap you in about a minute.

FATHER: You are really rude.

MOTHER: If you were a little girl, I'd put you over my knee and spank you.

FATHER: That's right.

When mother poses a tentative challenge, father supports her.

MOTHER: And that's what you're asking for right now.

FATHER: Turn around. I don't even want to look at you right now. Just turn around and think about it. (*He turns Judy's chair away from the table.*) Now, that's what we do to little kids. Turn them around and put them in a corner, right?

But when mother brings action into the present, father avoids confrontation by raising issues of shame, parental love, and rejection.

JUDY: Uh-uh.

FATHER: Sit there forever.

Daughter transforms transaction into a power struggle in which father is defeated.

JUDY: Yeah.

FATHER: I can't believe it.

MOTHER: That's just avoiding the confrontation of the problem, Judy.

Mother comes to father's defense, and the pattern repeats itself.

FATHER: That's right. You're avoiding it. Turn around. Come up here. (*He turns Judy's chair back to the table.*)

Father echoes mother's support, and it seems as if he supports her.

MOTHER: The food's still going to be there when you turn back. The problem is still going to be there until you learn to face it. It's not going to go away.

JUDY: I'm not eating it. (*Father starts to cut the chicken, and Judy holds his arm to prevent it.*)

FATHER: Judy, leave me alone, just leave me alone.

JUDY: I'm not eating it.

FATHER: Just leave me alone.

JUDY: I'm not eating the chicken.

FATHER: Don't touch me.

JUDY: I'm not going to touch you. I'm going to touch the chicken.

FATHER: Don't touch the chicken either. And if you mess this up, I will get all upset.

Father's response may indicate psychosomatic symptoms of his own: the "upset" could be physical, perhaps nausea.

JUDY: I'm not eating that, not after you touch it.

Daughter turns the avoidance of eating into an as-if acceptance transaction.

FATHER: Am I poison or something?

JUDY: Yes.

FATHER: I am. What's wrong with me?

JUDY: Poison with gravy on it.

Father accepts the detouring by activating an emotion-centered transaction.

FATHER: Well, we'll take the gravy off it then. (*He takes a paper tissue and dries the piece of chicken.*)

JUDY: I'm not eating it.

MOTHER: What's wrong with gravy, Judy?

JUDY: I don't like gravy.

MOTHER: You like gravy.

JUDY: No, I don't.

Mother intervenes when father proves ineffective. She accepts daughter's literalness, and together they go through the steps of pseudo-action.

MOTHER: You do, you're afraid that you will be fat if you eat gravy. (*Daughter makes her face look fat by inflating her cheeks in a mimicking gesture that is childish and dramatic in such an emaciated person.*)

FATHER: That's right. You're afraid you're going to get fat, aren't you? Huh?

JUDY: I'm not going to eat that bread. I'm not going to eat it.

MOTHER: You're afraid you'll look like other girls. (*Father tucks Judy's hair behind her ears.*)

JUDY: Don't pull my hair.

FATHER: Afraid you'll grow up. I'm not pulling your hair. I'm trying to get it out of your face. Come on. (*He arranges Judy's hair to try to push food into her mouth.*)

JUDY: No.

MOTHER: Come on, Judy, now put it in your mouth and eat it. (*Father puts a piece of chicken in Judy's mouth, which she chews and spits out.*)

JUDY: No.

MOTHER: Otherwise, Dad's going to force it in, and then you can spit it out and he'll put it in again and you can spit it out again. We could play this game for a long time, you know, until you decide to eat it.

Father joins with mother, repeating cycle.

Daughter then rejects the as-if acceptance.

Father manages in this transaction to repeat his usual pattern with daughter: he starts with a forceful statement and finishes with a stroke.

Mother again intervenes to defend father, putting him in the position of aggressor.

INTERVIEWER: Why don't you intervene?

MINUCHIN: I have been observing beyond the one-way mirror the endless repetition of ineffective patterns. The family members are caught in rigid, narrow transactions. Conflicts between two members are diffused by the creation of triads or the movement toward emotion-centered transactions. They're trapped in a no-exit situation. The only way to make them push for system transformation is to prolong the time in which they are involved in the usual transactions. This will result in an increase of the affective intensity among them and possibly force them to look for an exit.

MINUCHIN (*re-entering*): Maureen, I wonder if you feel you can do better than your husband?

Therapist's strategy moves to third step: the enactment of mother/daughter dyad around food.

MOTHER: No, I don't think I could.

MINUCHIN: You sit here and take your husband's position and try. You have had longer experience of dealing with children. (*Father and mother are now sitting one on either side of Judy.*)

FATHER: Judy, are you going to eat that? Is that what you're picking at it for?

JUDY: Yeah.

FATHER: Well, good. Good, honey.

JUDY: Leave that alone. My chicken.

FATHER: Good, it's yours.

JUDY: I'm going to throw it.

FATHER: Don't throw it.

JUDY: I'll throw it if I want. (*Mother is eating, and Judy eats some chicken from the tray.*)

> Therapist's new instructions seem to have encouraged a more cooperative mood in daughter. Perhaps after the intensity of previous scenario, all family members are ready for a change.

MOTHER: I know you hate to admit it, but it probably doesn't taste bad at all. That's a lot of fuss over a tiny piece of chicken, isn't it? Do you remember the little games we used to play when you were little? You know, flying it around the table?

> Mother's mood seems relaxed, since daughter has begun to nibble food on the tray.

FATHER (*laughing*): Yeah.

JUDY: I don't want my chicken. I had a big breakfast this morning.

MOTHER: Did you? What did you eat for breakfast?

JUDY: Never mind.

FATHER: You're being rude to your Mom, honey.

> Father intervenes to diffuse mother/daughter conflict, again raising values of harmony.

MOTHER: It's not necessary to be rude because it's not going to change how I feel. Would it be easier for you if I cut the chicken up?

> But mother remains on the track, accepting conflict and encouraging cooperation.

JUDY: No. I'm not eating the skin on it.

MOTHER: Leave the skin and eat the chicken.

JUDY: And I'm not going to eat all this chicken meat, either.

MOTHER: Would you like me to open your milk for you?

> Daughter is more cooperative with mother. Her refusal to eat is conditioned to circumstances.

JUDY: No. I'm not drinking my milk. It's sick milk.

MOTHER: What's wrong with it?

JUDY: I don't like whole milk. (*Judy picks up a piece of salad from the tray.*) What's this?

Again daughter uses concreteness to avoid confrontation.

FATHER: It's good. It's a chard, I think, Judy. Tastes like turnip greens or something like that. (*Judy nibbles the salad.*)

FATHER (*laughing*): This reminds me of a picnic, you know?

MOTHER: I can think of a lot prettier places to have a picnic, can't you Judy?

JUDY: I'd rather picnic by a little bubbling brook in the woods.

FATHER: Well, our new house is right across the street from a park.

MOTHER: We have a bubbling brook right in the backyard, Judy, right there.

FATHER: Kind of bitter? Try the noodles.

JUDY: No, I don't want the noodles. They're gross.

Mood of the session lightens. Although Judy has swallowed only two bites of chicken and a little juice, family members are all in collusion to declare this a victory and to leave it at that.

MOTHER: Well, she can work on the chicken. And there's plenty of bread and milk there. I'm sure if you ate enough, Judy, it wouldn't be long before you'd have those braces off your teeth.

JUDY: I don't care.

MOTHER: And you wouldn't have to keep worrying about them. One of the things that helps those teeth is the milk that you're refusing to drink.

JUDY: I don't want the milk. (*She begins pushing the food around her plate.*)

MOTHER: I know, you told me you didn't want it.

JUDY: I'm not drinking it. You don't have to keep bringing it up.

MOTHER: Does it bother you when I bring it up?

JUDY: Well, you're just going to keep bringing it up. I know you. "Drink your milk, Judy. Drink your milk."

In all, nineteen interactions take place around the offering and rejection of milk. It is through the transactions around such small events that family members play out the drama of mutual regulation and that the individual's sense of identity and sense of belonging are crystallized.

MOTHER: And it bothers you when I bring it up?

JUDY: You can bring it up. I don't care. I'm not going to drink it.

MOTHER: Because you don't think you need it?

JUDY: I don't want it.

MOTHER: I know you don't want it, but you don't think you need it either?

JUDY: I don't want it. I'm not going to drink it.

MOTHER: I didn't ask you whether you were going to drink it.

JUDY: I don't care if I need it.

MOTHER: You really don't care?

JUDY: No. I'm not drinking milk.

FATHER: You know I don't like to see you playing with your food, Judy. You know that bothers me. Are you going to eat that cherry?

JUDY: No.

FATHER: You don't like cherries, as I recall.

JUDY: I don't like cherries.

MOTHER: You like applesauce, though.

FATHER: That looks like good applesauce, too, Judy.

JUDY: I don't want it.

MINUCHIN (*re-entering*): I think your daughter will do anything that you tell her not to do.

FATHER: I know.

INTERVIEWER: Why did you come in then?

MINUCHIN: Once again the family has managed to deflect confrontation. The atmosphere is light and harmonious. When Judy chewed and swallowed one piece of chicken, everybody relaxed. The seriousness of her condition and the necessity for change have been forgotten in the warmth of family togetherness. A therapist may delude himself, as the family did, and accept

Daughter's refusal reaches a stressful level that activates father/daughter dyad. Father intervenes with a reference to his feelings which avoids conflict and requests cooperation: "If you want to see me happy, change."

Mother insists on the task. In general, she seems more able than father to deal with conflict and is more consistent in executive functions.

Judy's apparent offer of eating as if it were a real change. But swallowing one bite is not change. It is only another form of postponement. The family system has also remained unchanged. Therefore, I must return to continue the process of crisis induction to create conditions that will facilitate change.

MINUCHIN: I am interested in how absolutely rude this little girl is to you.

FATHER: She is. She's very rude.

MINUCHIN: She treats you as if you are—

FATHER: A peer?

MINUCHIN: No, no. She would not dare to treat a peer the way she treats you. She is much more respectful with a peer than she is with you. She is an inconsiderate, spoiled brat.

FATHER: And I don't know how to respond, frankly, at this point.

MINUCHIN: To an inconsiderate, spoiled brat?

FATHER: Right, I don't. I'm confused about my response, frankly.

MINUCHIN: Probably rarely have you been so meanly treated.

FATHER: M-hm.

MINUCHIN: How do you respond if somebody who is not an infant treats you like that? How would you respond?

FATHER: Well, I'm not certain. I would consider striking the person, probably. I'm not sure that I've had that happen. I don't know what my response would be, frankly.

MINUCHIN: You mean you've never been treated that way?

FATHER: That's right. No, I don't recall being treated that way.

MINUCHIN: She attacks your manhood. She attacks you as a total person.

FATHER: But, you know, this is new.

Therapist begins the fourth step in his strategy: the goal is to have both parents collaborate against daughter. This movement is extremely difficult, owing to the exquisite conflict-avoidance mechanisms used by both parents. Therapist is therefore relentless in challenging family members' behavior in such a way as to unbalance the system. Here he joins with father in a coalition against daughter. Father is triangulated: to gain therapist's support, he must change and accept conflict.

Father, frightened by demand for action, turns to the past for discussion.

MINUCHIN: It doesn't matter if it's new. It is—

FATHER: So I can reject her, I suppose, but I don't want to do that. (*Judy, meanwhile, has put her head on mother's shoulder. Mother strokes her.*)

MINUCHIN: You know, Mrs. Gilbert, I think you are incorrect when you respond to this little spoiled brat as if she's a grown-up person. You are really comforting her at the point in which I would be very indignant.

Therapist challenges mother. Because he wants to escalate conflict, he blocks her nurturance.

FATHER: M-hm.

MINUCHIN: I would be very, very indignant with somebody who is so absolutely inconsiderate. I talk about what she does to you as a person. About the way in which she treats you. Can you please sit here next to your husband? I'm wondering if she feels that she has your support. Because I don't know where she gets the gall to treat him like that. (*Mother changes chairs to sit beside husband.*)

MOTHER: No, she doesn't have my support to treat him like that. In fact, I bristle when I hear her talk like that to him, and I want to say to him, "Do something about it." But I can't do it for him.

MINUCHIN: You would like to slap her?

MOTHER: Oh, I would.

FATHER: Yeah, so would I.

MOTHER: If she said it to me, I would. Well, she knows that I have backhanded her before. On a rare occasion. I mean, I just don't really believe in hitting children.

FATHER: You know, I'm not a violent person. It's just that I don't know what else to do. It makes me bristle when she says something like that. It hurts me deeply. It hurts me in a way that I can feel the piercing arrows come driving in. But yet, at the same time, I don't want to destroy the source. I don't want to. And I know I could, you know. (*He puts his hands on the sides of his head.*) I feel like I'm not prepared to respond in the way I want to.

MINUCHIN: But, you do respond to her as if she deserved a response. You still treat her with respect even though she's disrespectful.

FATHER: Maybe I'm not really listening to what I'm hearing. I don't want to hear it, I suppose.

MINUCHIN: Oh, I think that this girl is treating you like a rug.

FATHER: Okay, that's fine. Okay, so she is.

MINUCHIN: No, no, no! It's not fine!

FATHER: No, no. I mean—I don't mean it's fine. But what am I supposed to do about it? Just completely disassociate from her?

MINUCHIN: You can't, because she's your daughter. But you shouldn't accept her behavior.

MOTHER: I cannot accept it. That's true.

MINUCHIN: But you do. You know, this is a mean little girl. I have very rarely seen such a level of disrespect.

FATHER: For what purpose though? Where are we going? Where are we today? That bothers me.

MINUCHIN: No, you see, don't ask yourself the whys. Just respond to the fact that it is.

FATHER: Yeah, but I'm sure that I've allowed it to happen.

MOTHER: I'm sure we both have.

MINUCHIN: She has the sense of utmost ridiculous power over both of you. You're talking about a nice girl, and I just don't believe that I'm hearing correctly. You have a mean little bitch.

FATHER: Yeah, she is.

MINUCHIN: And when you respond with all this love, it's very strange. It's very, very strange.

FATHER: Well, I like her as a person, but

I can't stand her behavior, is what I'm saying.

MINUCHIN: And the utmost attack that she is making on both of you is that she will die. She nibbles and then she spits and you accept that as if that is eating. She ate something like forty calories, and she needs four thousand. And, if she wins, she will die.

MOTHER: We know. We know this.

MINUCHIN: Okay, so I don't accept her as a grown-up, because she's not. She needs to eat, and she needs also to respect you. (*He leaves the room.*)

JUDY: By the way, this morning I had some cereal, some eggs, and some rolls.

MOTHER: Did you eat the whole egg?

JUDY: Scrambled. It was gross.

MOTHER: But, honey, you can't just eat one meal. (*She moves, so that parents are sitting on either side of Judy.*)

JUDY: I don't want any more.

MOTHER: Judy, you're not going to tell us that you're not going to eat any more. Now, do you want to put it in your mouth or do you want me to put it in there?

JUDY: Neither.

MOTHER: Well, it's going to be one or the other, hon.

FATHER: You want me to help you with it?

JUDY: No.

MOTHER: I don't care which one of us feeds you, Judy, but you're going to eat it.

JUDY: No, I'm not!

MOTHER: Yes, you are, and you're not going to talk like that to me again. Sit up! And eat the food!

JUDY: I don't want any more chicken.

MOTHER: I don't care whether you want it or not. You must eat.

JUDY: No.

MOTHER: Yes. (*She slaps Judy.*) Now, sit up and eat. You heard me. Sit up and eat.

JUDY: I don't want any more.

Therapist's interventions here may shock some readers, but they are designed to reach the goal of making daughter eat in the session. Therapist purposely dismisses the complexity of whole-family transactions, addressing himself solely to leading parents into scapegoating identified patient. This maneuver is distasteful to therapist, who would rather help children develop competence and self-esteem than attack them, but the rigidity of this family demands extraordinary measures. Though parents and child know that daughter's starvation may lead to her death, they still adhere to old, dysfunctional transactional patterns. It is essential to develop a crisis that will make change possible.

MOTHER: I didn't ask you that.

JUDY: I'm not eating any more.

MOTHER: You have got to eat the food. Do you understand that?

JUDY: M-hm.

MOTHER: Well, don't tell me no then.

JUDY: Uh-uh. (*Mother slaps Judy.*) I didn't say no.

MOTHER: Eat! (*She takes a spoonful of applesauce.*)

JUDY: I'm not eating applesauce. I'm not eating applesauce! (*Father and mother both hold Judy's head while mother tries to make her eat.*)

MOTHER: Come on. I'm going to slap you again. Judy, are you going to eat it yourself?

JUDY: No. I'm not eating applesauce.

MOTHER: What are you going to eat then?

JUDY: I don't want any more.

MOTHER: I know you don't want it, but you've got to eat. (*Mother gives her a piece of chicken.*)

JUDY: I'm not eating that bite.

MOTHER: What's the matter with that bite? It's not any different than any other bite. (*Father holds Judy's hands while mother feeds her.*)

JUDY: Yes, it is.

FATHER: No, it's not. (*Mother gives her another piece of chicken.*)

JUDY: Not eating that bite either.

FATHER: Oh, shut up and eat. (*Judy eats.*)

MOTHER: It's like feeding a baby. That's why I get this chair. It's where mothers get to sit to feed the baby, right? (*Judy spits out a piece of chicken.*) Stop it! Don't you take that out of your mouth. Did you hear me? Don't take the food out of your mouth. Put it in there.

FATHER: Open your mouth.

MOTHER: And I can let go of your hand. Now, chew it up. You know, this is going

Father and mother collaborate in making daughter eat. She eats some food and spits some out. She rejects some pieces and accepts others. She insists on not eating, but both parents remain glued to the task.

to be a long ordeal, Judy. There's a lot of food on that tray.

JUDY: I don't want that bite.

FATHER: There's a lot of food on this tray and you're going to eat it.

MOTHER: Don't give in to her, Gregory. Make her eat that bite.

JUDY (*crying*): No, I'm not.

FATHER: You're going to clean this food up. (*Judy is chewing chicken.*) Empty your mouth. Chew it up and swallow it.

MOTHER: You've forgotten how to chew. Didn't chew anything for so long.

JUDY: I'm not drinking any milk.

FATHER: Never mind what you're not doing, and stop telling me what you're not going to eat.

JUDY: You shut up.

FATHER: Oh, shut up yourself. Boy, I'm going to strike you down in a minute. (*He hits at Judy.*)

JUDY (*tauntingly*): Hit me. (*She covers her mouth with her hand.*)

FATHER: I will when I'm ready, and don't tell me anything like that.

MOTHER: You put your hand down then and keep it down, Judy. Keep it down. All right, you've chewed that food. You ready for another bite? You're going to get one anyway, so you better swallow fast. Swallow!

JUDY: I can't.

MOTHER: All right, put another bite in there, Gregory.

JUDY: I'm not eating that bite.

MOTHER: Yes. You're not going to play games with every bite.

FATHER (*stroking daughter's hair and then holding her chin to force her mouth open*): Judy, open your mouth. Open your mouth. Judy, open your mouth now.

MOTHER: Open it.

FATHER (*slapping her*): Now, do you want me to strike you again?

JUDY: No.

FATHER (*stroking her hair*): I'm not going to right now.

MOTHER: All right, Judy, open it up and eat. (*She starts to feed Judy.*) Are you going to feed yourself?

JUDY: I don't want any, Mommy.

MOTHER: I don't care whether you want any or not. You're going to eat it.

JUDY: You stink.

MOTHER: Keep going, and don't call me names because it won't make me change my mind a bit. Now keep eating.

JUDY (*sobbing*): I don't want to eat it!

MOTHER: Chew it up. Uh-uh-uh—don't you dare spit that out. Don't you spit it out! (*Dr. Minuchin re-enters the room and sits down.*) Don't you spit that out. NO! You chew it up and swallow it. (*Father and mother both hold her head.*)

MOTHER: Okay, you better have some milk to wash it down.

JUDY: No, I don't want any milk.

FATHER: Drink the juice then.

JUDY: No, I don't like that juice.

FATHER: One or the other.

JUDY: No.

MOTHER: Hold her hand down again Gregory. Come on, hold her hand down. Come on, drink one or the other.

JUDY: No. I'm not drinking the milk.

MOTHER: Hold her hand, Gregory. Don't let her push it away. Either milk or juice. Which is it going to be? Come on.

Mother develops an alternative.

JUDY: Juice.

MOTHER: All right, the juice. (*Judy takes a swallow and spits it out.*) I'll slap your face.

JUDY: Don't want it.

MOTHER: Yes, drink it. (*Judy takes some juice.*) Drink some more of it. That's not enough. (*Judy spits it out.*) Stop doing that. (*She slaps Judy.*) You know, you're going to have a mess over everything and everybody. (*Father is cleaning up.*) Just like a baby. Come on. I'm sorry I hurt your arm, but it's your own fault. If you wouldn't spit it up, it wouldn't hurt.

JUDY (*sobbing*): I don't want any more.

FATHER: Stop it. Goddamn it. (*He makes slapping motions but does not hit her.*) Stop it. Do you understand that?

JUDY: I don't like that juice.

MOTHER: Well, then, you can drink the milk.

JUDY: I don't like that milk either.

MOTHER: You don't like anything Judy. That's not the problem. It's you. It's not the food. Come on.

MINUCHIN: Let's wait a minute. I just want to ask you something. How much food do you think she needs to eat? Maybe you could discuss with her what it is that she will have, and once she has decided on that, she will eat all of it.

———

INTERVIEWER: Prior to this you have been stressing that the parents should make the girl eat, and now it seems as if you are supporting her not eating. Aren't you handicapping your therapeutic goals?

MINUCHIN: I enter here to begin to facilitate the development of negotiation. While my previous efforts were in the direction of eliciting conflict, I think that now there has been a transformation of family functioning. The parents are working together in an effective way; they are accepting the need to weather conflict to reach a goal; they are establishing clear boundaries between the parental and child subsystems; and the daughter is eating. She is probably experiencing herself as defeated by her parents. If the transaction does not move somewhat

so that she experiences the ability to negotiate successfully, the possibility exists that
she will revert to not eating after the session. I created a no-exit situation, and now
it is up to me to provide a way out.

――――

FATHER: We'll see if we can.

MINUCHIN: And, Mrs. Gilbert, you are doing very well. You are feeding her the way
you fed her when she was two years old.
You are responding to her crying, but there
is something more important that you are
responding to, and that is her need to
survive.

JUDY: Mother, I want to sit with you.
(*She pushes her chair next to her mother's
and leans on her shoulder.*)

FATHER: You want to sit with her?

JUDY: I—I want to sit with her. (*She sobs
while mother hugs and pets her.*)

FATHER: I've got a hanky, honey.

MOTHER: There's one in my pocketbook.

JUDY: I don't want any more to eat.

MOTHER: You have to, honey. You have to.

MINUCHIN: Your goal is for her to eat.
And what I want is that you should—

FATHER: Determine the portion?

MINUCHIN: Determine with your wife and
with Judy what it is that she needs to eat.
(*He leaves.*)

FATHER: How much of this—

JUDY: I'm not eating any applesauce.

FATHER: About two spoonfuls of applesauce?

MOTHER: Two bites of applesauce.

FATHER: Half of the bread. (*He cuts up
the chicken.*)

JUDY: No, no more chicken.

MOTHER: You must eat the chicken,
honey.

JUDY: Then, I don't want the skin.

MOTHER: All right, no skin, just the
chicken.

Here is the first instance in
which Judy selects what she
wants and then eats without
help.

JUDY: Let me pick it up.

MOTHER: Here, you can drink the milk. Yeah, that will help wash it down and then it won't be so dry.

FATHER: Put some in a cup. (*Judy spits out the bread.*)

MOTHER: No wonder you can't swallow it, it's too dry. You just take it all back.

FATHER: Put that back in your mouth. Put that back in your mouth.

MOTHER: Take a drink of milk, Judy. It will wash it down.

JUDY: I don't want any milk.

MOTHER: You've got to drink the juice then.

JUDY: Nope.

MOTHER: You must drink one of these— the juice or the milk. Which is it going to be?

JUDY: The juice. I don't want the juice. I don't like either of them.

FATHER: You're going to drink the juice.

(*For the next five minutes, parents and daughter fight and negotiate around her eating, daughter refusing and parents insisting. Sometimes parents push food into her mouth. Judy alternates between eating it and spitting it out. Occasionally she picks up a piece of food and eats without prompting.*)

MINUCHIN (*re-entering*): I will tell you what will happen from now on. I know that it's difficult for you, what's happening. But we will repeat it tomorrow and the day after tomorrow and on Saturday and on Sunday. You will come everyday to the hospital and we will start at 12 o'clock and we will finish at 2.

JUDY: I'm not going to eat anything.

MINUCHIN: Because we must make her survive. And that is a job for parents. Not a job for doctors, but a job for parents.

JUDY: I want to eat by myself.

MINUCHIN: I don't believe that Judy will
eat by herself.

JUDY: I do.

MINUCHIN: I don't believe her.

JUDY: You leave me alone.

MINUCHIN: I don't believe her. Mr. and
Mrs. Gilbert, I'm talking with you.

FATHER: We'll be here.

MINUCHIN: Tomorrow you come at 12
o'clock and we will go through the same
thing.

FATHER: Okay.

MINUCHIN: And I know how difficult it is
for you. But you have done very well, and
she has, for the first time in seven days, gotten some protein that she needs for survival.
And this is because of what you have done.

FATHER: Right.

MINUCHIN: She has absolutely buffaloed
us and we have not been able to be successful. You have, and we need your help. And
you will save your daughter. And so, we
meet again tomorrow.

FATHER: Good.

JUDY: Who says I won't eat by myself?

FATHER: Okay, we'll be here tomorrow.
Okay, thank you, sir.

JUDY: I'm never going to talk to you
again.

FATHER: And we're coming every day,
Judy, at noon, and we're going to feed you.

JUDY: And I'm not going to eat anything.

FATHER: Yes, you are.

MOTHER: It's your choice.

JUDY: Not if you're going to feed me.

MOTHER: Well, you have to eat yourself,
then.

Judy began to eat after the session, negotiating tensely with the
dietitian and nurses, but gaining weight. She was discharged weighing 70 pounds.

The family had moved into their new house, and Judy enrolled in
the eighth grade. Family therapy continued once a week. Judy's

weight was handled only between the therapist and the patient, who together left the parents during the session each week for the ritualized weighing-in. Much of the therapist's work was involved with disengaging Judy from the parental triangle and slowly moving her away from the little girl position between mother and father into adolescence and out of the family. To do so, the therapist formed a strong and respectful alliance with the father. Joining the mother was done largely by supporting her feelings of discontent over her husband's physical and emotional absence. The father was helped to become more assertive with both his wife and his daughter. The governing metaphor for the therapy was the reinstatement of this absentee father and husband back into family life by means of activities and endeavors that the father had to do with the children and his wife. As time went on and Judy began to improve both academically and socially, marital issues became more focused, and weekly sessions were conducted with the spouses alone and with Judy alone, as well as with the whole family.

Three months after Judy's discharge from the hospital, the situation was so much improved that husband and wife, with the therapist's help, decided that they should spend the summer alone together. Judy went to camp. It was hoped that she would be able to stay over 60 pounds, and because the camp was reluctant to accept anyone so thin, it was agreed that if she dropped below 59 pounds, she would come home. Unfortunately, she went down to 58½ pounds, even though she had done well there both socially and physically. The therapist discussed with Judy his feeling that, if she entered high school looking abnormally thin, she would be at a social disadvantage. Judy agreed, and with her consent she was hospitalized and started again on the behavioral program. She was discharged after five weeks, weighing 75 pounds and eager to start high school.

The therapist continued to meet with Judy and her family, occasionally at this point including her younger sibling as well. As soon as Judy's career at high school was going well academically and socially, the therapist began to taper the sessions off to once every two weeks and then every three weeks. Judy had his home phone number throughout treatment and could call him as needed. The formal sessions lasted one year.

At the six-month follow-up, Judy's weight was 94 pounds. At the two-year follow-up, she and her family were continuing to do well in every way. Three years after the termination of therapy, Judy was having success as a senior in high school and was looking forward to going to college and getting a degree in early childhood education. In the summer of her junior year she had worked in the conservation corps full time. She was very popular, had a boyfriend, and was president of the church youth group. She bought a used car. At 5 feet 2 inches and 105 pounds, she was an attractive girl. Her parents were very pleased with her. Her father, who had become more involved in the family, commented that he had grown firmer about establishing rules for the children.

The Priestman Family

10

Miriam Priestman (case no. 2 in outcome tables, ch. 7) is a fourteen-year-old Jewish girl from an upper middle class professional family. When she was six, her mother died of cancer. As far as the father remembers, there was no anorexia or emaciation associated with the mother's death. The father and only daughter lived with the father's parents for about two years, until the father remarried. The stepmother has two children from her previous marriage, Rebecca and Sally. Thus, Miriam's family is composed of her father, stepmother, and stepsisters. The father's work keeps him away from the home two or three nights a week, leaving the mother responsible for settling most of the problems at home. The father has relinquished these responsibilities to her, but he criticizes her for being incompetent and disorganized.

A year before the onset of anorexia, the family pediatrician recommended an evaluation by a child psychiatrist because Miriam was emotionally immature, verbally and socially inhibited, and lacking in self-confidence. She was seen in individual psychotherapy for ten months with some improvement. Occasionally, her parents were seen separately for counseling sessions. Four months after she stopped therapy, she began to diet because she thought her hips and thighs were too heavy, although she was not overweight. In four months, she went from 112 pounds to 85 pounds. At this point, her parents telephoned the child psychiatrist, who arranged for hospitalization to evaluate the child's medical status, and to try to effect a weight gain by separating her from the family. Hospitalization revealed no medical causes for the anorexia, but all attempts to stimulate weight gain failed completely. A month later, after Mir-

Note: The author of this chapter is Ronald Liebman, M.D.

iam's discharge from the hospital, her weight had dropped to 72 pounds. At this point she was again hospitalized.

Miriam resembled a World War II concentration camp victim. Her emaciated, skeleton-like appearance was repulsive. When the therapist first saw her, she was lying in bed, whining and continually wiping her mouth with a tissue to avoid swallowing saliva because she feared that too much liquid could cause her to gain weight.

Periodically during this hospital stay, the therapist ate lunch with Miriam. At these times, he told her that when he was hungry, his stomach hurt and he felt light-headed. He said that it felt good to eat and be satisfied. No attempt was made to get the patient to eat her lunch. Sometimes the therapist asked Miriam's permission to eat some of her food, such as a piece of carrot or celery. Then he would offer to share part of his lunch with her. This procedure provided an opportunity to relate to her around the issues of sharing food, while avoiding a power struggle over the act of eating. During these meetings, information regarding her family, her peer group and school relationships, and her past history and mental status was obtained in an informal fashion.

On the second day of hospitalization, the pediatrician explained to Miriam the behavior modification program that would be put into effect on the third day by the pediatrician and his nursing staff under the supervision of the psychiatrist. Miriam would be allowed to discuss the details of her menu with the pediatrician, nurses, and dietitian. She could add or subtract certain foods as long as she ate a balanced diet at each meal. She could have three regular meals or five to six smaller ones. The goal was to give her an increased sense of autonomy and responsibility for her physical status.

For the first three days after the start of the inpatient behavioral program, Miriam's weight stayed at 72 pounds. On the morning of the fourth day, she gained her first pound; nine days later, she weighed 79 pounds. She then developed a viral gastroenteritis with nausea and vomiting which lasted for three days. On the morning of the sixteenth day, she weighed 76 pounds, a net gain of four pounds. That afternooon, the first family therapy lunch session was held.

The family lunch session includes the patient; her parents, Solomon and Ruth Priestman; the pediatrician, Dr. Baker; and the psychiatrist, Dr. Liebman. The siblings, who were invited, could not attend because of school examinations. The session marks the beginning of the transition from the inpatient to the outpatient phase. It also demonstrates that the psychiatrist and the pediatrician can work together in a mutually supportive way with the common goal of helping the patient and her family. At this time the patient has not eaten a meal with her parents in six months.

(*Drs. Liebman and Baker and Mr. Priestman are waiting for Mrs. Priestman and Miriam, who have not yet arrived.*)

FATHER: We're going to have a food session?

LIEBMAN: Yes, we're going to eat lunch together.

BAKER: Time is so hard to come by, we thought we'd eat and talk simultaneously.

FATHER: My field's in the throes of exploding all over the place. I wish I were twenty years younger, to be honest with you.

LIEBMAN: Are you talking about the changes in the techniques?

Therapist joins with father to alleviate his obvious anxiety about session.

FATHER: Techniques and not only that. If I told you what it costs to learn it, you'd die.

LIEBMAN: Do you usually send out bills, or how does it work?

FATHER: With me, my personality comes through.

LIEBMAN: You never send a bill?

FATHER: I never send a bill. In eighteen years, how do you like that? And I'm out less than $300. That's my personality.

LIEBMAN: You've only been out $300 in eighteen years?

FATHER: Right, that's 97.9 percent of the people. I have no problems. (*Mrs. Priestman and Miriam enter the room.*)

MOTHER: Is there any special place we should sit, Dr. Liebman?

LIEBMAN: Yes, Mrs. Priestman. You sit here next to your husband, and Miriam will sit in the blue chair. (*Miriam shakes her head and remains standing with her back to her parents.*)

FATHER: Well, where'd you like to sit?

MIRIAM: I don't know.

MOTHER: She'd rather not sit here at all.

LIEBMAN: Well, you're her parents. It's not up to us, it's up to the two of you. You're her mother and father.

Therapist attempts to establish generational boundaries to differentiate daughter from parents.

FATHER: Why don't you join us? I haven't seen you since Sunday.

MOTHER: I'd like to have you here, Mimi. We'd like to have you. We haven't visited with you this way for a long time. (*Miriam does not respond.*)

LIEBMAN: Well, the two of you are going to have to make a decision about your daughter.

MOTHER: I felt very happy because I thought I didn't have that decision to make. I thought that you or Dr. Baker would tell us what to do. Mimi said that you would make her eat. I was very happy that I didn't have to make the decision. Are we just going to eat, or are we going to discuss?

Mother, overwhelmed by tenacity of daughter's symptoms, relinquishes appropriate parental control of daughter's behavior to therapist. Parents must become aware of their potential to help daughter and regain control of executive action in family.

LIEBMAN: Both.

FATHER: Both. Grab a seat, Mimi.

MOTHER: So I thought it would be better if you're here, because if Mimi doesn't eat—

FATHER: Mimi! Sit down.

MOTHER: We're avoiding the problem. We're here, and Daddy took off work and I took off. Why shouldn't you be here? If there is a problem, shouldn't you try to solve the problem? If we say, "okay, you can go," then we're avoiding the problem. Maybe it would make life more pleasant.

Mother pleads with daughter to join parents.

MIRIAM: No!

MOTHER: But—(*Miriam starts to move toward the door.*)

Daughter responds in negative, confronting fashion.

FATHER: Stay here.

MIRIAM: No, I don't want to.

MOTHER: You're staying.

MIRIAM: No, I don't want to.

FATHER: What's the difference?

MOTHER: Well—

FATHER: Mimi, it's like staying in music class. If you—

MIRIAM: I don't want to.

FATHER: That's my analogy.

MOTHER: Well, do something.

MIRIAM: I don't want to.

MOTHER: Well, be polite. Daddy and I have the day off. Okay, let's pretend we took the day off and we went out for lunch. Okay?

MIRIAM: No, I don't want to.

FATHER: How can we have a discussion if you're not here?

MOTHER: Mimi, let me ask you this. Why don't you want to? Are you afraid that we're going to sit and stare and watch you eat? Is that what you're afraid of?

MIRIAM: I don't know.

MOTHER: Why not?

MIRIAM: I don't know.

MOTHER: Is it because you're afraid that I'm going to watch you eat?

MIRIAM: I don't want to.

MOTHER: But why?

MIRIAM: Because.

MOTHER: Mimi, there has to be a reason. What reason?

MIRIAM: Uh uh.

MOTHER: Why? Because you don't like me?

MIRIAM: Uh uh.

MOTHER: If we weren't going to eat, would you sit?

MIRIAM: I don't know.

MOTHER: It's just the eating, right? You don't want to eat. I'm not going to watch you. I don't care. It's the eating, right?

MIRIAM: Yes.

MOTHER: It's not the sitting.

FATHER: What about the eating?

MIRIAM: You know.

FATHER: Do you? I don't know.

MOTHER: I'll tell you. Do you mind, Miriam? You don't mind? Because she said out there, I think that she doesn't want everyone looking at her. The thing is that the problem is always focused on the food, so that at the dinner table I was always watching.

LIEBMAN: What happened at dinner?

MOTHER: There was always a problem at dinner. It would either be manners, you know, or "Don't use your fingers," or something. Sometimes Mimi doesn't have the best table manners in the whole world.

LIEBMAN: Oh, that makes two of us!

MOTHER: Yes?

LIEBMAN: I was afraid to order a big sandwich with lettuce and tomato because I was going to make a pig of myself. (*Miriam takes her assigned seat.*)

MOTHER: Yes. So the point is that it would depend on how I felt. If I had a good day and I was reasonably relaxed or whatever, I mean maybe it wouldn't bother me. But then maybe if I was tired or something really annoyed me, then I would look at it and say, "For Pete's sake, you're at this age already, do you have to eat with your hands?" But I mean at this point I don't care if she eats with her feet because, you know, it's not worth it really.

LIEBMAN: Look, she's trying to talk to you. We noticed that there was a marked difference between Miriam's behavior here with the family and Miriam's behavior when she was not with her family. She was a relatively mature, very pleasant girl to be with when I saw her at the hospital. But when she was upset and trying to talk to you, she had a hard time getting her point across to you. Now, I don't know whether she didn't say it loud enough, or what it was. But there was some kind of problem between the two of you. Talking to each other may be a prob-

Mother shows the power of symptom to organize and control the behavior of entire family.

Therapist attempts to join with identified patient by sharing her symptoms, a technique which decreases the centrality and power of daughter in the family.

Therapist redefines problem, not as anorexia, but as a problem of communication between parents and teenage daughter.

lem, I don't know. You need to really talk and listen to each other. Mimi, Mother will listen to you. You just need to talk to her.

MIRIAM: I don't want to.

MOTHER: Why?

MIRIAM: Because I don't want to.

MOTHER: Why?

MIRIAM: Because.

MOTHER: Because I'll look at you?

MIRIAM: Yeah.

MOTHER: But why?

MIRIAM: Because I just don't want you to.

MOTHER: I know you don't want me to, but why?

MIRIAM: Well, that's the reason. I don't want you to.

MOTHER: Are you afraid you won't be able to eat? And you won't gain weight?

MIRIAM: Yes, I don't want to sit with you.

LIEBMAN: Excuse me. Can you hear Miriam? I can't.

MOTHER: Yes, she says she doesn't want to sit with me.

LIEBMAN: Maybe you could try, Sol. You're like the heart in the family. You're kind of the way I am. Why don't you help your wife out in any way you can.

FATHER: Oh, may I?

> At this point the relationship between mother and daughter is clearly dysfunctional, with daughter having great difficulty expressing herself. Father functions as a detached observer. Now therapist tries to involve father directly, in order to decrease his peripheral position, to increase support for mother to talk effectively with daughter, and to further the differentiation of daughter from parents.

LIEBMAN: Yes, but don't get in between the two of them. Just whisper your suggestions in your wife's ear. Give her an idea to help with Mimi, and then sit back and see how it works. Okay?

FATHER: Okay, okay.

LIEBMAN: And if you think you need some help, I'll be available to you. Maybe you need

> Therapist attempts to change the family system of communication by realigning family members in a goal-directed, concrete process.

to talk about something other than the eating, Mrs. Priestman. Anything at all. Just have a conversation. But listen to her. And Miriam, you speak up so that Mom can hear you.

MIRIAM: I'd rather eat by myself.

MOTHER: But over in the hospital, when they serve the food over there, then do you eat it with everybody? Do you like it better?

MIRIAM: I don't know.

MOTHER: Aren't you ever going to eat with me again? Ever?

MIRIAM: I don't know.

MOTHER: I wish you would. Mimi, how about if I weren't here. Would you be eating with Daddy?

MIRIAM: Yeah.

MOTHER: You would eat with Daddy, but not with me. Why?

MIRIAM: Because.

MOTHER: Mimi, we have to—something is wrong. Should we try to correct it? Hmmm? (*She sighs. Dr. Liebman whispers to father, "Tell your wife to ask Mimi why Mimi won't eat with her." Father leans forward and talks softly in his wife's ear.*)

MOTHER: Mimi! Mimi, why will you eat with Daddy and not with me.

MIRIAM: I don't know.

MOTHER: Suppose we were just going to sit and talk. (*Miriam shrugs.*) It wouldn't matter then? Is it the food? Is it the eating?

MIRIAM: Yeah.

MOTHER: It's the eating. And you, you would eat with Daddy but not with me. Can you think of why? Why?

MIRIAM: Because.

MOTHER: There has to be a reason why.

MIRIAM: It bothers me.

MOTHER: Okay, it bothers you. When you eat, it bothers you when I'm here. Okay. Now, can you think of one reason why? Tell me.

In continuing to plead with daughter to explain her eating problems, mother manifest's a role reversal: she asks her symptomatic teenage

MIRIAM (*shrugging her shoulders*): I don't know.

MOTHER: Isn't it just me? Miriam, would you eat if I weren't here and Dr. Baker and Dr. Liebman and Daddy were here? Would you eat then?

LIEBMAN: I am hungry. My stomach is growling and I have a headache. I am going to eat before my sandwich gets cold. (*After he begins to eat, Dr. Baker and father also begin eating, while mother and daughter continue to talk about* not *eating.*)

MIRIAM: I would eat if—

MOTHER: You would eat if Daddy and I were here but not Dr. Liebman and Dr. Baker?

MIRIAM: Yes.

MOTHER: Well, that changed.

MIRIAM: I changed my mind.

MOTHER: Why? Is it the food or the discussion?

MIRIAM (*crying and whining*): I don't know.

MOTHER: Now it changed, Mimi. So now I guess in a way I feel better, but now I'm more confused than ever. You mean if Dr. Baker and Dr. Liebman weren't here, but Daddy and I were here, you would eat? Better that she should hurt your feelings than mine, Doctor.

LIEBMAN: Yes, but she's an artist at hurting your feelings. Both of you get hurt. Doesn't that get you upset? Watching Miriam cry, whine, and refuse to eat?

MOTHER: Yes.

LIEBMAN (*looking at parents*): So, whose feelings is she hurting? The two of you.

FATHER: Right.

LIEBMAN: She's a princess, an artist at doing that. Can I have one of your carrots, Miriam? You know, I'm a carrot freak. Thank you. (*He reaches to take a carrot from Miriam's tray and eats it. Shortly*

daughter for help when it is the responsibility of parents to provide limits and direction for daughter.

Therapist tries to change the process of dysfunctional dialog between mother and daughter by announcing his intention to eat, hoping that others will follow his lead.

Therapist separates daughter from parents in a negative way, to emphasize need for distancing in this family. He then shares food with daughter, symbolizing need to establish a therapeutic rela-

thereafter Miriam begins to eat a carrot as Dr. Liebman continues talking to parents about communication.)

MOTHER: This is our problem with the communications now. It's been hard for her to articulate because I talk a lot and I talk very fast.

LIEBMAN: Yes, but you're a pretty smart woman, you know. You say a lot of things that make a lot of sense. I don't know whether you know that or not, but you certainly do. See, the problem is one of communication. The problem is one of you being able to talk to Mimi and Mimi being able to talk to you and your husband as parents. The other, secondary problem is the two of you as parents being able to control Mimi. It's not the eating. Eating is a byproduct.

FATHER: We always had an undercurrent of fear. Fear.

LIEBMAN: An undercurrent of what?

FATHER: Of fear in communication.

LIEBMAN: You have to pardon me, but I am really hungry and I want to eat lunch. (*He continues to eat.*)

MOTHER: I—I would like somebody—I would like somebody to give me a program.

LIEBMAN (*talking to parents*): The two of you need to help one another. Don't you? I mean, you're the mother. Although Miriam's mother died when she was six, you are the mother now—.

FATHER: Right.

LIEBMAN: —and have been for several years.

MOTHER: I always felt that Miriam looked upon me as a mother. I mean, maybe emotionally I haven't always acted right, but I don't think there's ever been the ambivalence—

FATHER: No.

tionship aimed at alleviating the patient's symptoms and the family's dysfunctional relationships.

Therapist makes another attempt at redefinition, moving the problem away from eating to communication.

LIEBMAN: You are not the stepmother kind of figure.

FATHER: You're right.

MOTHER: Well, I think Miriam may have wanted more from me than she got, but I don't think so. For instance, last night they told me from 5:30 on when her stomach hurt, she kept calling for me, you know?

LIEBMAN: She loves you. But you'd never know it.

FATHER: One of the biggest shocks was when this whole problem started.

MOTHER: But maybe she feels that I don't love her. (*Miriam mumbles to herself inaudibly.*)

BAKER: I think Miriam is trying to say something.

LIEBMAN: If you're going to say something, you have to say it loud enough so that we can hear you, Mimi. (*Miriam continues to mumble inaudibly.*) Don't eat, or eat. Do what you want. You're a big girl now. (*Father coughs, stands up, walks over to Miriam, gives her a handkerchief, and then returns to his seat. Dr. Liebman puts his hand on father's shoulder.*) You remind me of my grandmother. My mother's mother, from Russia. She was a very warm, sensitive, concerned—overconcerned person. If I were crawling around on the floor, she would watch me as if under a microscope. You know, Sol, you are like my grandmother. You're the heart. You've got all this heart. It's wonderful.

MOTHER: And maybe I don't have enough heart?

LIEBMAN: I don't know. Do you believe your wife doesn't have all that heart? (*As he engages parents in conversation, Miriam starts to eat her lunch.*)

FATHER: No.

LIEBMAN: I don't believe it either. I think she does.

Whereas therapist has tried verbally to separate daughter from parents in conflict over eating, father re-establishes contact in a dramatically non-verbal fashion. In order to prevent father from engaging daughter, therapist likens his behavior to that of an anxious, overprotective grandmother.

MOTHER: Yes, but I'm not as outgoing. I get upset when people express their innermost emotions.

LIEBMAN: You know, innermost emotions are private.

FATHER: I will say this: my wife will avoid discussions.

LIEBMAN: But you see, your wife doesn't have cold eyes. Look at her. She has very pretty eyes, very warm, tender blue eyes. Now then, a woman with those kind of eyes can't be cold. I mean, she might say she's cold, but is she cold to you?

FATHER: No sir.

LIEBMAN: As a wife?

FATHER: No, as a woman, and as a wife, and any other—

LIEBMAN: As a woman, a wife, a mother, she is not cold.

FATHER: No problems at all between us.

LIEBMAN: Then I don't know why in this family the myth is that mother is so cold. That's a big bugaboo. A woman with those eyes can't be cold.

MOTHER: But no,—

LIEBMAN: Why do you think that you are cold, Mrs. Priestman?

MOTHER: Because people are demonstrative, like hugging. Do you know what I mean? With physical contact. That's what we're talking about.

LIEBMAN: Physical contact.

FATHER: Demonstrative, physical, outward show of affection.

LIEBMAN: Well, that's kind of private. What do you mean? With a little child? With a teenager?

FATHER: I am much more physical than my wife.

LIEBMAN: What are you talking about? I don't understand.

FATHER: Expressions of affection.

To further the process of disengagement, therapist directs father to concentrate attention on wife instead of daughter.

Therapist modifies mother's image in family, enabling daughter to identify more positively with her. He also draws husband closer to wife by "competing" with him for wife's attention. Finally, by occupying parents, he keeps daughter in relatively conflict-free position where she can eat spontaneously because power struggles over eating do not develop.

LIEBMAN: Oh, you mean like at home in the morning or evening.

MOTHER: That's right. I do have this feeling that I like to kiss everybody goodnight at night and I like to kiss them when they go away in the morning.

LIEBMAN: My wife gives me hell for not doing that.

MOTHER: But—

LIEBMAN: But what? So what's the matter with that? You kiss him goodnight. Do you do that because your husband has given you that as a chore, or because you want to do it?

MOTHER: No, I feel better when I do it.

LIEBMAN: You want to do it?

MOTHER: Yes.

LIEBMAN: Then do it if you want to.

MOTHER: I do.

LIEBMAN: So, that's an outward display of emotion. Why do you still think you are a cold person?

MOTHER: And I always felt that Mimi needed a lot of affection. She likes to cuddle. And I think Sol is very affectionate. I think that Mimi is very affectionate also.

LIEBMAN (*putting his hand on father's shoulder*): We've established the fact that your husband is the heart of the family. There's no doubt about that. I mean, we don't even have to debate that issue. You know it, Mimi knows it, Becca and Sally, your husband knows it. Your husband is the heart of the family. Right? Why can't he share some of that with you? Why does he have to be so selfish? Sensitive people like your husband and me sometimes get selfish. We hog everything, all the attention, all the affection. We give it and we want just as much back.

MOTHER: That's true.

LIEBMAN: So that excludes other people. I get so involved with my children sometimes —we light the fire, especially on the weekend. That's when I don't have to run around. We watch TV, or I put on the stereo and the kids run around and the dog barks. I get so involved with the kids that I nearly exclude my wife from having anything to do with them. Not in a mean way, but just because I'm so involved. (*During the course of this conversation, Miriam has been eating her lunch spontaneously without being involved verbally with the therapist or her parents.*)

MOTHER: I don't feel as though I'm cold. I feel as though I'm strict.

LIEBMAN: That's understandable.

MOTHER: I feel that my idiosyncracies are what Mimi is talking about when she says that the house is stiff, because I'm compulsively neat. Physically, I feel better if the papers in the living room are stacked up and there aren't any papers on the floor and clothes are neatly in the drawer. I know that it's like a neurotic kind of thing.

FATHER: But who's there, who's there to see it?

MOTHER: It's me. It's the same reason that I get up on a Saturday when there's not a person around and just put my makeup on before I go have coffee. I know it's a neurotic kind of thing.

FATHER: You're a fastidious person, that's all.

LIEBMAN: That's a neurotic kind of thing? I disagree with you.

MOTHER: Well, that's what everybody says.

LIEBMAN: Who says that?

MOTHER: I say that it's neurotic to want everything to be neat.

LIEBMAN: But you'll be able to teach Mimi and Becca and also Sally how to dress well, how to keep the house or apartment in reasonable shape. You're a big plus. I

Having noted that as long as he holds parents' attention, daughter will eat, therapist continues to track conversation and build on the content provided by parents. Parents are able to triangulate therapist instead of daughter, freeing her to eat. Therefore, the content is used to keep the process going in the session.

Therapist refuses to accept mother's definition of her idiosyncrasies as neurotic pathology, because that would permit husband to

don't know why you look at it as a negative when it certainly can be a positive attribute.

MOTHER: Mimi didn't you learn from me? I don't know if it is good or bad. Your drawers, for instance they are always neat. Did you get that from me? (*Miriam nods.*) Her drawers are neat, she got that from me. The other kids didn't get it from me yet.

LIEBMAN: So you helped Mimi with that already, and you didn't even know it. Maybe you and Sol can help her in other ways?

MOTHER: Yes, maybe we can, but I don't know. Well, yes, because when Mimi says that our house is stiff, I mean, I think this is part of what Mimi means. I don't know.

FATHER: I don't know either. I'm very confused.

MOTHER: After this morning, I don't feel too good. You know, I feel inadequate.

LIEBMAN: You feel inadequate? How do you feel inadequate?

MOTHER: Something I'm doing is wrong.

LIEBMAN: What are you doing that's wrong?

MOTHER: I don't know.

LIEBMAN: You mean that you are the cause of Miriam's problem?

MOTHER: Yes, that's right.

LIEBMAN (*turning to father*): Do you agree with that?

FATHER: No.

LIEBMAN: I don't see how it's possible. How can one person be the sole cause of somebody else's problem? Especially in a family.

MOTHER: I may not be the sole cause, but I didn't help it.

LIEBMAN: What didn't help it?

MOTHER: My personality didn't help her problem.

LIEBMAN: Your personality didn't help whose problem about what? That's a very involved question. Your personality—you're

criticize her and would make daughter's identification difficult, both of which would split the spouse dyad.

Therapist includes father to stabilize spouse dyad and fix generational boundaries separating parents from children. He also shifts conversation away from examples of parental ineffectiveness and toward more positive, constructive ways for parents to help daughter.

a very nice person. What personality are you talking about? Do you mean that you're a mean devil?

MOTHER: Well, now wait. I'm not that bad.

LIEBMAN: Why don't you be like Cinderella's stepmother, be a wicked witch? (*He turns to father.*) Is that what you want your wife to be? A wicked witch?

MOTHER: Yeah, but when I say I'm not—

LIEBMAN: Wait a minute. I asked your husband a question. Relax. (*He again turns to father.*) Do you want her to be a wicked witch?

FATHER: No.

LIEBMAN: Why does she have this desire to be a wicked witch?

MOTHER: I don't feel I'm accepting enough when it comes to other people.

LIEBMAN: You are not accepting of yourself. That's what I think.

MOTHER: I didn't say that.

LIEBMAN: I thought you did.

MOTHER: No.

LIEBMAN: What did you say?

MOTHER: I always think I'm accepting of myself. I don't think I'm accepting enough in the house, maybe, or about things people do. Do you know what I mean by that, Miriam?

MIRIAM: What? No, I didn't hear it.

MOTHER: I said, I'm not accepting enough about things people do. Do you know what I mean by that?

MIRIAM: Well—

MOTHER: What do I mean by it, Mimi?

MIRIAM: I—

LIEBMAN: There's some milk. Do you want some milk, Sol?

FATHER: It gives me diarrhea. It gives me gastritis. I double up on the floor.

LIEBMAN: Does milk do that to you? You must be allergic to milk?

Therapist confronts mother's negative self-image by comparing her to stereotypical stepmother, which gives her the opportunity to see herself less harshly. He also solicits father's agreement that wife is not as negative as she imagines.

Confronted by her view of herself as sick and responsible for daughter's problems, mother resists change by seeking daughter's agreement about her inadequacy.

Therapist addresses father in order to block the dialog between mother and daughter.

FATHER: I love it, but I can't drink a glass of milk.

LIEBMAN: Well, we all have our problems. I think Mimi started to tell you something.

FATHER: And I interrupted. I always do that.

LIEBMAN: Your husband and I—we will just sit here and listen.

MIRIAM: What? I don't know what she's talking about.

MOTHER: Not, you know, accepting people. Being accepting.

MIRIAM: Yeah. What should I say?

MOTHER: What should you say? Whatever you want. I was just asking you what was your idea of a person being an accepting kind of a person. You know, what does that mean to you?

MIRIAM: Oh, You mean separate things?

MOTHER: Um-hum. That other people do. Even though it upsets you. (*Long pause.*) Do you know what I mean?

MIRIAM: Not really, no.

MOTHER: Tell Daddy how to be an accepting person.

LIEBMAN (*turning to Miriam*): Excuse me, are you going to drink your milk on your tray? Can I have your milk? Do you want to get it for me? So, you really want to talk to her, but there is something that—I don't know—kind of blocks you in this communication problem. (*Miriam hands him her glass of milk.*) Thanks very much. You don't mind if I drink it, do you? There's something that blocks you. What do you think it is? Sol, do you have any idea what prevents your wife from talking with Mimi? Because there's nothing the matter with your wife. There's nothing the matter with Mimi. But something happens when they try to talk together. I don't know what it is. It's a curious thing.

Therapist again interrupts conversation between mother and daughter to prevent daughter from being triangulated between parents and to shift focus of dialog away from daughter.

MIRIAM: Can you see a problem? What is it?

LIEBMAN: I think you know better than I do because I just met your family.

FATHER (*turning to mother*): I can understand Mimi's personality and I think I have a good understanding of yours. I think there's a basic thing. You'll repeat an incident over and over again, and people get angry with you.

MOTHER: I never thought too much about that.

FATHER: No, it's not a criticism, believe me. Primarily, I think it's your emotional make-up. You're—

MOTHER: I'm a teacher. I talk a lot.

FATHER: The whys aren't important.

MOTHER: Is it because maybe Mimi takes a long time to say something?

FATHER: No, I think you're that way with all the kids. I think you're that way with everybody.

LIEBMAN: Is she that way with you?

FATHER: That's a very good question. I don't know.

LIEBMAN: That surprises you.

FATHER: I don't know. I happen to be a very happily married man so it's hard for me to be critical. In my relationship with Ruth, I could make one or two points. Is she that way with me?

LIEBMAN: Yes, that's what I am asking.

FATHER: Yes. But it's not a criticism. Believe me, I'm being objective. It doesn't bother me.

LIEBMAN: You know, with the problems you have with your children—Becca with her friends, Sally fainted a couple of weeks ago and had to be taken to the hospital—

FATHER: Right.

LIEBMAN: —and Miriam has this problem talking and expressing herself—so with

Therapist returns identified patient to child subsystem of family by stating that all three children have problems. He also shifts focus away from children's problems and onto the effect that their problems have on mother-father relationship.

these kinds of problems, I wonder if it affects your marriage.

FATHER: Yes, it has, but this problem has existed from the day I married Ruth.

LIEBMAN: What problem?

FATHER: Something I feel about my wife.

LIEBMAN: What is that?

MOTHER: But I don't think he has that big a problem with Becca and Sally.

FATHER: I have certain feelings and I have them for two reasons—love and gratitude.

MOTHER: What kind of feelings?

FATHER: I think it's hard for you—I don't know what the hell the word is. Give me— no, I can't express that.

MOTHER: You mean, oh, because I never say I'm wrong.

FATHER: Right. This is something I happen to be sensitive about, and the second is communications. I wonder if you really hear the kids half the time.

MOTHER: Oh, I certainly do.

FATHER: Yes, you do, intellectually you do. But emotionally I don't know if you feel it.

MOTHER: But I don't see that we have that tremendous a problem—

FATHER: I don't have it.

MOTHER: —with Becca and Sally.

LIEBMAN: Excuse me, but when the two of you talk, you don't look at one another. You look down and Ruth looks at the pictures on the wall. How do you know what's going on with each other?

Therapist again diverts conversation away from mother/daughter to mother/father. Daughter, who has continued to eat, now finishes her lunch.

FATHER: Simple. My brain is functioning.

LIEBMAN: Yes, but your eyes, expressions, faces—

FATHER: I bring a personality into the conversation by—

LIEBMAN: You have a lot of personality.

FATHER: I do.

LIEBMAN: You overflow with personality.

FATHER: Yes, yes. That's why I had to get psychiatric care.

LIEBMAN: That's why you had to get psychiatric care? Well, then, you ought to be an excellent therapist for your wife. I mean, if you think she doesn't have enough of it and you have too much of it, you could share some of the heart and the personality with her.

When father volunteers information about his psychiatric status, therapist uses the data to explore the marital relationship further and to encourage parents to talk to each other.

MOTHER: I don't see why you say I don't listen to you. I listen to you.

FATHER: You do. Yes, you do.

MOTHER: All the time. All the time.

FATHER: Again, Ruth, what can I say? The one thing I learned from psychiatric care was to trust my instincts, and that was the hardest thing as a human being I learned.

LIEBMAN: And is that true? Can you trust your instincts?

FATHER: Yes, I do.

MOTHER: I want to tell you something we never discussed, but this—Sol is a loner. Do you know what his human instinct is?

LIEBMAN: Tell him directly. I'll listen to every word you say.

MOTHER: I'll tell you, Sol. You don't like anybody.

FATHER: No, I don't. I have a mortal distrust. When I try—

MOTHER: You don't like—you don't trust —you don't like anybody. (*Miriam stares at mother.*)

Mother asserts herself to criticize husband in a departure from family norm, which surprises and perhaps even frightens daughter.

FATHER: That's right, that's right.

LIEBMAN: Is your wife saying that you are a suspicious person?

FATHER: Suspicious? I wouldn't say that's the word.

LIEBMAN: Cynical?

MOTHER: Very cynical.

FATHER: Cynical, very good.

MOTHER: Very, very cynical and terribly pessimistic. I hate to tell you about anybody who has any kind of illness because the first thing you will tell me is that they are going to die.

FATHER: You know, that's one thing— when I married you, I told you that I never met a human being who has more capacity to enjoy life, either eating a lousy steak sandwich or going out to dinner. I never met anybody more—

MOTHER: My problem is, I cannot stand to be not happy.

FATHER: That's right.

MOTHER: I like to arrange things so that I am happy.

FATHER: And I am the reverse.

MOTHER: I can't stand being not happy, and your general state is that things are usually miserable.

LIEBMAN: I don't think this is relevant in communicating with Mimi, although everything you have said makes sense.

MOTHER: Well, I don't know.

LIEBMAN: Could you find out from the heart of the family why the heart of the family is so pessimistic and cynical and—

MOTHER: Well—

FATHER: Why I am that way?

MOTHER: You tell me.

FATHER: I'll tell you.

LIEBMAN: I don't think your wife knows, Sol.

FATHER: I have a number of reasons.

LIEBMAN: Well, tell your wife, and we'll all listen. Mimi and I and Dr. Baker will listen together.

FATHER: May I? Can I just list them right down?

LIEBMAN: Go.

FATHER: Number one, I'm bitter about my background, the problem I had with my mother and the fact that it affected me organically and I had to go through massive psychiatric care. Secondly, I'm very, very bitter about the death of my first wife with

The attitudinal differences between parents having been elucidated, therapist can help couple to deal with them directly.

Therapist uses content to establish boundaries between patient and parents, who are encouraged to talk to each other, leaving daughter out of dialog.

this needless, tragic, lousy medical care from top physicians. It was misdiagnosed CA and the needless, horrible, tragic death. There was my relationship with my family and my failure to break with them. It's not your fault. It was a missed opportunity in my life that I didn't walk out of the whole situation.

LIEBMAN: How long ago was that?

FATHER: I'm fifty-one. How long? When I got out of the army, I was twenty-six or twenty-seven years old. It's affected me; it affects me every day of my life. I can't help myself. I can't control it. It bothers me when I eat.

MOTHER: But right now, I feel that that's all in the past, and so why should these past things—if now things are reasonably better, why shouldn't you enjoy what you have? And why should all of this still affect how you feel?

FATHER: But one reason—you're not distinguishing—you're using the human brain. I live by the emotions. These waves of feelings creep over me. They come over me—I can't measure it—a couple of times a week.

MOTHER: But one of the reasons, you know, when I married you, I felt, well, things have been bad and now they're going to be better. But I feel—

LIEBMAN: Aren't they better?

MOTHER: Well, yes, but you see, the thing is that I feel sometimes oppressed. I try to make things better, but every now and then I feel that, well, I can't cope, because obviously, you know, whatever I do or however things are, you're not going to be any happier because you're basically miserable.

LIEBMAN: How do you feel you could help your husband with these uncontrollable waves of emotion?

MOTHER: Well, I never really thought about it specifically, but just by being there

The father having declared himself a "patient," therapist directs wife to help husband, implying that she has the necessary competence and strength.

and having things running, you know, somewhat smoothly and, you know, having things that maybe weren't there before. I thought that this would be enough. Maybe this is not enough. I don't know. But also I feel sometimes that I shouldn't have to do more.

FATHER: Right. You resent it at times.

MOTHER: Yes, I mean, I feel that—

FATHER: I'm aware of all of this. I've already expressed my gratitude. I verbalize how I feel.

LIEBMAN: Okay, let's feel this out now. Twenty-six years ago some things happened that got you kind of cynical and upset. Lots of things. Now that's roughly half your lifetime.

FATHER: Right.

LIEBMAN: Approximately half your lifetime. So, you're fifty-one.

FATHER: Right.

LIEBMAN: So we've got at least twenty-five years left on this earth, depending on how you compute it. So for the next twenty-five years, do you want to be as cynical as the past twenty-five years?

FATHER: I wouldn't know how to be any other way. If you want honesty, I'll give it to you. I'm really not scared. I know what it is to talk to the doctor honestly.

LIEBMAN: For twenty-five years you've wrestled with the waves of emotion when they come over you. Right?

FATHER: Right.

LIEBMAN: It's a problem for Ruth, too. You've been married how long?

MOTHER: For nine years.

LIEBMAN: Nine years. Okay. I think I have a solution. It would involve the two of you cooperating. Is it usually at home when you get these waves of emotion?

FATHER: It follows no set pattern. Usually, when I am at rest at night, prior to going to bed.

Therapist implies that it is possible for people to change their behavior. He is pushing parents and daughter to consider alternate ways of relating to each other that are not based on symptoms.

LIEBMAN: At home?

FATHER: Yes, they keep rising when the massive problems of the day are off.

LIEBMAN (*putting his hand on father's shoulder*): It may be that that would be a good time for you and your wife to be intimate with one another and love one another, and that would probably instantaneously take care of all of the waves of emotions and feelings.

FATHER: It's not that simple, and you know it isn't. But certainly, I'll go along with it. I'll give it a try.

LIEBMAN: You say it usually occurs at night prior to bedtime. That's interesting, isn't it Dr. Baker? (*Dr. Baker nods.*)

FATHER: Right.

LIEBMAN: And that's a good time anyhow, instead of getting all obsessed and preoccupied and upset with all of this.

FATHER: I'm not aware of it half the time.

LIEBMAN: Well, now, we've already eliminated the problem by 50 percent because half the time you don't even know it happens. Okay, that only took a minute, so to cure the other 50 percent, why don't the two of you try being intimate with one another and—

MOTHER (*looking at the two doctors*): But let's talk about this. You know, it sounds interesting.

LIEBMAN: We are flattered, but don't talk to us. Talk to Sol. He's got all the heart.

MOTHER: You constantly complain. You get up in the morning and you're tired; you go to bed at night and you're tired—

FATHER: Ruth, I resent my very existence. You know that. I'm a hustler. I'm used to rushing.

MOTHER: That's true.

LIEBMAN (*looking sternly at father and sitting closer to him*): Sol, you know something? Your wife is trying to help you, and

Father agrees to work on problems with wife, establishing a mutually acceptable therapeutic goal for parents which is separate from problems of daughter.

Mother accepts the challenge and the possibility of changing the way in which spouses relate to each other.

Mother also accepts therapist's cue to talk to husband.

she starts to make a suggestion. She didn't even get it out. And you say that you dislike your very—

FATHER: I resent my very existence.

LIEBMAN: You resent, you resent. That means you resent your family, your children, your wife, your work.

FATHER: Do you want to know something? You're right.

MOTHER: You do. You do resent all of us.

LIEBMAN (*looking at mother*): What would you like to do with this situation? He resents you. Imagine that.

FATHER: Yes, wait a minute. To me, there's no humor in these thoughts that go through my mind.

LIEBMAN: Why are you having those thoughts?

FATHER: Maybe a type like me should never have been married and shouldn't have all of this responsibility. It gives me high blood pressure.

MOTHER: In other words, you resent the fact that you do have a lot of responsibility. And after all, marrying me gave you two more children, and that's three kids.

FATHER: Ruth, my feeling is equal, believe me. When I was married with one child and my wife died and I left the one child with my mother—this feeling has been a con-sistent thing.

LIEBMAN: One child? Who's the one child?

FATHER: Mimi.

MOTHER: But, I mean to say that this is the way it always is and it has to be and whatever. You know, you hate what you do. You're in a profession that you hate. You hate all the members.

FATHER: It's not that.

LIEBMAN: Your husband is a master of self-pity.

MOTHER: Well, it is. It is rather self-pity, because—

Marital problems emerge spontaneously, setting the stage for potential resolution in the future. There is hope for change in this system, because its members have affect, humor, intellect, and spontaneity. They are likable people, and it seems possible to work with them.

LIEBMAN: Do you have one of those arm cushions? Whack! No, just hit him with it.

MOTHER: There was one—it sounds kind of dumb, but I think it was the rabbi—I hate to tell you, but in his sermon, he once said, "Life is very short and so that each day you should find one good thing that happened—"

FATHER: I'm going to throw up.

MOTHER: Isn't that nauseating? But one good thing that happened for that day so—

FATHER: You've said this to me about twenty or thirty times.

MOTHER: But you are saying that each day is going to be such a lousy day. You know, you get up tired and you go to bed tired, and you know, I don't feel very useful to you.

FATHER: That's a lie. You really are.

MOTHER: And there are many times when you come for dinner that everybody—do you know what the kids have said? Is Daddy coming home for dinner? Because when you get—

> Mother probably tries often to activate children to support her criticisms of husband.

MIRIAM: That's not true. *You've* said it sometimes!

MOTHER: Me?

LIEBMAN: Look, Mimi, you can say something of a critical nature toward your father. He isn't going to collapse. Miriam, you've got to understand it, and you, too, Ruth, and next week the other kids will have to be here so they can understand. (*He puts his hand on father's shoulder.*) Sol has been upset for twenty-five or twenty-six years. The man is as strong as a rock. No man can be upset and miserable as you have been for twenty-five years and still be as functional, as intelligent, alert, and as ambitious as you are. You are a rock, and you give everyone the impression that you are putty. You aren't putty. You are a rock.

> Here for the first time daughter makes an assertion that challenges mother. The disagreement represents an attempt to differentiate herself from mother and from problems that exist in marital relationship.

> Therapist redefines duration of father's symptoms as a manifestation of strength and the ability to cope with problems for the purpose of moving parents to a more positive, competent level of functioning compared to the mutual ineffectiveness that they displayed at beginning of session.

MOTHER: Well, I do have a lot of confidence in his sickness.

LIEBMAN: In his *what*?

MOTHER: In his sickness. No, wait a second, Sol. Every time you get sick, you always say, "I haven't been sick for a long time." (*She laughs.*) And to me, it doesn't seem so long ago since the last time you were sick.

LIEBMAN: Your husband is a rock. You don't have to pamper him. You're the one who needs to be pampered a bit. You've got three kids, the house. Do you work full time?

MOTHER: Yes, but we have a housekeeper, and that's one of the things that concerns me. None of my kids think I can cook, and Sol gets very angry because I say, "I used to make" something. I kind of, you know, got out of the habit of cooking.

FATHER: That's right. The last time you made a meal, where did I end up? I was really sick.

MOTHER: You see, I have to do a lot of preparation for the teaching, and there has been a conflict. Sometimes I am marking papers when maybe I should be with the kids. I have a lot of responsibility with the work. Now maybe that's an excuse for not doing other things, or perhaps I could manage better. I don't know.

LIEBMAN: You know, one other thing which just came up—and it comes out here—when you talk a lot to your husband, he talks at the same time, either with you—

FATHER: Yes.

LIEBMAN: —or since I'm here, he talks with me. I think that's why you have such a need to try to say what you are going to say and drive it home because he certainly doesn't give you a chance to relax and think and say what you want. It comes out in terms of your communications with Mimi. You know, you're trying to say something and it's as if, if I don't get it out within two

Therapist labels father's tendency to interrupt and intrude a contributing factor to communication problem between mother and daughter. Thus parents and daughter are again involved in a mutual problem, but now one of communication, not anorexia.

seconds, somebody's going to jump in and prevent me from finishing it. And that's what happens between the two of you.

MOTHER: I also think that—

LIEBMAN (*looking at Dr. Baker*): I think it's kind of sad, to tell you the truth, but you know, we'll have to figure out something to do to help them? (*Dr. Baker nods.*)

FATHER: I didn't realize it. She's trying to talk, and I constantly interrupt.

LIEBMAN: You see, is that what happens at home?

MOTHER: But if Mimi has something to say, it's very difficult for Mimi to get in here, because Mimi's voice is physically lower and—

LIEBMAN (*leaning toward mother*): Do you think you could help Mimi with her speech problem?

MOTHER: We have tried.

LIEBMAN: No, you. You alone. Not doctors and the entire family. Just you can help Mimi, because you have no trouble talking. You say things very succinctly and explicitly, so that they are easily understood. Your husband and I get too involved with feelings and the profundity of problems. We get off on tangents. So maybe you could help Mimi with the speech problem. With thinking about what you want to say, or formulating it, and then saying it, you know. And saying it in such a way that it's heard and understood.

MOTHER: Yes.

LIEBMAN: Because, you know, you're a teacher and you can do this. So teach her what you already know so well.

MOTHER: Well, one of the problems in teaching your own children is that there is a certain resentment. Of course, we may not have always done it the right way, because when Mimi tries to say things, we'll say, "Come on, say it," you know, and that sort of thing. And the other thing is, Mimi, part

Therapist and pediatrician further agree to help family with the new problem of communication.

Therapist wants to change relationship between mother and daughter from dysfunctional and frustrating to constructive and functional. The task he assigns to mother presents her as competent and effective, providing an appropriate identification model for daughter.

of this comes out in school. Because all
through school we have had this: "Mimi
does not participate enough." And part of
that comes out in school because even if
she does know an answer and does have
something to say, she will not say it, will
not have a loud voice, is not aggressive
enough. She goes to school where, I'm sorry
to say, there are large classes, and—

MIRIAM: French. I'm good in French.

MOTHER: French. Right, you're good in
French. But all through school, we've had
this: "Please help Mimi talk."

MIRIAM: You're right.

MOTHER: You're not aggressive enough.
You give up too easily. Or there have been
times when you come home from school,
and two or three people know the same
thing, and you'll start and somebody else
takes the story away, and then you get
furious.

MIRIAM: Right.

LIEBMAN (*looking at father*): Do you
think that it would be all right for your wife
to help Mimi with this communication
problem? Because that really seems to be
of primary importance, as you can obviously see.

FATHER: I think my wife has helped an
awful lot in the past.

LIEBMAN: I know, but would it be all right
if she continues to help, but in a way that's
better for a fourteen-year-old girl?

FATHER: Of course.

LIEBMAN: You're sure of that? Without
ambivalence.

FATHER: Emotionally, I answer you 100
percent yes. I'm totally uninvolved. No
problem at all.

LIEBMAN: No, no. You need to be involved. You need to be involved in order to
permit it to occur.

FATHER: What do you mean, "I need to be

Patient wants to see herself in
a more positive, competent
fashion.

Therapist underlines im-
portance of father's role in
order to prevent him from
undermining relationship
between mother and
daughter.

involved"? To do anything verbally or
physically?

LIEBMAN: No, just so that it's okay with
you. Emotional consent.

FATHER: Yes, sure. No problem at all.

LIEBMAN: All right, we have traveled a
long journey and we have only about ten
minutes, so maybe Dr. Baker, our medical
expert, can tell us about the prognosis.

Therapist shifts emphasis to
pediatrician, who will pre-
pare family for discharge
from hospital and for transition to outpatient therapy.

BAKER: She might be able to go home
some time next week, I would think. When
she goes home, we will have another program set out for you in terms of weight. As I
explained to Mimi, the eating is her business, and what we're interested in is just
like a checking account kind of thing. Deposits and withdrawals, and then you have
a certain net amount at the end of the
month. Relative to weight, it's calories in
and energy expended. The eating is the calories in and that's her area exclusively, in
which we are not going to interfere. She
should get nutritious, well-balanced meals,
and we can talk about planning menus and
so on later, and get some clues from the
dietitian.

LIEBMAN: Did you want to say something?

MIRIAM: I don't believe I can walk to
school and all that.

MOTHER: You're worried about expending
the energy.

MIRIAM: That's going to be a lot, a 20-
minute walk to school.

In thinking about returning
to school, patient indicates
desire for a more normal
life-style.

BAKER: Well, that's something we're going
to have to talk about in terms of what energy she should be allowed to expend.
That, again, will be keyed to what the net
balance is.

FATHER: There'll be a medical checkup on
her somewhere?

BAKER: Oh, sure. We're going to be in very
close contact with Dr. Liebman throughout
therapy.

LIEBMAN: Dr. Baker and I work together.

BAKER: We keep in very close contact. If she gains a certain amount of weight, she's allowed out of bed. If she gains more than that, she's allowed to go to the snack bar or something like that.

MIRIAM: What about my blood tests today? Do I have to have more of them?

BAKER: Okay, so there's a certain allowance made for that. You don't have to gain as much tomorrow to get out of bed. We are making those allowances.

LIEBMAN: She can probably make up for it by having a couple of snacks.

BAKER: Yes, she can do that, but we'll make some allowance for it. That's not a major thing. The same thing will pertain when she's at home—a certain amount of weight gain means that she can participate in normal activities. More than that means a couple of extra treats in terms of things that might require energy. If she's not gaining weight, then there might have to be restrictions, although I don't think that will be a problem.

MOTHER: I think Miriam should say something. Miriam, I don't know, I haven't heard from you. But you said before to Dad and me both that you like it here. That you don't want to live with us. That you would rather stay here.

MIRIAM: No, that's what I said—that was before we had lunch.

MOTHER: Maybe you will feel differently about it.

MIRIAM: No.

MOTHER: Listen to me.

MIRIAM: No, no. That wasn't anything. No. Forget what I said.

MOTHER: But Miriam, I just mentioned it now because—not that I want to say what you said or whatever, but just that I am

Therapist and pediatrician emphasize their collaboration, which serves as a model for a mutually supportive relationship between parents in their approach to daughter's behavior.

Pediatrician lays groundwork for the outpatient behavior conditioning program that will be assigned to parents. They will be told that if they work together in a mutually supportive way, daughter will be able to eat and gain weight, instead of dividing and conquering family.

Daughter manifests ambivalence about giving up symptoms of anorexia and leaving hospital.

Daughter's ambivalence is matched by mother's anxiety that it may not be possible for them to change.

concerned for the total picture when you do come home because of what happened before you came to the hospital.

LIEBMAN: Well, we'll be in very close contact so that—

MOTHER (*looking at Miriam*): It's your life. Everybody has problems, so you learn to live with them, and adjust, or arrange, or make them better.

LIEBMAN: You know, you treat Mimi the same way you treat your husband? With kid gloves. Don't you think you should see your daughter as a fourteen-year-old teenager?

MOTHER: That's true. You are right.

LIEBMAN: Who runs your house? Are you the mother of the house, or is Mimi?

MOTHER: Now, the problem is that. Lately Mimi's been running our house, and I resent it. I resent it.

MIRIAM: I don't run it. Not now. I'm not running it any more.

LIEBMAN (*looking at mother and talking in a humorous tone*): I think you ought to let it happen. I think you ought to move out of your bedroom, move out of your kitchen, give her your checkbook, your car—

MIRIAM: No, not now, I'm not.

MOTHER: Yes, you are, because—because you're here, we have to change. We've got to manage. You know, we have to come down here and do whatever we have to do to change. Becca and Sally said, "When Mimi comes home, do we have to act the same way as we did before she went away? Because the whole house was depressed." That really got to me.

LIEBMAN: The whole family was upset.

MIRIAM: That was before. That was before when I didn't feel good. I feel better now.

Therapist tries to decrease daughter's ambivalence and mother's anxiety by suggesting possibility that daughter will be able to change if parents are willing to treat her in a more age-appropriate fashion.

Patient expresses willingness to vacate her central controlling symptomatic position in the family, enabling her to resume the normal developmental tasks of an adolescent.

Therapist exaggerates the problem of role reversal in order to stress the need for differentiation and change.

LIEBMAN: You no longer feel that sick, do you?

MIRIAM: No.

LIEBMAN: I think Mimi's going to be a healthy, normal person, and so is everybody else in the family. Becca and Sally will also be able to work out their problems. (*He turns to father and mother.*) That is, if you want your house back. I don't know if you want your house back or not.

MOTHER: I feel that I should really watch myself, and listen to what people have to say.

LIEBMAN: Nobody can be perfect all the time. Just some of the time. (*Laughs.*)

MIRIAM: I'm not going to be turned away. (*She looks at mother.*) I'm not going to need your help. You don't have to tiptoe around the house for me.

Daughter would like to change her image in family from that of a sick, frail, vulnerable, precarious person.

LIEBMAN (*talking in a humorous and sarcastic tone*): Oh, no, you're going to fall apart, my dear. Absolutely, you're going to fall apart if Mother looks at you the wrong way. God forbid she should tell you that you have to eat dinner, or you have to clean your room, or you have to help Becca do something. You have not been an equal member of the family.

Therapist paradoxically supports daughter's desire to change her status in family from that of "patient" by returning her to child subsystem, where she will share equal responsibility with her siblings.

MOTHER: But if problems were caused because people acted some way, don't we have to make changes?

LIEBMAN: Yes, but I'm not concerned with the past. I'm concerned about right now and the immediate future. You have to be concerned about yourself, your marriage, your three children, and how to live.

MOTHER: Well, that's it. How to live. That's a good idea.

FATHER: I agree. Let's do it.

The session ends on a more positive, hopeful note, expressed by both daughter and parents.

———

INTERVIEWER: During the session you were involved in a number of issues relating to the parents and their marriage. You didn't address yourself to the anorexia problem, and sometimes it seemed that you were not taking the situation seriously. Yet the patient ate her lunch and by the end of the session was acting much more competently. Can you discuss why?

LIEBMAN: My approach to this family followed a series of steps, all directed toward the goal of decentralizing the patient and redefining the problem. First, early in the session I used the process of deamplification. Deamplification is a technique in which the therapist states that he has problems with himself or with his own family similar to those of the anorectic's family. This approach makes the patient's and family's behavioral patterns seem less deviant, which decreases their defensiveness and resistance and facilitates their acceptance of the therapist and therefore of his interventions. In this particular case, I deamplified by allying with the patient around the issue of table manners, which defused the potential explosiveness and negativism associated with food and eating and gave me control over the family's area of manifest symptoms without having to focus on them.

I furthered the therapeutic alliance with Miriam by asking her permission to share small portions of her lunch—a piece of carrot, a sip of milk, and so on. I had already done so with her in the hospital, using the eating and sharing of food to establish a therapeutic relationship. Although the technique always startled her, she gave her permission, which was a step toward following my lead and eating. By sharing Miriam's food, I also forced her to compete with me for her lunch.

In the session I also treated Miriam as though she had no problem with food or eating. I purposely avoided including her in the various topics of discussion, leaving her in a conflict-free area, protected by her own individual boundaries. This kept her from being triangulated by the parents and prevented the development of a power struggle over eating. Because eating was not the problem area and the atmosphere was not stressful, Mimi was able spontaneously, and perhaps even without cognitive awareness, to eat. By the end of the session she was able to defend her competence in school and to indicate her determination to change from the symptom-ridden family problem into a more normal teenager.

During this time I was also building a strong relationship with the parents. I used primary-process spontaneous associations to join and engage them on an affective and cognitive level. I found myself functioning as a magnet to draw the parents' attention to me and away from their daughter's eating. In fact, I took her role and allowed myself to be triangulated by the parents, leaving her free to eat. The process of the session, with the goal of having the patient eat, was much more important than the content. In other words, I used my position as leader of the group to begin a process of eating, covertly directing the other members of the group to follow my lead.

In addition, I used some of my personal and family experience to gain entrance into the family system and to establish a therapeutic relationship with the patient and her parents. The goal was to provide the family with an entirely different experience around the issue of eating. The patient behaved in the same way as all the other people in the room; that is, she ate her lunch without any difficulty. This was different from and in marked contrast to what had been occurring at home during the six months prior to referral. Therefore, the family saw that

change could occur, and this realization provided them with a more optimistic, hopeful
attitude. I experienced the session as stimulating, but equally draining.

On the morning of the first family lunch session, Miriam weighed
76 pounds. Over the next six days she gained 11.5 pounds, achieving
the weight required for discharge. There were no episodes of bu-
limia. During this six-day period she was allowed to eat in the
hospital cafeteria, accompanied by family or nursing staff. She
seemed happier and talked about leaving the hospital and returning to school. At the second family lunch session, attended seven
days later by the entire family, Miriam was told that she could be
discharged from the hospital. At first she said that she was "not
ready" to go home, but when all of the family members indicated
that they wanted her to rejoin the family, she agreed to go. She had
been in the hospital for twenty days and had gained a total of
15 pounds. No medications were used.

In the outpatient phase, the family psychiatrist assumed primary
responsibility, with the pediatrician functioning in a supportive
consultative way. This was the reverse of the system used during
the inpatient phase. The four general goals of the outpatient phase
were: to eliminate the symptom of refusing to eat and to stimulate a progressive weight gain, which had top priority in order to
prevent the family from concentrating on Miriam's symptoms as a
way of avoiding or detouring family conflicts; to elucidate and
change the dysfunctional patterns in the family that reinforced the
patient's symptoms; to improve the executive and marital functioning of the parents by establishing age-appropriate generational
boundaries between parents and children; and to strengthen the
relationships of the siblings with each other and their respective
peer groups.

The initial weight gain and family lunch sessions had started the
process of changing Miriam's role as the family's scapegoat. This
process was continued by the assignment of an outpatient behavior
modification program, which provided the parents with something
concrete to do at home, decreasing their anxiety and sense of helplessness in dealing with their "sick" child. The outpatient program
was defined as an interpersonal process. The parents were told that
it was their responsibility as parents to enforce the program, and

that if they worked together in a mutually supportive way, they would be successful. Miriam was told that it was her responsibility to herself and to her parents to follow the regimen. The family was advised that Miriam must gain a minimum of 2 pounds a week in order to maintain normal activities. If she gained less than 2 pounds from Friday to Friday, she was not allowed out of the house on the weekend, and she could not have friends come to the house. In addition, one member of the family had to stay at home with her at all times on such a weekend. This plan was designed to produce a great deal of stress in the family system, causing the members to join together to ensure that Miriam ate. If she gained between 2 and 2½ pounds, she was allowed to be active on either Saturday or Sunday, but not both days. She was given the choice of day and the choice of activities. If she gained more than 2½ pounds in the preceding seven-day period, she was allowed to be active on Friday night, Saturday, and Sunday.

During the first two weeks following discharge, Miriam tested her parents by gaining less than 2 pounds. With the therapist's support, the parents were able to make her stay home on both weekends. In the third week, Miriam gained the required 2 pounds, a pace she maintained thereafter. She was also told that she must weigh 112 pounds to go to summer camp with her siblings, a weight that she attained by mid-June. Thus, she had gained 25 pounds in the three months following discharge from the hospital.

Once her weight was progressing in a gradual fashion, family therapy concentrated on trying to influence the different subsystems of the family. The strategy used was to assign different tasks to the family. These tasks were directed toward changing the structure, organization, and functioning of the family as well as the quality of interpersonal relationships in the family.

Miriam's symptoms resulted from and were a manifestation of dysfunctional patterns in her family system. The parents were ineffective, disorganized, rigid, and incapable of resolving conflicts finding solutions to problems, or dealing with stressful situations. Miriam was emotionally close to her father and more distant from her mother, siblings, and peer group. The marital relationship was weak and inadequate, allowing Miriam to be inappropriately involved in parental affairs. The family's pattern of functioning was characterized by constricting parental overprotectiveness, lack of privacy for individual members, denial of the existence of any problems except for Miriam's symptoms, and a lack of resolution of spouse conflicts which remained submerged by parental concern for and preoccupation with Miriam. The patient served as a detour for family conflicts, with the parents united around concern for their sick child.

The first goal of outpatient therapy was therefore to help Miriam free herself from this detouring position, and the first intervention was the assignment of the behavioral program. Because this program was a task to be enforced by the parents, it separated Miriam from the spouse subsystem and its conflicts, returning her to the child subsystem of the family. Thus the behavioral program helped to establish generational boundaries and to increase the executive functioning of the parents.

Another important area for change was the relationships between the parents. The father and mother were given the task of discussing privately, each evening, any problems associated with the children or the behavioral program. These discussions were not to end until a plan of action had been formulated. While the mother was given the responsibility for dealing directly with the children, the father's task was to coach her, but not to undermine or criticize her in any way. The therapist directed his major efforts to the father, supporting him to help his wife assume more responsibility in a competent fashion.

Two months after the beginning of outpatient therapy, the parents stated that eating was no longer a problem. The problem, as they now defined it, was Miriam's poor interpersonal relationships, manifested by her lack of friends and outside interests. This transition indicated to the therapist that the family was ready for further change.

With the permission of the older sister, Rebecca, the parents were instructed to send Miriam along to the parties and other activities that the sister attended. The patient was told she must go, which she did, though initially with reluctance. The parents were told to reward themselves for having become competent parents by planning to go out for a social evening alone at least once a week. At the end of the third month of therapy, the parents went away for a weekend alone for the first time in their marriage. They also planned a two-week summer vacation by themselves, to be taken while the children were in camp. A closer relationship between the parents, within which their needs could be mutually satisfied, began to develop, freeing the children to develop relationships among themselves and with their peer groups.

The children went to summer camp for July and August. Miriam had an enjoyable summer, making many friends and volunteering for flood relief work in Pennsylvania. She developed obvious secondary sexual characteristics, grew about two inches in height, and let her hair grow longer. She was spontaneous and relaxed when talking and joking with her siblings. In general, she appeared to be attractive, confident, and genuinely pleased with herself. She talked enthusiastically about the new school year, looking forward to seeing her previous classmates and developing new friendships.

After the summer vacation, therapy resumed because the parents stated that more "work" needed to be done. However, the format was changed. The children and parents came to the clinic on different days in order to underline the disengagement process. Periodically, a family session was held to assess the transactional patterns between parents and children. During one of the family sessions, the parents stated that they were now more concerned about Miriam's older sister, because they believed that Miriam, having grown stronger, demonstrated better judgment than Rebecca. Clearly, the role and status of the former patient in the family had changed.

Shortly after therapy resumed, the therapist showed the family a videotape of an early session which clearly demonstrated how the mother had focused on some problem of the patient or her sister to decrease the peripheral position of her husband by stimulating his concern about the particular problem. This videotape, which was reviewed in detail with the entire family in order to point out the relevant transactional issues, served as a turning point. To reinforce further the disengagement process and the establishment of generational boundaries, three more tasks were put into effect: the sisters were allowed to go on weekly unescorted shopping trips with their friends and to use public transportation to keep appointments with the therapist that did not involve the parents; Miriam was allowed to babysit for the neighbors and to go to the movies unescorted with her friends, and Rebecca, at age sixteen, was allowed to begin dating.

The parents were supported in their efforts to give the children gradual increases in freedom and responsibility. The rationale offered for the separation was that the parents would be able to have more time and energy to satisfy themselves if their children could function in a more independent fashion. Instead of being concerned about the children, the parents could now concentrate on their concern about each other. The remainder of therapy dealt exclusively with resolving marital problems; the children no longer participated. The therapy lasted fifteen months in all.

After a five-year follow-up period, Miriam continued without symptoms. Her eating patterns and weight were normal, and she appeared to enjoy her physical attractiveness. She had done well academically and was attending college away from home. She was invested in age-appropriate peer group activities and heterosexual relationships. The siblings had not manifested any significant problems, and the parents had been able to sustain the marked improvement in their marital relationship and parental functioning.

The Menotti Family

11

Loretta Menotti, now sixteen years old, is an Italian American girl who comes from a lower class family. Her parents came to the United States from a village in southern Italy after their marriage. Neither of them completed grammar school, but they are both competent and intelligent people. The father is an unskilled civil servant. The mother is a housewife. Both families of origin also have settled in the United States, and both live near the Menottis. There is daily contact with the mother's family, but Mrs. Menotti has quarreled with her mother-in-law. Loretta likes her paternal grandmother, with whom she often stays after she has had a serious fight with her mother.

At fourteen years of age Loretta Menotti was admitted to a large city hospital with a severe pain in her left lower abdomen. A laparotomy was suggested to determine if she had a twisted ovarian cyst, but it was not performed. The patient remained in the hospital for two months, not eating at times because of the intense pain in her abdomen. The diagnosis, after intensive medical examination, was that the patient had "psychological problems." She refused to see a psychiatrist.

A year later Loretta was seen by a psychiatrist because of a preoccupation with swallowing and choking. She had continued to lose weight and was obsessed with this problem. The doctor diagnosed her condition as "simple schizophrenia with superficial depressive features" and prescribed Thorazine.

Three months later the patient was hospitalized for the second time with a diagnosis of anorexia nervosa. On admission she weighed around 80 pounds. She remained in the hospital for six weeks. Her eating improved, and she gained weight. The continuation of therapy on an outpatient basis was recommended, but the family did not follow through.

Four months later the patient was admitted to the intensive care unit of another hospital, then transferred to the previous hospital, where she remained for two months with little improvement. The patient was signed out by the family against medical advice. She weighed 75 pounds.

The mother contacted a community mental health outpatient clinic, where Dr. Minuchin conducted the initial interview. At the time of the interview, the patient was sixteen years old and weighed 85 pounds. She was amenorrheic, depressed, and had not attended school for two or three months prior to the interview.

MINUCHIN: First, I want to understand what has been happening. I understand that Loretta has been losing weight for the last three years. Is that correct?

LORETTA: Right.

FATHER: Two years.

> First transaction between father and Loretta signals identified patient's inferior position in family. Father indicates that his memory of Loretta's experience is better than hers.

MINUCHIN: When did it start, Loretta?

> Therapist challenges this sequence, initiating messages of differentiation and individuation.

FATHER: Two years.

> Father insists on indicating that father knows best.

MOTHER: It started at the beginning of Lent. I take her to St. Francis Hospital because Loretta, she don't feel too good. She got pain all over. So they want to take picture inside Loretta's stomach, but I say "no." I say, "I take my daughter home."

MINUCHIN: Do you remember that, Loretta? (*Loretta nods.*)

> Mother claims the position in family as a good parent, one who will challenge the outside world in the protection of her kin. In the process, both parents preempt Loretta's response. When therapist questions daughter, she only nods.

INTERVIEWER: In the first actions in an interview, do the family members always define themselves?

MINUCHIN: Not necessarily. Quite frequently the family presents its "public image" in the first encounter with the therapist, who in some way represents the "public." The therapist stores this first "tableau" for later exploration. He will have to see whether it is congruent with other family scenarios.

MOTHER: So I take Loretta home because I don't want nobody to touch my daughter. So I take her home, and next day Loretta throws up. She cries. She has a pain. So I call the car service, put Loretta in the car, and take her to Dr. Smith. He calls Tenafly Hospital, and from there we go straight to Tenafly Hospital. Loretta stay in bed two weeks there in the hospital.

MINUCHIN: I would like to know from your point of view, Loretta. What was it that you were having?

LORETTA: The first night that I went to St. Francis Hospital was because I was having strong pains in my abdomen and my back and they found it was a kidney infection and they gave me intravenous since the pain was so great.

MINUCHIN: Okay, so you went then for something very, very specific. And when you went to the Tenafly Hospital, was it a continuation of the same issue?

LORETTA: I don't know. I mean, they never actually said anything there.

MINUCHIN: Since Mother is the memory of the family, she will tell, but you will need to check it, because it's your life that she is describing. Okay?

MOTHER: So I take her to Tenafly to my doctor. For two weeks they check Loretta. Loretta, she doesn't eat enough, and the doctor told me, "Take your daughter home and bring her to a psychiatrist."

Mother presents herself as an effective manager and a mother tigress.

Therapist feels mother's power but persists in his message that Loretta owns her own experience. He is also signaling at the start of session that he will control the flow of communication and establish the rules.

Therapist's previous interventions, all directed to Loretta, have been variations of the same message: she owns her own experiences and has the right to challenge parents on this subject.

MINUCHIN: Hold it a moment, because I want to check something. Loretta, when you were in the hospital, you did not eat anything?

Therapist challenges mother, insisting on the same message.

LORETTA: For a while, they put a sign up on my bed that said I wasn't supposed to eat anything because they didn't know what was causing the pain. And then I didn't have any appetite. So I had the IV's from the first time until I went home.

MINUCHIN: Okay. Do you know that this happens to many people? If they are two or three days without eating, they lose the appetite. It was at this point that you stopped eating, and this was when? Two years ago?

Therapist joins with Loretta and makes a normalizing statement. Unwittingly he has also accommodated to parents, accepting their statement that it all started two years ago.

LORETTA: Right.

MOTHER: So, I stay two weeks with Loretta in the hospital.

MINUCHIN: You stayed in the hospital with her?

FATHER: Yes, she spent many nights with her.

MINUCHIN: But, Mr. Menotti, didn't you miss her?

FATHER: Well, I did miss her, but we managed to go on, you know—

A pattern has emerged: mother claims the right to control contact with identified patient. She is the family switchboard. Therapist experiences that unless he can somehow establish control over mother, therapy will be handicapped by her insistence on regulating daughter's interpersonal contact.

MINUCHIN: What about the little ones? Who handled Giuseppi and Enrico?

SOPHIA AND MARIA (*in unison*): Both of us.

MINUCHIN: Both of you? I have the feeling that you, Maria, are a manager. Who is the one who takes the responsibility when Mama is away?

Therapist makes contact with two other teenage children.

MARIA: We share it.

MINUCHIN: Does Sophia try sometimes to boss you around a little bit?

MARIA: Yeah.

Therapist's question carries the implicit message, which will be elaborated many times throughout the session, that there are different hierarchies and different levels of power at different developmental stages.

MINUCHIN: You know, I thought so. She wanted to boss me around. She said, "You should sit there in that chair." I thought it

Therapist employs a trivial incident between himeslf and one family member to indicate other transactions. This

was great. That's wonderful. It means that you are this kind of person. You are active and you like to do things.

SOPHIA: Yeah.

FATHER: Yes, she does.

MINUCHIN: That's wonderful. Okay, and Mother stayed two weeks in the hospital. My goodness. That's an Italian heart for you.

MOTHER: One day, my husband told me to come home to see the kids and, "If you still want to go tomorrow, I'll take you in there." So, I said I would see what I can do. So we go home. When I go home, I got a funny feeling. Loretta, she doesn't feel good, so I say to my husband, "You better take me back to the hospital. I have a funny feeling about Loretta." He say, "Oh, no, you stay here." I say, "You take me or I go." So my husband take me there. When I go back, I find Loretta all black and blue. She has pains. She's screaming, "I have a pain all over here, I have a pain over there." She is screaming. I say, "We will call the doctor." So they say nothing is wrong with Loretta. And I say, "What do you mean nothing is wrong with Loretta? She's all black and blue." "That's all right, don't get nervous." So they give her needle, and Loretta, she sleep all night.

———

INTERVIEWER: Is this description of continuity between mother and child similar to what Hilde Bruch describes as occurring between mother and infant?

MINUCHIN: No doubt. It is unusual to get so graphic a description of fusion between mother and adolescent daughter in non-psychotic people. I think that the position of the mother in this family is buttressed by the role of the mother in the peasant culture of southern Italy. While both parents have been in the United States for over twenty years, they still maintain the cultural mores

strategy of framing a small event to suggest a pattern of interpersonal contact collapses time and facilitates the positioning of therapist as a long-time member of the system.

of the old country. As a result, the adolescent children are caught between two cultures. Loretta is caught between her parents' idea of what a good daughter should be and what her peers expect of her.

MINUCHIN: That means, you had the feeling—

MOTHER: Loretta could die.

MINUCHIN: Do you have the same sense about Maria?

MOTHER: Yes, with everybody. All my kids.

MINUCHIN: I don't think Maria sends vibes. I think she is a very self-sufficient kind of girl. If Maria has a pain, I bet you don't know.

MOTHER: If I kiss her, I do.

MINUCHIN: What do you think, Maria? If you have a pain, do you think she knows?

MARIA: Yes.

MINUCHIN: She does! What about Father? That's a special gift. Does Daddy have that?

MARIA: Yeah.

MINUCHIN: Is that so, Carlo? Can you experience the pain of your kids as your wife does?

FATHER: Well, I can see by just taking a look at them. If they don't look good, then I assume there is something wrong, you know.

MINUCHIN: That must be just the kind of thing that happens when a family is concerned with children. You look at them a lot.

FATHER: Right.

MINUCHIN: But Margherita says she can hear vibrations from the hospital.

FATHER: I brought her back from the hospital, right? The minute that we were home, she says, "I want to go back." When

Therapist tracks Maria and differentiates the two daughters.

Therapist challenges mother's claims of owning her children's pains.

But therapist is disqualified.

Father implies that he has no magic, but he does not challenge the magic of mother.

Therapist frames magic as a normal transaction.

she got back, Loretta was in bad shape.

MINUCHIN: I'll tell you something, that feeling is very, very important when the kids are young. That's essential. Let me ask you a little bit, Loretta. You are sixteen now?

LORETTA: Yeah.

MINUCHIN: That kind of sensitivity that Mom and Dad have toward you is very helpful because if you have a problem or a care, then they respond, but when you begin to be a little bit grown up, as you and Sophia are, does it sometimes bother you that Mother still is so sensitive to you?

LORETTA: Sometimes.

MINUCHIN: What about you, Maria? Do you feel sometimes that Mother doesn't know that you are thirteen, that she still thinks you are twelve or eleven?

MARIA (*sighing*): I don't know. No-o-o.

MINUCHIN: Sophia, what's your feeling? Sometimes she forgets that you are fifteen. She treats you as if you are younger?

SOPHIA: Yeah.

MINUCHIN: This always happens. When you are very sensitive to the pains of the younger kids, there is then a problem of how to become the mother of older children. A good mother of younger children sometimes becomes a difficult mother for older children. So, you are still a very good mother for Maria, Giuseppi, and Enrico, but I think there is some problem with Sophia and Loretta. I think that you are too much for them.

MOTHER: No. (*Father laughs.*) How?

Therapist tracks the family's mystical feeling of togetherness and joins them by accepting the reality of the experience, but he challenges them by rejecting the usefulness of this mode of transaction in the present case. He continues to differentiate children according to their stages of development.

Being a mama is a significant part of the mother's identity. Therapist confirms her in that function, but challenges her approach to adolescent children.

Father joins therapist in challenge of mother. Though father's move is tentative, therapist registers it and stores the information to use later in his challenge of mother. Mother's question acknowledges the challenge.

INTERVIEWER: How clear is it to you that the husband may affiliate with you if you challenge the mother?

MINUCHIN: I start with the knowledge that the spouse subsystem always encompasses areas of unstable balance. To unbalance a family system in order to achieve family transformation, I search for areas of disagreement between family members. I am always alert to and probing for possible areas in which they will affiliate with me in a challenge to the usual transactional patterns. In effect, I search for co-therapists among them. The husband's mild affiliation with me suggested a possible avenue for later probes to change the wife's central position in the family.

LORETTA: You always have arguments with me and Sophia. Always.

MINUCHIN: Carlo, help the two girls to talk, because Mama is too strong and they are in the hot spot. Help them to say how they would like Mama to be sometimes.

FATHER: Why don't you express yourselves about what the doctor is saying? At fifteen, you should know how to say a few words by yourself, huh?

SOPHIA: I don't have too many fights with Mom.

FATHER: We are talking about how you wish Mom treats you from now on, since you have become fifteen.

SOPHIA: I don't know. She doesn't treat me bad.

FATHER: Do you think Mom needs to be changed to somehow make you feel better?

LORETTA: I think that's not the point, Dad. It's not the point of changing.

FATHER: What is the point?

LORETTA: Dad, you really can't change.

Loretta also challenges mother after therapist and father have done so.

Therapist enlists father as a co-therapist, enacting a father/daughter coalition against mother.

Sophia disaffiliates from the coalition.

Loretta qualifies her challenge to mother, challenging father instead. Clearly neither daughter trusts that father can be an effective ally.

Once you are the person you are, you have to try and then compromise a little.

FATHER: But you wish that Mom could change toward you somehow.

LORETTA: I am not saying change totally. I'd rather have her worry less.

MINUCHIN: What you are saying, Loretta, is that it's not a total change, but you would like your mother to be less worried about you and about the other kids.

Therapist pays heed to daughter's signal but tries to maintain the thrust of his challenge to mother while accommodating to a softer approach.

LORETTA: M-hum.

MINUCHIN: Do you think that Mama has too big a heart and that sometimes that makes her worry more than is necessary?

FATHER: Well, what I've seen, Mama does herself much of the things that the girls could do by themselves. She makes it too easy for them. Now they find it a little hard to begin to manage by themselves and try out this situation.

Father disaffiliates from two daughters and stands alone, challenging them and mother alike.

MINUCHIN: That's a very interesting and very sensitive view. Can you say it again, because I think Margherita is deaf in this ear?

Therapist joins with husband, supporting his strength and using humor to increase intensity in a sensitive area.

FATHER: I am sure Margherita understood already what I'm talking about.

MINUCHIN: Do you understand what he says? What do you think about that?

Therapist challenges directly.

MOTHER: Why do I have to think? I am a mother. The things they can't do, I do.

But therapist finds a brick wall.

MINUCHIN: If the kids say do something, you do.

MOTHER: What am I to do—let the kids down?

MINUCHIN: Now, what about what Carlo says, that you do more than what they need?

Therapist challenges mother, using father's statement as a vehicle.

FATHER: You've been doing, and you don't mind doing anything for them, right?

Husband challenges wife. There are implications that she sacrifices her wife function to mothering.

MOTHER: I don't. I help my kids all the time in all ways. If they want help, my kids, I give it to them. That's what I do for my kids, then, all the time.

Mother hears the challenge and establishes clear priorities as a mother.

MINUCHIN: I think that you still did not hear clearly what your husband has said, and what Loretta said. Loretta also said something which you did not hear. So say it again, Loretta, so that Margherita can hear it.

Therapist tries to re-establish a father/daughter challenge to mother.

LORETTA: That you worry too much. And you've got to try to worry less, because I am sixteen and she is fifteen and she is thirteen and you worry too much, as if we were ten and not sixteen, or fifteen. And let us try to do some things by ourselves. Because if we want to try something, you say, "No, let me do it. It's better if I do it."

Loretta's challenge to mother repeats the developmental message that therapist suggested previously. This accommodation of Loretta to therapist suggests a good prognosis for Loretta's ability to explore alternatives.

MOTHER: Wait a minute, Loretta, I give you the chance—

LORETTA: In certain things that are easy to do. But in other things, you don't dare give us a chance.

MOTHER: Well, sometimes it has to be no.

LORETTA: But it's no to the things that are new to you. To things that you already know about, everything is yes. But to things that are new to you, it's always no. You don't want to hear about it.

MOTHER: When it have to be no, it have to be no.

LORETTA: But, you don't care to listen about it either. You just say no and that's that. You don't want to talk about it or nothing. You just say no and that's final.

Loretta's challenge seems effective and appropriate. Therapist feels impressed by its quality and wonders why Loretta is involved in anorectic behavior, since she does not shun interpersonal conflict in other areas.

MINUCHIN: Loretta, I just want to congratulate you. I think you are very good. Sophia, do you help her sometimes?

Therapist explores organization of sibling subsystem vis-à-vis mother.

SOPHIA: In what?

MINUCHIN: Do you help Loretta? Because she took the leadership position to defend all three of you. Do you sometimes join her?

SOPHIA: No.

MINUCHIN: So, Loretta, you are the only fighter?

LORETTA: Yes.

MINUCHIN: Carlo, you have a lovely wife. You children have a lovely mother. But I think that she can become a problem for the children that are growing up.

FATHER: Yeah, I thought that, too. In the situation of these two girls, now that they wish to do things but they are not really prepared to do, just because—

MINUCHIN: They didn't have any experience. Yes.

In finishing father's phrase, therapist functions in synchrony with father. This indication that therapist is caught in the family transactional patterns could be dangerous, since he might lose his freedom of action.

LORETTA: Yeah, but there has to be some point where you have to begin.

Loretta joins in a coalition with father against mother.

FATHER: And that causes more worry for my wife, you know, when the two girls are willing to do something that we might consider unusual.

MINUCHIN: What kind of things? I am interested in your point of view.

FATHER: Say, Sophia wants to go out at night, and my wife will find whether or not to let her go out.

SOPHIA (*laughing*): I think it's the other way around.

MOTHER: I think so, too. I'm sorry. I don't agree with that.

FATHER: You think it's the other way, too. Who's most worried, me or Mamma?

SOPHIA: Oh, she's worried about it, but she's willing to let us go, while you're—you know.

Sophia diffuses conflict by defending mother.

MOTHER: Thank you, Sophia. Thank God.

Mother acknowledges the stress.

FATHER: What I wanted to say is she's the one who worries; she worries too much. So she might prefer not to let her go in order to worry this much when at ten o'clock she hasn't come home yet.

MINUCHIN: What about with Loretta, who is sixteen now? Do you let her go out?

MOTHER: I give her the permission. If she wants to go out, at ten o'clock she has to be home. If she comes a little late, she has to call me.

FATHER: Well, so far, we've never had this problem really. We'll have this problem to manage when one of them goes out. This hasn't happened yet.

MINUCHIN: Do you have a boy friend, Loretta?

LORETTA: No.

MINUCHIN: Sophia, do you have a boy friend?

SOPHIA: No.

MOTHER: No. Sophia, she already asks me, "Ma, somebody asked me to go out and what am I to do?" I say, "Go out." And then my husband say I worry. I told her to go out.

FATHER: You don't understand. You'd worry if they went out and weren't back on time.

MOTHER: I don't know what kind of boys she meets afterward, but with the school boys, they don't bother me. I'm a mother, right? So I say, "You have to watch yourself and at ten o'clock you have to be home." What's wrong with that?

MINUCHIN: I don't know that anything is wrong.

_____

INTERVIEWER: What happened there?

MINUCHIN: I felt somewhat lost, as if I had been unfair with the mother. And I questioned my right to push my value systems at the expense of theirs.

INTERVIEWER: When you feel like this, isn't it an indication that you are too close? Wouldn't it be helpful, at this point, to have a co-therapist who took over for the moment so that you could regain your ability to use a wide lens?

MINUCHIN: To your first question, the

While the rules have theoretically changed for the older daughters, they have not yet tested the new boundaries, thereby avoiding conflict.

answer is yes. It is clear that I have been sucked into the web of family patterns. But this could be an advantage. I am experiencing what other family members experience when they challenge mother—a sense of disqualification and guilt. My ability to disengage from this transactional trap and to find alternative ways to deal with mother can provide directions for therapy. To your second question, therefore, my answer is no. A co-therapist might free me from the trap but might also rob me of the possibility of finding alternatives. To work alone, a therapist needs to feel comfortable while working in proximity, to know how to survive while enmeshed, and to have the necessary techniques to disengage and become invisible.

———

FATHER: You know, the news has been too bad. We don't want these kids getting into any of this kind of trouble. Like drugs, you know, and sex and—

MINUCHIN: Loretta, can you disagree with Mother?

LORETTA: I can disagree, but it gets into an argument. Sometimes I don't even bother, because I know already that the situation is going to turn out to be an argument.

MINUCHIN: Can you disagree with Father?

LORETA: No, neither one of them is easy, because should I disagree with one, then they get together and the two of them think one way.

MINUCHIN: They join.

LORETTA: Right. The two of them think one way. Perhaps in a situation where my mother may say no whereas my father may say yes, I'll give my mother some time to speak to my father. And they'll both say no. You know, they both change. And then I have the two of them against me, and I don't have either one to help me.

Therapist disengages from mother by contacting identified patient, which is probably a common transactional pattern in the family, rendering Loretta vulnerable.

MINUCHIN: Do you remember any specific situation in which you had disagreed with them?

LORETTA: I can't think of one.

MINUCHIN: What about you, Sophia? Can you disagree with Mom?

SOPHIA: No.

MINUCHIN: Can you disagree with Dad?

SOPHIA: I don't think so.

LORETTA: You do once in a while, though, Sophia.

MINUCHIN: But you think you can't. Okay. What about you, Maria, can you disagree with Mom?

MARIA: Not really. She always wins.

MINUCHIN: She always wins. And what about with Dad? Can you disagree with Dad? (*Maria sighs.*) Sophia, let's say you want something very, very strongly. Can you convince Mother?

SOPHIA: I don't think so.

MINUCHIN: Then you have an uphill battle now. How can you grow up in the family and introduce new things?

LORETTA: It's a pretty hard battle, and I'm not getting anywhere.

MINUCHIN: You feel defeated. Carlo and Margherita, talk with Loretta about that, because that is a very important issue—the issue of how to help each other. And I think that since you are from the old country and they are from the new country, they have different ideas. And I think that they don't know how to talk with you.

MOTHER: They know how to talk to me. I am of the old country, but I grew up over here, too.

MINUCHIN: The girls feel that you are too strong for them.

MOTHER: No.

MINUCHIN: They said yes.

MOTHER: With Sophia, there are no problems. She never asked me thing do I have

While the session has shown that Loretta can be effective, able to enter successfully into interpersonal conflict, her self-perception is that she will be ineffective and will always lose.

Therapist decentralizes Loretta as a patient by exploring experiences of the three teenagers in family and emphasizing their similarities as subsystem members.

Therapist frames conflict in idiosyncratic terms: to give a cultural explanation for the conflict takes away the blame involved.

Mother disagrees with therapist.

Therapist disagrees with mother.

Mother denies.

Therapist affirms.

Mother denies and qualifies.

to say yes or no. We have a little problem with Loretta.

MINUCHIN: Margherita, you are not hearing.

Therapist disqualifies mother. The pattern of family conflict seen here between mother and therapist is typical. The content is irrelevant, because it is only the ammunition in a family power operation.

LORETTA: I would like to interrupt for a minute. It is a big problem with my parents coming from the old country and us being raised and educated and born here, because we use certain words, but they don't understand them.

Loretta interrupts to diffuse conflict.

MOTHER: Oh, Loretta.

LORETTA: Like, right now, you're getting kind of angry because I'm saying this, but it's true. We use certain words and you don't understand them. You know your own meanings for them and you misunderstand what one of us is trying to say to you, and when we explain to you what the real thing is, you don't want to hear about it and won't unless it was the way you said it.

Loretta enters into conflict with mother.

MOTHER: Well, this is—Loretta—

LORETTA: Even now it's happening. You don't understand sometimes what Daddy's saying or the doctor is saying or even what I am saying now. You're getting angry at me.

MOTHER: No, I don't get angry with you. I want to know when I disappoint you.

Mother uses self-sacrifice as diffuser of conflict.

LORETTA: I am not saying you disappoint me, Mom, but it's time you let loose a little bit.

Mollified, Loretta becomes gentler.

MOTHER: I lose all the time. You win all the time in the house. Not your sister, not the other sister, not your brother, not your father. You win, Loretta.

As if to confirm Loretta's content, mother confuses the word "loose" for "lose" and accuses Loretta of differing from other family members by winning.

LORETTA: You know why? Because I'm the only one who fights back. The others just sit back and take—

MOTHER: Why do you fight back then? Why do you fight back and you stop eating?

Mother equates assertiveness with anorexia. By framing the anorectic behavior as self-

LORETTA: That's another thing. You are always bringing up eating. That's what makes me even sicker.

assertion, she maintains symptom as an appropriate avenue of independence for patient.

INTERVIEWER: It seems to me that what mother is saying is similar to what you said in the Kaplan and Gilbert families, that noneating is a rebellious act. If so, how can that interpretation be a symptom maintenance mechanism instead of a symptom repair strategy, as in the two previous families?

MINUCHIN: In the previous families, the strategy of equating noneating with rebellion was used by the therapist to increase stress, to detriangulate daughter, and to increase spouse subsystem cohesion. It was also used to relabel daughter as a rebellious adolescent and to decentralize eating. In this family, the concept has already been incorporated without any system transformation. On the contrary, mother uses the statement to maintain closeness—"How can you do that to us?"—and she supports noneating as a legitimate adolescent strategy for winning. Therefore the therapist will have to find another strategy for the detriangulation procedure, one that will allow Loretta to assert adolescent individuation through more functional interactions. The dilemma illustrates the difference between a dynamic interpretation and a structural maneuver. The dynamic interpretation (in this case, the mother's) brings knowledge. The structural intervention brings family transformation.

MOTHER: That's why we're here. I told you this morning—

LORETTA: Mom, I am the subject in this case, and that's why I'm scared.

MINUCHIN: Loretta, you are wrong. You are not the subject, the family is the subject.

LORETTA: Yeah, but none of us would be here if it wasn't on account of me.

FATHER: She thought she was the focal point, and that's why—

MINUCHIN: I am interested in the family.

LORETTA: I realize that.

Loretta joins with therapist.

MINUCHIN: To me, it is very important what's happening now. That the girls are growing up and don't know how to grow up.

FATHER: Right.

MINUCHIN: Carlo, you think that Margherita is too easy and that it's not helpful to the girls. Can you change seats to sit near her so that you can talk to her in such a way that she can hear? I want you to defend the girls. They are fifteen and sixteen and Mama needs to change a little bit.

Therapist continues strategy of supporting father to decentralize mother. Therapist also wants to enact a husband/wife dyad in order to probe for alternative transactional patterns between spouses.

MOTHER: Tell me something. Why am I to change?

MINUCHIN: Carlo will—

MOTHER: Come on, say it.

FATHER: Well, really, I don't know the ways she needs to change.

MINUCHIN: The things that you were saying. That she is too easy—

FATHER: You see, I have a problem. There is a misunderstanding between me and my wife and Loretta.

Husband rejects therapist's strategy of enacting husband/wife dyad and focuses on father/daughter dyad or mother/daughter in coalition against father.

MINUCHIN: M-hum.

FATHER: Loretta was assuming that I was the odd father—the one who said no all the time. If I see a situation in which she wanted to do something, I would let her do it. My wife blames me that I was going to say no even when I didn't know anything about the situation.

MINUCHIN: Let me understand. Sometimes you feel that Margherita and Loretta are together in something and that you are the bad guy.

FATHER: In their own mind, they assume that I want to stop whatever they are planning to do, you know.

MINUCHIN: Do you know what your father is talking about?

LORETTA: I know what he's saying, but that's another misunderstood situation.

MINUCHIN: Do you know what Carlo is saying, Margherita?

MOTHER: What about, Carlo?

FATHER: What about? Just about everything. When she wanted to go out, you assumed I was going to say no, right?

Father frames husband/wife conflict around issues of parenting in which Loretta is triangulated.

MOTHER: Wait. When Loretta was asking me, "Ma, I want to go out," I say to Loretta, "Yes."

FATHER: You say, "Loretta, yes," before telling me, then?

MOTHER: Yes. I say, "You go out, Loretta. I tell Daddy." When you came home, you asked, "Where is Loretta." I say, "Out." "Where?" "With a boy." "Who?" you say. I say, "I know the boy. I know the mother. Don't worry about it. She's okay." I gave Loretta until ten o'clock to go out because Loretta stay one month at the hospital and the doctor say, "You have to give freedom to your daughter." I do what the doctor say.

Mother's ability as an infighter should not be underrated. She brings up on her side:
1. The authority of the doctor.

FATHER: But this is not the point.

MOTHER: That's the point, Loretta went out.

2. The actuality of the event.

FATHER: The point is that you two undermine me.

MOTHER: I'm sorry because you say one day, "If Loretta go out with a boy, I'll break her neck because she is too young."

3. The husband's past "misbehavior" in the same area.

FATHER: That was when? When she was ten years old or eleven years old.

MOTHER: No, thirteen. She tells me, "I'm afraid to tell Daddy because I will go out with a boy and Daddy don't want me to go out!" And I say, "Forget about it, don't worry about it." Loretta wants to go out with a boy, I say yes. I told you, Carlo, please don't work in the nighttime no more. I want you in the daytime. I want you at the

4. The lack of accommodation by husband in other areas.

table with the family because I told you I'm tired to take care of seven people, go shopping, go for the bills. I'm tired.

FATHER: Let's come to my point, right? She claimed that I was going to stop her and all of the things that you have been planning to do. Assuming I was going to stop her. And I don't understand why you wanted it that way.

MOTHER: Loretta told her mother because you told Loretta if she goes out, you break her legs.

FATHER: Loretta should tell me—

MOTHER: No, Carlo, because you're her father. She comes to her mother.

FATHER: No, what you did was wrong. You taught her wrong about me.

5. Guilt-producing self-pity.

6. Further accusations about the past.

7. And finally, cultural stereotypes.

INTERVIEWER: You describe "anorectic families" as conflict avoiders. How do you square this definition with the Menotti functioning?

MINUCHIN: It is an interesting question, but despite all the intensity of affect that is transacted in the session, there is really an avoidance of conflict. I know, because I experienced it. When I was involved in a disagreement with mother, I experienced frustration and helplessness, but never anger. When wife challenged husband, he avoided conflict and tried to elicit pity. The same occurred when Loretta challenged mother. In the end, mother elicited guilt. When one member insists on open disagreement, the other becomes an avoider. Loretta also diffuses conflict by interjecting herself to form a triad when the conflict between two family members reaches unacceptable thresholds.

MINUCHIN: I want to talk with both of you, Loretta and Sophia, because your father says that you two don't know him.

Having observed mother's power with daughters and experienced it himself, therapist by now sympathizes

That if you would talk with him, you would find that he is a person who can understand and can compromise. And he is saying that you don't know him because you go and talk with Mother about him instead of talking directly with him.

LORETTA: May I say something?

MINUCHIN: Yes.

LORETTA: I've tried talking to him before. That's why, at this point, I went to my mother. I tried before. I mean, when we were younger, the set rule was nobody goes out until they are sixteen, otherwise you have a broken leg. And he was very strong about it.-

MINUCHIN: But he says that he has changed and that you don't know he has changed.

LORETTA: The only reason both of them have changed is because they feel sorry for my being in the hospital, and they figure that this will help. But that's the only reason why they changed, because had this not have happened, it wouldn't have been so.

FATHER: When did I say that I was going to break your leg if you went out? Do you remember how old you were?

LORETTA: Since we were little, you were saying nobody goes out until they are sixteen. And I said, "All right, I am almost sixteen. What's going to happen?" And you said, "We'll talk about it then." It was never a subject that was discussed. And when it did happen this summer that I wanted to go out, Mommy was there at first because you were working. So I asked her, and she said yes. Then I said, "Well, then we have to ask Daddy." And she said, "No, don't worry about it. You go out."

FATHER: Now wait a minute.

LORETTA: Wait a minute, Dad. "You go out, and then I'll tell Daddy." Now, I felt very uncomfortable going out without your

strongly with the depowered husband. While the strategy of bringing father between mother and daughter is probably correct, therapist proposes it because he too is stymied by mother's imperviousness to his input and finds it difficult to support her. He thus unwittingly moves husband/wife conflict to father/daughter conflict, accepting family rules.

Therapist helps the enactment of father/daughter dyad.

Daughter pictures father role as "male" in just as concrete and primitive terms as mother pictures her own traditional female role.

Loretta elicits conflict.

knowing it. I was very uncomfortable all the while I was out. All I was thinking about was not telling Daddy and what would happen if I went home and he found out. I did not say that I didn't want to tell you, but had I gone to you first, it would have been "No," because you had expressed your belief on this subject very strongly before. And the only reason why you or Mommy have changed your opinion on this subject totally is that I was in the hospital. Because the doctor said, "Let her have some freedom and go out," Mama thought it would help me get better. So she says, "Here, Loretta, go out."

FATHER: All right.

LORETTA: That's the *only* reason why you let me out, not because you believe in it at all.

FATHER: If you believe it that way, Loretta, that means it's part my fault. It's my fault that you think that way about me.

By taking a down position, father flashes a yellow light, indicating a dangerous threshold.

Loretta acknowledges warning light.

LORETTA: No, I'm not blaming anybody for anything. I'm just saying this is the way it really is.

FATHER: Loretta, you know that I am your father, but you still insist that you ought to do things exactly the way you planned. Maybe I don't speak English as well as you do, but I have a good mind up here and occasionally I can be very understandable, you know, can manage any situation from time to time. You may not know that.

Father continues to replace conflict between spouses by father/daughter conflict.

LORETTA: Look, you are getting into an uproar. Like right now. I want to sit down here and talk like two human beings and you want to start yelling and screaming. Every time I start talking to you nicely about something and the minute you hear that it is something you disagree with—into an uproar. You yell and you scream, and Mommy gets into it too, and I have to be the only one to stand up for myself. I have

Loretta diffuses direct confrontation with father by casting herself as her sisters' champion: "I am alone against both parents, who are unfair. I am alone defending my siblings, who are ungrateful."

nobody on my side and nobody wants to sit down and listen to me. These two don't ever help me, and if I did get an opportunity to express my points and I made it clear, then they take advantage of it. It's an easy road for them because Loretta went through all the hardships making this possible, and then they just sit back and take advantage. That's why everything that they discuss with you is all right, but when it comes to me, I'm the bad person because I stood up and talked for everyone and I made it easy for them because they didn't have to argue about it anymore. It's already done, so it's all done for them.

FATHER: Why don't you let them speak for themselves?

Father collaborates with Loretta, moving confrontation to sibling subsystem.

LORETTA: They wouldn't speak for themselves. Just because they agree with you when they see what I'm going through.

Loretta replaces mother as overprotector.

FATHER: Who told you that they would never speak for themselves?

LORETTA: Now, look—see how they're talking.

FATHER: I mean, if they want to talk, since you assume that you say what they wanted to say.

LORETTA: No, I'm not assuming.

FATHER: You stop them from expressing themselves. I still think they want to talk.

LORETTA: No, I asked them before even talking to you. "Come in and be with me and tell Daddy how you feel about it too." And, "No, you do it. We don't want to have any part of it." Just now. They were being asked questions. "I don't know." "I don't want to talk." So, there's your example.

MINUCHIN: These arguments are good. Loretta needs to be able to express her mind to you, and you need to be able to tell her what you have in mind. What your father said about Sophia and Maria are true. He

Therapist continues supporting father. His therapeutic strategy requires mobilization of the peripheral father, so as to move mother out of her central controlling position. Therapist also continues

said that Mother does that with you, and now he is saying that you do that with them. He has an eye for the process of growing. He knows that to grow up, one needs to struggle. And he says when you take the job of fighting for Maria, she is not growing up.

LORETTA: I know, but I'm not struggling for her. I'm doing it for myself, is what I'm saying.

MINUCHIN: Loretta, your father says that if you say to him, "Father, I am sixteen years old and I have a date and I want to go out," he'll say, "Yes." Carlo, talk with Loretta. Because she needs to know you, and she needs to know how much power she has.

FATHER: You find it hard to believe that I'm flexible at the time it is necessary to be flexible. But if I see that things are unimportant, I don't see why Mama has to give—

LORETTA: But they may not be important to you, but to me, it may just be that important. Just the other night, it was a little thing—nothing important—some movie on TV. "You can't see it. Absolutely not." What are you trying to hide by saying no? I am sixteen.

FATHER: But you know, at the time you wanted to see it, there were two little kids who wanted to see the movie. Now, since they're kids and you're grown up, you should please the little kids. That's my idea. If this is wrong, then I don't know.

LORETTA: You can't always please the little kids. The little kids watch television all day, and that time, it was time for them to be in bed already. You don't tell them to go to bed. You tell them, "Stay there," and I can't watch the movie. And I have to grow up.

FATHER: I should deprive these two little kids of watching what they are watching and please you and let you watch that kind of movie? That would be right for you?

stressing the theme of age-appropriate functioning. Each time he uses this concept with parents and three older daughters, it becomes more familiar to them, until it will eventually become accepted as a universal truth.

Therapist uses daughter as a means of communication, directed toward increasing father's flexibility.

Father, then daughter, accommodate to therapist: the theme of age is here used either to justify or to challenge other behavior.

LORETTA: Mommy was already in bed. They should have been in bed. But you didn't tell them or express any feelings of having them go to bed. "Just stay there."

FATHER: If they don't listen, I'm to beat them up, put them to bed, and let you see the movie.

LORETTA: I didn't say beat them up, but you didn't even at least say, "Kids, it's time to go to bed." You didn't say that at all. You just let it go.

FATHER: But, you know, when I say once, nobody listen, right?

LORETTA: Well, you have to learn to—

FATHER: In this case, at nine o'clock, ten-thirty, I have to make these kids cry, right?

LORETTA: No, you didn't have to make them cry. I'm not saying that.

FATHER: And force my way and put them in bed and please you to watch the television, okay?

MINUCHIN: I think she's right, Carlo. She is saying she's sixteen and in your home there is no difference in the rights of a sixteen-year-old and the rights of a twelve-year-old. I think you are saying that.

LORETTA: Thank you.

MINUCHIN: Now, convince your father that you really are saying that you have different rights because you are the oldest. He can understand that.

LORETTA: Of course, he can understand it, but he doesn't want to let anything change by it.

MINUCHIN: No, your father says that he is here because he wants the situation to change. (*He looks at his watch.*) It's 12:15. We can make a break now and have something to eat, because I think Loretta's problem is related to what we are talking about. Loretta, I think you are a good fighter. I am impressed by you.

FATHER: She is, yes.

The seemingly authoritarian position of father in family contrasts with his actual functioning. His power is limited to the fact that his rules are not openly challenged. When he needs to implement authority, he falls back on declaring himself a good or a helpless father. Like Mr. Kaplan and Mr. Gilbert, only his bark is powerful.

Therapist, having gained affiliation with father, tries to use his affiliation to break the family pattern of argument and increase proximity between father and daughter. According to the pattern, members of the dyad in conflict, whether husband/wife, father/daughter or mother/daughter, assume symmetrical positions. There is no search for a resolution to the argument, just a maintenance of the balance of power.

MINUCHIN: I am concerned about what she feels, because if she feels that she cannot fight and win, then she will probably starve herself. But she is fighting for you, Sophia, and she is fighting for you, Carlo, and she is also fighting for you, Margherita. She is saying that she will help you become a mother of adolescents, and that can be a very helpful thing for you. If you need to work only for the three small ones, it will be easier. If you let both of them grow up, the two older ones, then the other little ones will.

MOTHER: She is big enough to do anything she wants to do. Sophia the same thing.

(*The food is brought in.*)

INTERVIEWER: Why did you break for food at this moment? It really seemed unnecessary since you had been able to elicit conflict in other areas.

MINUCHIN: The why of the particular moment to interrupt the sequence and call for lunch was simply practical. I prefer to have lunch in my first session with anorectics, and I use the first part of the session to join with the family members and create affiliations so that I can work with them later in a situation of stress. I saw that it was 12 o'clock, and I waited for an appropriate moment to interrupt, and after fifteen minutes I decided I would just announce lunch. In relation to the locus of conflict, I think it is necessary to work around the area of food. This area has become the center of Loretta's fantasies and the coin of transaction for many interpersonal sequences among family members. The cessation or substitution of the symptom requires that we work in this area invested with high affective intensity. After the symptoms disappear, we will continue to work with other areas.

INTERVIEWER: In the two previous cases, you used the introduction of food as the signal to induce a crisis. What were your ideas in this case?

MINUCHIN: I was impressed during the previous hour with Loretta's experience of self as helpless, hopeless, and controlled—very similar to Deborah's and Judy's. But, unlike the other two girls, Loretta also demonstrated a capacity for demanding and defending her individual turf, which indicated normal adolescent strength. To put the parents in control of her eating even for one session didn't seem appropriate. It would have strengthened her angry dependency on them instead of encouraging a safer area for claiming adolescent autonomy. I decided, therefore, to minimize food as a signal, not paying attention to her eating, and to continue with the theme of family development.

(As the food is brought in, Loretta gets up and runs out of the room, crying that she will not eat. The therapist goes after her, and after five minutes they return together.)

INTERVIEWER: What happened in the hallway?

MINUCHIN: I talked with Loretta. I had already decided that my strategy during lunch would be to de-emphasize food and to continue the discussion of the necessity for autonomy. Loretta's leaving was a test of my commitment to support her autonomy. It was also, as usual, a use of food to communicate her need for individuation. So I followed her out, and in the corridor we agreed that she would return, but she would not eat. We agreed that she had to be able to negotiate with her parents and win. I said that I would help her win. She was to come back, not to eat but to negotiate with her parents, and she was, with my help, to win.

MINUCHIN: Loretta, how old does your mother think you are?

LORETTA: I don't know. Apparently, not sixteen.

MINUCHIN: I absolutely agree with you. If you are not sixteen, you will not begin to eat. Because Loretta is fighting a battle for winning. She is fighting in the area of food and she says, in this area, "I will win."

MOTHER: She wins me all the time, my daughter. Do you know by what? Because I say something, "Loretta, we have to do this." "Oh no, Mama, we have to do this." I say, "No." Loretta then she stop eating, because we have to do it Loretta's way all the time. If we don't do it Loretta's way, we have to put our hands in the air; we have to stop everybody. I have to stop Sophia. I have to stop my husband. I have to stop the phone ring. I can't talk to nobody because Loretta, she nervous. She do anything to send me, my husband, her sister, her brothers, any way she wants. We say, "Yes, Loretta." We have to do anything you want and everything will be okay. If we do something we don't have to do, forget about it. Loretta, she say, "No."

> Mother's experience of the tyrannical power of the "sick" Loretta over every aspect of family life is quite at odds with previous transaction that showed identified patient as hopelessly controlled. Both transactional aspects are activated at different moments and experienced with different intensity by family members.

MINUCHIN: Can you answer your mother, Loretta? Carlo, let Mama sit near Loretta. Loretta, talk with Mother, because she says that you are controlling the house.

> Therapist begins strategy of challenging identified patient's self-experience.

LORETTA: I am not controlling nobody, Mama.

MOTHER: You're controlling your father, you're controlling me, Sophia, Enrico, Maria, Guiseppe. Why, Loretta?

LORETTA: I'm not controlling nobody. It's just that somebody has to do something.

MOTHER: No, you do not. That's me and your father's job. You have to do something by yourself. You are not to interfere with Sophia, Maria—

> Mother's challenge to Loretta incorporates therapist's previous comments.

LORETTA: I want to stand by myself and you are stopping me.

MOTHER: No, Loretta, Mama never stopped you.

LORETTA: Yes, Mama. You may not realize this sometimes, but you're doing it anyway.

MOTHER: But sometimes, Loretta, you put us in the world in a way that we can't do nothing. We have to agree with you. We have to do what you want. But sometimes we can't. And if we don't get what you want, you start crying.

LORETTA: No, I'm not saying that, Ma.

MOTHER: Screaming. Pulling the chair. Pulling anything the way you want.

LORETTA: No, Mama.

MINUCHIN: Does she do things like that?

MOTHER: Yeah. I'm sorry to have to—

LORETTA: I pull the chair?

MOTHER: She get nervous so forgets about anything that she does. She pulls the chair, she throws her shoes, her clothes, everything—

LORETTA: Since when?

MINUCHIN: She has temper tantrums? Like little children?

MOTHER: Oh, she got the temper, Loretta. I'm sorry—

MINUCHIN: Like little children, she does?

FATHER: Well, she perfectly all right when she's cool. When she blow the cool—

MINUCHIN: You agree with your wife that Loretta is the one that drives the house?

FATHER: Well, I—she's not really—

LORETTA: I don't throw shoes around. Why are you saying I throw chairs around?

MOTHER: Plenty you have pulled the chair—

LORETTA: I don't throw anything around, Ma.

MOTHER: No, Loretta, I don't lie. I want to tell the truth like he—

Instead of emphasizing the sick aspect of identified patient, as in the beginning of the session, mother, who has been challenged as incompetent in mothering, now labels Loretta's behavior as bad. This operation could strengthen boundaries between mother and daughter.

Therapist, having supported Loretta's competent behavior, begins process of challenging it by framing certain aspects of her interpersonal transactions as childish.

LORETTA: That is not the truth. You're making me sound like a bad person.

Loretta objects to reinterpretation of her behavior, because being sick is acceptable in family and activates family members' concern and protection, but being bad is experienced as deviant from family values.

MOTHER: No, you're not bad person. You're—

Mother accepts daughter's objection.

LORETTA: Well, that's exactly what you're doing.

MINUCHIN: She is saying that you have temper tantrums. She is saying that you are childish.

LORETTA: I am not childish.

MINUCHIN: That's what she's saying.

LORETTA: I may yell. I may scream. But I am not childish. I don't ever throw things around.

MOTHER: Loretta, I don't say that—

LORETTA: If anything, you throw shoes at me or whatever it is that's in your way. You're trying to make me sound like a bad person.

The same mother/daughter transaction begins again: daughter requests acceptance into family fold.

MOTHER: No, Loretta, you are not a bad person.

Mother acknowledges.

LORETTA: I am the bad person in the family. I'm the black sheep of the family simply because I stand up and say what I feel. The other children are always good. They're always your little sweethearts because they don't open their mouths.

Loretta relabels her bad behavior as corrective behavior for family's improvement and reinstates herself in the system as unfairly treated Cinderella.

MOTHER: No, Loretta, nobody is sweetheart—

LORETTA: They agree about everything with you and Daddy. Whatever you say is all right with them.

MOTHER: When you want something that I can't buy you, you cry for three days. I have to tell the truth—

LORETTA: But, this is what you and Dad always bring up. Money. That's all you talk—

Loretta is already back on the attack.

MOTHER: We have a money problem.

LORETTA: I'm the bad person, right?

MOTHER: No, Loretta. Anything you want I can't buy because we are seven people in the family—

LORETTA: But this is always what you bring up. For you, the issue is always money. For me, it's not.

MOTHER: Because, you see, Sophia, she don't cry—

LORETTA: Sure, because they agree with everything you say.

MOTHER: Sophia tells me, "Don't do these things. You're killing yourself." Now you, Loretta, you tell me this, see? How many aspirin? I'll get them for you, because when you get nervous, you stop eating. Right away, no food. Not get up from the bed. You don't want to see nobody. You don't want to talk to nobody. And Mama cries.

> Mother signals an end to the conflict by introducing her role as a good, hurt mother.

MINUCHIN: Is your mother saying that you are blackmailing them? That your not eating is a way of controlling them?

> Therapist insists on conflict.

LORETTA: That's not—

MINUCHIN: That's what she's saying. She's saying that you are controlling her by having temper tantrums and not eating.

> Therapist increases stress between mother and daughter.

LORETTA: I don't have temper tantrums.

MINUCHIN: That's what she's saying.

LORETTA: Well, she's wrong, because it's not true.

MOTHER: Why you do the same thing to the hospital? You blackmail the doctor. You don't want to eat. You don't want to get the tube out. The doctor told me, "Your daughter say she eat. I'm sorry, Mrs. Menotti, your daughter, she don't eat." So then I have to tell the doctor the truth.

> Mother again uses therapist's language to challenge daughter. In a system in which parents and identified patient see themselves as having equivalent power, every conflict creates a need for coalitions. Therapist, now part of the system, is being used in familiar pattern.

LORETTA: I don't blackmail nobody.

MOTHER: That's what they told me. You don't eat. They bring food in and you give it to somebody else.

LORETTA: It always turns out that I'm the liar.

MOTHER: Now, you have to tell Dr. Minuchin you stay almost two months and no food in the stomach. The tube in the nose, but they don't get no food in you, did they? Only that kind of food they give you through the tube. You cry. Mama cries outside in the hallway when they put the tube in the nose. Mama cries.

LORETTA: I'm not going to feel sorry for you, Ma. I'm sorry because you're wrong. I am not a liar.

MOTHER: I don't feel sorry for you because you do that way—

LORETTA: Well, I don't blackmail no one.

MOTHER: I lose a daughter if you do that way.

LORETTA: Well, you have to be compromising, too. If you're losing her, it's because of you too. It's not because—

MOTHER: No, Loretta, I want you. I want all my kids healthy.

LORETTA: Well, then help. Then don't insist—

MOTHER: You are cooking, but you don't eat it. You want to make this, then don't eat it. Oh my, you make a cake for me to eat. I don't want to eat it. You start screaming. Why? Because I make—I tell you all the time, I don't need cake. You ask your sister eat it. Somebody say no. You right away say, "You don't eat it because I make it." Bloop, everything goes up.

LORETTA: What goes up? Don't lie, Ma, I'm tired of hearing it.

MOTHER: No, Loretta. I'm over here. Your sister don't go to school today because we want to help you.

LORETTA: And this is going to be repeated a hundred times. "Your sister didn't go to school. Your father didn't go to work. For

Identified patient again rejects the label of badness, according to family values.

Mother begins process of reestablishing enmeshment.

Similar to other anorectic cases, the "family metabolism" is expressed in Loretta's fattening other members of the system while starving herself.

Daughter and mother are now comfortable in their oft-repeated "balanced" conflict. The balance is maintained

you. For you. For you." If you want to help me, you don't have to be stubborn like you're being now. You're making a liar out of me, which is not true.

MINUCHIN: Do you think that the arguments that you are having with Loretta are the same arguments that you were having at home?

MOTHER: My Loretta, she cooks for everybody. Oh, she likes to cook, but she don't touch it. But we have to eat it. Not Loretta. I don't really argue with Loretta. All I say— Loretta, eat it because the doctor at the hospital they told me your daughter is in danger. She could die. I see she don't eat nothing. Now, this morning, she get up and she come over here. Not even a glass of water. There's nothing in there. I have to worry about her.

MINUCHIN: I think that Loretta feels a loser in your family. You say that Loretta is a winner. I think she is a loser.

MOTHER: No, she's a winner.

MINUCHIN: I saw, just now, that she was a loser.

MOTHER: Because she cries?

MINUCHIN: Because she feels absolutely helpless to defend herself. I don't know. You are very powerful. Do you know that?

MOTHER: Might be because my daughter lose weight. Everyday I told her she have to eat.

MINUCHIN: The issue is not eating. Loretta will begin to eat when she is sixteen and when you treat her as if she is sixteen.

MOTHER: You see, I can't do anything with Loretta. Loretta, she say, "You don't love me because you don't want to get this." I have to do what Loretta say. If I don't do what Loretta say, what I have to do? Loretta, talk.

either by repeating one's own view without increasing intensity and attempting to change the "opponent's" view or by changing the content and starting again with continued "low-intensity" weaponry.

Therapist tries to unbalance the conflict.

MINUCHIN: I know that she feels that you are very powerful. I don't think that you let her feel that she is sixteen.

In maintaining a constant content—"You are not letting her be sixteen"—therapist is caught, like all members of the system, in a no-win, low-intensity conflict.

MOTHER: No, she is the winner. Loretta, Mommy don't tell you you are sixteen?

Mother triangulates daughter.

LORETTA: Yeah, you tell me, but you don't make me feel it; you don't treat me like sixteen. You treat me like I was two years old.

With daughter's response, pattern of conflict recurs.

MOTHER: No, Loretta.

LORETTA: Yes, Mama.

MINUCHIN: Margherita, you do so many things for your daughter that she becomes an extremely childish, incompetent person.

Therapist uses a technique of complementarity that he learned from his grand-mother: he challenges daughter's behavior, but puts responsibility for her actions on mother's behavior.

FATHER: Right, I have to agree with you.

MINUCHIN: And at some point your daughter needs to grow up. And your wife needs to start to grow up first, so that your daughter can grow up. Your wife needs to be able to let her lead her own life. I am still doing your job, Loretta. It's very difficult to fight your mother because she is a very lovely person and a very lovely mother. Carlo, how can you help your daughter to become sixteen? Because she will begin to eat when she's sixteen. Not before.

Therapist's request that parents grow up so that children can do so too is syntonic with the concept of complementarity. This concept may be carried further by asking children to help parents grow up.

FATHER: I wish she'd make herself clear with me what she wanted to do. I wish she'd be reasonable to understand that sometimes things are not so easy, or not possible to do the way she finds them. Do you know that?

MINUCHIN: You know, sometimes Loretta is very childish and she needs to grow up also. Sometimes her demands are too childish because up to now, she has not been helped to grow up. You have a very incompetent daughter—a very childish person. But I think the family, and particularly you, Margherita, support her being childish.

Therapist repeats the message: Loretta is childish, and mother supports her being childish. Then, after supporting the daughter as a way of challenging the system, he will switch, focusing on Loretta's participation in the maintenance of her symptoms and challenging her to change.

MOTHER: How? How, Loretta?

MINUCHIN: When you tell her *how* to move her chair, you are treating her as if she's six. That's how. It's very simple how. When you say to her that she can go out with a boy friend without asking her father because you will protect her from her father's anger, that's how. You keep her as a little child.

MOTHER: No, because I—

MINUCHIN: That's how. Because, Loretta, you need to be able to talk with your father, not have your mother protect you. That's how your mother keeps you a little girl, and then you become a very incompetent child. You have temper tantrums and you do all kinds of things. Will you help your wife, Carlo? You need to help her.

FATHER: When the tempers rise between the two of them, it's not possible to understand Loretta. Most of the time, even a little thing creates a situation that becomes impossible because of tempers.

MINUCHIN: I think you need to talk to your wife about keeping her a little girl.

FATHER: I'll be yelling many times that she is doing just too much and won't let these girls do things that they could do. Even when they were younger. And I don't think much has been changed in that area.

MINUCHIN: Can Margherita hear you or is she deaf?

MOTHER: No, I hear my husband, I hear what he say, but I want to tell you something. Loretta, she grew up a long time ago. When she wants to be, she's a young teenager. She knows it.

MINUCHIN: No, Loretta, I don't think you are a grown-up person. I think you are very much tied to your mother, unable to make decisions, to take initiative. You are fighting a battle for growing up in the worst possible ways, by killing yourself so that you will

Therapist resumes his attempt to increase proximity between father and daughter in order to separate mother from daughter. Ultimately it will be impossible to make this separation unless there is a concomitant increase in husband/wife affiliation.

Mother absolves daughter's behavior and rescinds her own responsibility for it.

Therapist challenges identified patient. He frames her behavior not as autonomous but as controlled by mother, signaling that her rebelliousness is a fake.

demonstrate to Mama that she is wrong. I think you can be a winner, but I don't know yet that you want to. You will eat when you are sixteen. But I don't think you feel, act, or think like sixteen. And I think this is because the family, especially Mama, is always doing things for you. Mother is moving your hands; she is moving your arms. (*He takes Loretta's hands and arms and moves them.*) You don't have anything for your own. So, I think you should not eat now, but you will eat at the moment when you are sixteen.

INTERVIEWER: You seem to like concrete images. Earlier you said to Deborah Kaplan, "They take your voice." Here, you move Loretta's arms and hands. You ask people to change seats. Don't you rely on the power of words?

MINUCHIN: I feel that using a physical movement gives emphasis and intensity. A concrete metaphor such as this one can be seen and understood by all family members regardless of age, but while the meaning will be clear for everybody, each person will give it a different affective intensity.

MOTHER: She fight me before, because Loretta, she's a nice girl, but she's stubborn.

MINUCHIN: At this point, she's not a nice girl. At this point, she is just a stubborn person and you are a stubborn person and both of you are fighting.

MOTHER: Yeah, I fight all the time with my daughter because—

MINUCHIN: You are not helping! You are fighting for her, but you are not helping her. You are not helping her. Loretta, do you eat with your family?

MOTHER: Loretta, she don't—

LORETTA: What do you mean, I don't eat?

Thinking that intensity of mother/daughter transactions around food supports the symptom, therapist begins to devise a task that will separate daughter from family when she eats. But as soon as he asks the first question,

MOTHER: You want the truth, I give you the truth.

LORETTA: Just because I don't eat *with* you, it means I don't eat? No, don't worry, I'm better off eating without you.

MOTHER: Wait a minute. You told the doctor we eat our lunch together. Now stop it.

MINUCHIN: I don't want that argument. Do you argue with Mother every day about food, Loretta?

LORETTA: Of course, because if she doesn't see me eat in front of her, I didn't eat. She can't take my word for it.

MOTHER: I don't mention it.

LORETTA: Yes, Ma, if you don't see me eat —yesterday, I went out to eat. And if you don't see me eat, I don't eat.

MINUCHIN: No, no, no. I want you to fight about anything, but not about food.

LORETTA: Yeah, but that's what it is everyday in the house. Food. And if relatives come over, "Oh, Loretta, did you eat? Did you eat?" I'm hearing it everyday.

MINUCHIN: Loretta, what is your weight at this point? Write it down on this napkin so that nobody sees it. Keep it secret. I also want you to write what is your height. (*He gives identified patient a napkin, on which she writes that her weight is 82 pounds.*) Okay now, I want you to help me, Carlo. I don't want any arguments at home about food. What would be the best way? Would you like to eat alone for one week?

LORETTA: It doesn't matter.

MINUCHIN: I want you to make a decision. Would you like to eat with some family members, or alone, or would you like to sit with them at the table, but eat alone? Select one alternative. Which one would you prefer? Which one would make it more comfortable for you?

LORETTA: It really doesn't matter as long as nobody bothers me about what to eat or how much.

mother and daughter go at each other in another redundant, meaningless sequence of unresolved bickering.

Therapist emphasizes that patient's weight is not a public family matter but a part of the bond between patient and therapist. With this secret, he increases the strength of identified patient's body boundary.

Therapist offers alternatives as another concrete way of challenging the experience of being controlled and helpless.

MINUCHIN: Loretta, you need to understand their point of view as well. If you eat with them, then they will look at what you eat and what you don't eat because you will make their situation uncomfortable. Just for one week, I want you to eat in your room. Could you do that? Because I don't want your family to know what you eat.

MOTHER: Can I say something? In the morning I bring the big kids to school. Loretta, she is alone. She can eat anything she wants. If she want to eat alone, if she want to eat in her room, in the kitchen, anyplace—

MINUCHIN: Beautiful. That's okay. Then, for a week you will eat by yourself. Okay?

LORETTA: On Sunday, I want to eat with them.

Patient exercises right to alternative behavior.

MINUCHIN: Fine, on Sunday you want to eat with them. Now, for the next week there will be no fights with Loretta about eating. Carlo, you will be the foreman of that. I think that your wife is very concerned and she is not objective because she's a mother hen. She vibrates with the kids. Now, do you think you can do a thing like that?

FATHER: Yes.

LORETTA: I don't want to be weighed. It's better for me not to know.

MINUCHIN: Loretta, I will weigh you because I need to know if you can maintain your weight, but this will be between you and me.

The weighing-in can be a kind of ritual between identified patient and therapist, during which issues of autonomy and belonging, among other matters, are discussed.

LORETTA: Okay.

MINUCHIN: You see, there are negotiables and nonnegotiables. In order to work with you, it is necessary to know that you will not die.

LORETTA: Well, I can be weighed, but I don't want to know it. I don't want to hear about it. I don't want to know my weight.

MINUCHIN: If that's how you want to arrange it, okay, but if you lose weight, I will tell you.

LORETTA: Okay.

MINUCHIN: Because then other things need to be done, but I want you to learn how to grow up, how to be able to fight with your mother differently. I want you to be competent. I think you're a very incompetent person. Do you know what I am saying?

LORETTA: I know it, but I am not accepting it.

MINUCHIN: Okay, so that is something you, Carlo and Margherita, can be relaxed about. We will check her weight. Meanwhile, she needs to learn to handle you two and you need to learn to handle her. When she has temper tantrums, what do you do?

MOTHER: Oh, I stop her. I have to stop her. Loretta get too angry.

FATHER: You should stop her before—

MOTHER: Every time *I* stop her. All the time *I* stop her. Why didn't you stop her the other day when Loretta get angry with you and yell at you, "Why don't you get out of here?"

FATHER: No, because I say to her, "Instead of staying home all the time, why don't you go out and see if you can't find a job. You know, do something that's—"

LORETTA: That's not what you said.

FATHER: No? What did I say?

LORETTA: You said, "If you don't like it here, leave. Get out of here, because I don't want to put up with you anymore."

FATHER: That's not what I said.

LORETTA: That's what you said. Don't be innocent now.

FATHER: That was among the other things.

LORETTA: Yeah, among the other things. That was the first thing you said.

FATHER: Yeah, but I've forgotten what the argument started from. I can recall what I said, but I don't know what the argument came from. Well, we stopped the argument. I don't know.

LORETTA: The only reason why I get mad

Therapist, having completed his transaction of disengaging Loretta from family, now wants to increase affiliation between parents by supporting their rights against Loretta's control.

But spouses go through another bickering sequence.

Spouses' bickering is replaced by a similar sequence between father and daughter.

First father, then daughter, expresses the hopelessness of a pattern that keeps them united in an argument that, like Sisyphus' work, is never resolved.

and the only reason why I scream and yell is because I don't know what to say anymore. I've had it. It's been years since this business and I can't take it anymore. I'm tired of it. Absolutely tired of existing and the whole situation. And that's why when I say something, I don't even know what I'm saying, and when I think about it, I'm sorry I said it.

MINUCHIN: Loretta, this was a perfectly good argument. Okay? Now, I want you to tell your father that you have been looking for a job without making it an argument. I want you to win this one.

Therapist, aware of the approaching end of the session, tries to break the pattern and finish a transaction in a mood of cooperation.

LORETTA: He knows it already. There's no point in saying it anymore.

MINUCHIN: I want you to hear what he says if you say it without it being an argument.

LORETTA: I've been looking for a job and haven't found anything yet.

FATHER: That's more like it.

MINUCHIN: Carlo, answer in such a way that she hears and she knows that you have heard what she said.

FATHER: So, why have you been looking for a job?

LORETTA: Because I don't want to stay in the house all day long and have nothing but arguments. That's all.

MINUCHIN: Loretta, say it nicely. What you said is correct, but the way in which you say it makes your father angry. And you, Carlo, answer her, but in a nice way.

FATHER: What did you say before? I didn't hear that.

LORETTA: I said I didn't want to stay home all day long and have arguments. That's why I was looking for a job.

FATHER: What are you arguing on?

A familiar sequence begins again between father and daughter.

LORETTA: Dad, all day long there's arguments about food. I've had it.

FATHER: With who?

LORETTA: With all of you.

MINUCHIN: Carlo, she said something that was nice. She said she is looking for a job. She says she is looking for a job because she wants to be out of the house. And this is important for a young person. You want that, also. Why are you making that an argument? Answer her without making it an argument.

FATHER: If it is possible, can you tell me what kind of a job you are looking for?

LORETTA: Anything that I'm able to do.

FATHER: Anything, like what?

LORETTA: Office work or help around the office. Straighten out papers and what not. Nothing so difficult that I won't be able to do it.

FATHER: That will make you happy if you find something to do like that?

LORETTA: Yes, it would.

MINUCHIN: Could you help her? Could you help her with that?

FATHER: She never asked me before. If it's possible, why not?

MINUCHIN: Could you talk with her about some of the ways in which you could help her?

FATHER: Well, if she had told me exactly why—

MINUCHIN: She is telling you now. Don't make an argument out of it.

FATHER: You want me to help you find a job?

LORETTA: Yes, I'd like that.

MINUCHIN: Okay. It's possible, but it is difficult. You have been involved in many fights. And I think you need to fight, Loretta, but with arguments suited to teenagers. I think that you should not start eating with the family until you are sixteen. How old are you now?

LORETTA: Sixteen.

MINUCHIN: When was your birthday?

Therapist controls the sequence.

LORETTA: Last week.

MINUCHIN: Last week, but you are not sixteen yet. I would say to avoid fighting about food. And since Loretta will not start eating until she is sixteen, I want Loretta to eat alone. At the point in which she begins to eat, she will be exactly sixteen. Then, she will come back because then you will not fight with her about food. I think, Loretta that you should not put too much weight on because your face looks rather nice long. But you need to gain probably ten pounds. But, this is for you to decide. Because at sixteen, you will need to do things on your own. At home, I want you, Carlo, to talk with your wife, and then talk with Loretta, about what rights does a sixteen-year-old have and what obligations. Can you help your wife to think like that? That a sixteen-year-old has obligations?

FATHER: I will try.

MINUCHIN: Can she hear?

FATHER: Margherita, did you hear what I said?

MOTHER: I hear good.

FATHER: Do you think you need that doctor to tell you?

MOTHER: I think so.

MINUCHIN: Okay. Carlo, you will need to talk with Margherita. I think she has run the house for too long alone, you know. You will need to talk with your father about jobs, Loretta. Maybe he can help you with this and other things. Carlo, can you begin to let Loretta know you—

FATHER: What I want for Loretta—excuse me for interrupting you—is to think different about me. She has to think about me not as an obstacle course.

LORETTA: Well, I can't think it, Dad, unless you show it.

FATHER: I have to show you before you will believe me, huh?

LORETTA: Well, so far you haven't proved
anything to show me that you are any different. You say it here, but when we go outside,
it's no different.

MINUCHIN: For this week, before you return again, I want you, Loretta, to talk to
your father twice for a half an hour. Carlo,
you will select two evenings to talk with
your daughter. Today is what? Friday? Talk
with him during the weekend one time and
talk with him next week, Loretta. If she
doesn't do that, you make a time, Carlo, and
you say, "I want you to know me." And you
talk no more than half an hour.

FATHER: Okay.

MINUCHIN: No more than half an hour
and twice during this week, Loretta. I want
you to talk with your father. Maybe the first
time you tell him something about you.
Okay? So that he will know you. The second
time, I want you to tell her something about
yourself, Carlo. I think she needs to know
you and that will be a help. Carlo will take
over more of helping Loretta. Will that be
a help, Margherita? Loretta, when your parents argue, you do not enter. Okay? Margherita, she will start eating at the point in
which she is sixteen, and she will not die of
that. If she loses weight, then we will think
differently. If she maintains the weight
which she has now, it's safe for the moment.
So, you don't worry about that.

After this consultation interview, the Menotti family continued
in treatment for four months. Loretta gained 21 pounds during the
first three months, whereupon her weight stabilized at around 105
pounds.

The therapy focused on issues of individuation and age-appropriate autonomy. A follow-up one and a half years after the initial interview found Loretta working as a waitress, a job that she had
occupied for the last six months. She had re-enrolled in school and
was planning to finish high school. She had many friends and maintained a stormy relationship with her mother.

Psychotherapy
for a Small Planet

12

Anorexia is an illness with great dramatic appeal, whose impact stretches far back into history, evoking images of ascetics and martyrs. It recalls the victims of the concentration camps, as well as the government-rocking "passive" protesters—the suffragettes, Gandhi. Today the drama is played out in the setting of a society seduced by the angular. In contrast to the Romans who taught *mens sana in corpore sano*, we have switched our enthusiasm for the curves of Rubens and the *Maja Desnuda* to an admiration for the angularity of Modigliani and Giacometti. We idealize the woman in the television commercial who drinks only diet sodas: aesthetic without effort.

Ironically, in a society in which the new women's consicousness promises a change in the relationship between the sexes, we are seeing more and more anorectics.[1] Young women willfully deny their bodies the energy necessary for development. In a strange way, anorexia still represents the triumph of the will over bodily needs, bringing back centuries of learned argument on the dichotomy of body and soul. It also remains, in a changing society, an expression of the patriarchal society's feminine ideal of passivity and obedience.

Anorexia nervosa has had great impact in the mental health field. These pathetic hunger-strikers have attracted the attention of healers throughout history. Today we are treating them in the revivalists' tents of the Midwest, on the analysts' couches of Manhattan's Upper East Side, and before the one-way mirrors of family therapy clinics. Each of these therapists claim eloquently that his view of man and man's needs is the correct one.

In our own work with anorectics and other psychosomatics in

their family context, we produced results that appeared to underscore the necessity for reevaluating the scope of psychotherapeutic services and enlarging the focus from dysfunctional people to people in dysfunctional situations. But when we began to present these results to the mental health field, the response was: If your results are so good, then you cannot be treating true anorexia. Or if these patients are true anorectics, then they must be very young. Or if they are true anorectics and not very young, you must be seeing them very early after the onset of the illness.

Challenges to the linear model are still regarded by many therapists as anomalies of the normal science of anorexia nervosa. Therapists, like other human beings, are a product of their society. They are, as Kuhn stated, members of a guild who are trained by the same methods, read the same books, and transmit similar ideas. Anorexia nervosa has for the last three hundred years been described and treated by investigators trained in the linear paradigm. The idea that the patient contains her own pathology retains its grip on modern therapists, who defend their interventions eloquently. In the field of helping people, beliefs speak with a clearer, sharper voice than results. The tragic consequences for the anorectic are shown by the case of Ellen West, who was treated in the first quarter of this century.

The beginning of the twentieth century was a time in which man believed that the new technology would help him create a better world, that man could wrest from the earth the infinite products necessary for the betterment of humanity. In this new world of unlimited, machine-produced resources, man would conquer, regardless of circumstances. In such an ambience, the concept of man as a hero could still prevail. During that time, Ellen West grew up in Switzerland and developed an "obsession with being thin." Her case is significant because the expression of her suffering, and the way in which the physicians who treated her selected and organized the "relevant data," incorporate a conceptualization of man in which selfhood is disconnected from the context for being.

The case begins: "Ellen West, a non-Swiss, is the only daughter of a Jewish father for whom her love and veneration know no bounds. She has a dark-haired brother four years older than she, who resembles her father, and a younger brother who is blond. Whereas the older one 'has no nerves' and is very well adjusted and cheerful, the younger is 'a bundle of nerves' and is a soft womanish aesthete. [The] father is described as an externally very self-controlled . . . man of action, internally, however, as very soft . . . The mother . . . likewise of Jewish descent, is said to be a very soft, kindly, suggestible, nervous woman who underwent a depression for three years during the time of her engagement." Thus writes Ludwig Binswanger in describing the history of a woman who was under psychiatric and medical care from the age of twenty until her suicide at the age of thirty-three.[2] Although Ellen West's case history is extremely detailed, not much more is known about her family. She married her cousin when she was twenty-eight years old, but this too is almost all that is known about her marriage.

Her illness, according to the record, starts at the age of twenty when, "at her father's wish, she breaks her engagement to a 'romantic foreigner.'" She is at the time on a trip to Sicily. She experiences "a definite dread—namely, a dread of getting fat . . . At once she begins to mortify herself by fasting and immoderate hikes. This goes so far that when her companions stop at some pretty spot Ellen keeps circling about them. She no longer eats sweets . . . and skips supper altogether."

A year later, she is "constantly tormented by the idea that she is getting too fat and, therefore, she is forever taking long walks." She complains that "she does not find the activity she is seeking . . . that she feels a veritable torment when she sits still, that every nerve in her quivers, and that in general her body shares in all the stirrings of her soul." She is depressed, feeling worthless and useless.

At twenty-three, Ellen West has an unpleasant love affair with her riding teacher. During this period "she watches her body weight and reduces her food intake as soon as she threatens to gain weight. But now dread of getting fat is accompanied by an intensified longing for food."

At twenty-four, she becomes engaged to a student, and her parents demand a temporary separation. Although her involvement with this student lasts for three years, nothing more is known about the relationship. While she is on a trip to the seashore, "a severe depression sets in again . . . She does everything to get just as thin as possible, takes long hikes, and daily swallows thirty-six to forty-eight thyroid tablets! Consumed by homesickness, she begs her parents to let her return. She arrives completely emaciated, with trembling limbs, and drags herself through the summer in physical torment, but feels spiritually satisfied because she is thin."

Ellen West's case is never diagnosed as anorexia nervosa. But her symptoms through the years, with idiosyncratic variations, are characteristic of the anorexia syndrome. She loses over 30 percent of her body weight, dropping from 160 to 99 pounds in three years, and develops amenorrhea. She takes long hikes, often twenty to twenty-five miles a day. After her marriage to her cousin, she "becomes intensely preoccupied with calorie charts . . . She demands of those around her that they eat much and well, while she denies herself everything. She develops great skill in not letting them know that she is eating almost nothing by filling her plate like everyone else and then secretly emptying the greater part of the food into her handbag." She herself notes her obsessive concern with weight and food: "Since I acted only from the point of view of whether things made me thin or fat, all things soon lost their intrinsic meaning." In a letter to her husband, she adds: "My life's ideal, to be thin, continued to occupy me more than all else. I shall really become a wife only when I have finally given up my life's ideal." When writing this description of her interpersonal transaction with her husband, Ellen West, at the age of thirty-two, is hopelessly involved in the context of sanatoriums and doctors, with a concomitant concentration on food ideation. She has lost her anchor to all previous life and exists in a context where "being" is restricted to "being a patient."

At the age of thirty-three, she is hospitalized again. She has begun a second analysis, her first one having been interrupted after six months of treatment. She writes in her diary: "I wanted to get to know the unknown urges which were stronger than my reason and which forced me to shape my entire life in accordance with a guiding point of view. And the goal of this guiding point of view was to be thin. The analysis was a disappointment. I analyzed with my mind, and everything remained theory. The wish to be thin remained unchanged in the center of my thinking . . . It was no longer the fixed idea alone which embittered my life, but something far worse was added: the compulsion of always having to think about eating. This compulsion has become the curse of my life, it pursues me waking and sleeping, it stands beside everything I do like an evil spirit, and never and nowhere can I escape it."

After thirteen years of illness and a number of hospitalizations in rest homes and clinics, she makes a series of suicidal attempts. Kraepelin, when consulted, diagnoses melancholia. Ellen West's analyst considers this diagnosis incorrect and continues the analysis based on his own diagnosis that the patient is suffering from severe obsessive neurosis combined with manic-depressive oscillation. Later Bleuler is consulted, who makes a diagnosis of schizophrenia. Subsequently a foreign psychiatrist labels her condition a "psychopathic constitution progressively unfolding." The upshot, according to the director of the clinic where she is now staying, is "that no definitely reliable therapy is possible. We therefore resolved to give in to the patient's demand for discharge."

Ellen West leaves for her home. Her weight upon discharge is approximately the same as upon arrival, namely 104 pounds. "On the third day of being home, she is as if transformed. At breakfast she eats butter and sugar; at noon, she eats so much that—for the first time in thirteen years!—she is satisfied by her food and gets really full . . . She takes a walk with her husband, reads poems by Rilke, Storm, Goethe, and Tennyson, is amused by the first chapter of Mark Twain's 'Christian Science,' is in a positively festive mood, and all heaviness seems to have fallen away from her . . . In the evening she takes a lethal dose of poison, and on the following morning she is dead. She looked as she had never looked in life—calm and happy and peaceful."

The case of Ellen West, noted Edgar Z. Friedenberg, "illustrates clearly enough the depth and commitment of existential psychiatry to the client's real sense of herself. It is better, she decided—and her physicians and husband accepted the decision—to feel your real selfhood for one, fatal day than to go on for years, in the ordinary way, trying to carry on metabolism as though one had not died at all."[3] But who was that "self" whom Ellen West reaffirmed in her act of death? So little is known about her life circumstances. She was rich enough to afford thirteen years of different treatments through a variety of sanatoriums. She was married, and her husband was at times in the sanatorium with her; they hiked together, and she wrote letters to him. But very little else emerges about the nature of their relationship in five years of marriage. What was Ellen West's position in her family prior to the marriage—in this family who broke two of her engagements and accepted her marriage to her cousin? What was her relationship to her parents, whom "she begs to let her return" home after they demand a temporary separation from her fiancé? What was the nature of her transactions with her siblings, with an older brother who "has no nerves" and the younger "womanish aesthete" brother? What concept of man permits so detailed a history of a patient's torments, fantasies, and taste for poetry and literature, yet tells so little about the patient's social context?

Man, regardless of circumstances, could only be conceived in a world of infinite resources where it would be possible to wrest from his context whatever was "most correct for the development of his separated self." This concept created psychotherapeutic procedures that have in common, regardless of their differences, the idea of helping the self to actualize itself. Thus Binswanger describes the dynamic of Ellen West:

> The dread of becoming fat . . . has thus to be seen anthropologically not as a beginning, but as an end. It is the "end" of the encirclement process of the entire existence, so that it is no longer open for its existential possibilities. Now they are definitively fixated upon the rigid existential contrast between light and dark, flowering and withering, thin equaling intellectual and fat equaling the opposite . . .
>
> The "way" of this life-history is now unmistakably prescribed: it no longer runs into the expanse of the future but moves in a circle. The preponderance of the future is now replaced by the supremacy of the past . . . That the direction of circles in a present closed off from the future, ruled by the past, and therefore empty, is dramatically expressed in her truly symbolic act in which she keeps circling around her girl friends who have stopped at a scenic point . . . She offers the picture of a lioness imprisoned in a cage, circling along the bars, vainly looking for an exit.

In this description there is no concern with what exists outside the cage, who keeps the keys to the door, or even who makes the bars to the cage. This is a description of people in a world that they should be able to control.

How different the conceptualization of man offered by Ionesco in his play *The King Dies*, in which a vigorous king has a magnificent palace in a vast kingdom populated by courtiers. Bit by bit the king, through mismanagement and lack of military skill, loses the parts of his kingdom until only the palace remains, and gradually the palace declines in splendor and dies. In this parable, Ionesco describes the aging of the king through the changes in the external context of the king. There is no separation between time and space. People are their circumstances.

The concept of man as successfully confronting his ecology for the survival of self could exist only in a world that had not yet discovered the limitations of its own resources. Binswanger's description of Ellen West's tormented life during her last thirteen years, as well as of the therapeutic procedures that were instituted which certainly contributed to her death, could only derive from a linear conceptualization of people that sets them apart from their ecology. Ellen West's "self," as described in a world without space, is the product of a philosophical conceptualization of man, positioned nowhere, beating his fist against his chest and proclaiming, "I am, I am."

But in this quarter of the twentieth century, we are learning that resources are not infinite, that if man won his battle with nature, he would be, as E. F. Schumacher pointed out, on the losing side.[4] Context therapists share with modern ecologists, ethologists, economists, geographers, and philosophers an awareness of the constraints of ecosystems:

> Every spring in the wet meadows I hear a little shrilling chorus which sounds for all the world like an endlessly reiterated "We're here, we're here, we're here." And so they are, as frogs, of course. Confident little fellows. I suspect that to some greater ear than ours, man's optimistic pronouncements about his role and destiny may make a similar little ringing sound that travels a small way out into the night. It is only its nearness that is offensive. From the heights of a mountain, or a marsh at evening, it blends, not too badly, with all other sleepy voices that, in croaks and chirrups, are saying the same thing.[5]

Ecologists and writers are saying what the mental health field is taking far longer to discover. Man is not a self within himself. Man is not a closed system impervious to the universe.

Roy R. Grinker defined the meaning of this view, as compared to the linear view, for psychosomatic studies:

> Our assumptions that the human organism is part of and in equilibrium with its environment, that its psychological processes assist in maintaining an internal equilibrium with its environment, and that the psychological functioning of the organism is sensitive to both internal needs and external conditions, bring us to the realization that a large aspect of psychosomatic organization has been neglected by most observers . . . [The] focus has been on unidirectional, linear causal chains . . . [But] the actual functioning of the organism

cannot be understood except by a study of its transactional processes as occurring in a total field . . .

It has become the contemporary task of biological science, advanced by the borrowing of field theory from physics, to study integration in a more sophisticated manner than as a simple relationship between parts. The use of system foci in transaction within the total field requires that more than two systems be studied simultaneously. Physiologists have been accustomed to studying modes of integration . . . enzymatic, hormonal, nervous. Psychologists have focused on intrapsychic systems, sometimes in relationship with total or specific somatic processes or symptoms and sometimes with social or cultural processes narrowly defined as "life situations" or as "reality." Anthropologists have concerned themselves with culture as an influence on somatic or personality patterns and with social forces affecting psychological states. However, often the psychosomatic field has been sharply broken into fragments which have been then artificially correlated with other fragments far removed in space and time, and structure and function. Today we have come to realize that both the genetic and the transactional approach require for analysis and synthesis the concepts of a field of theory.[6]

Our study of anorectic and other psychosomatic patients supports and gives specificity to the contextual model. We have seen how people form part of "field structures." The "permeability of boundaries" and the "interdependency of all parts in the field" have been fleshed out in the powerful helplessness of Deborah Kaplan, in Mr. Gilbert's impotent pride, and in Mrs. Menotti's maternal extrasensory perception. We have learned from these families the tremendous power of the social system—how it constrains and governs, how family members accommodate to it without any awareness, how in some families simply to express one's being can be an abrogation of contract. And in our research we have been able to document the power of family rules by measuring their effect on the FFA in the bloodstream of the diabetic. The soft data of transactional patterns have been given scientific confirmation.

Linear thinkers treated the anorectic as a closed system, responding only to her internalized context. After our experience in the family sessions, this approach has become impossible. Anorexia nervosa is a disease of the child in the family.

The marvel of these sessions has been to see how the psychosomatic patient can be freed from the death-threatening symptoms by actualizing, in therapy, healthy alternatives in the family system. What the systems paradigm offers is the recognition of a systemic interconnectedness. When people are understood in their ecosystems, every system member can be seen as responsible for the creation and maintenance of the psychosomatic symptom. And every part of the system can offer a route to health-giving change.

APPENDIXES

NOTES

INDEX

The Family Task

APPENDIX A

Recorded Instructions

1. Suppose all of you had to work out a menu for dinner tonight. You would all like to have your favorite foods for dinner, but in putting this menu together you can have only one meat, two vegetables, one drink, and one dessert. We'd like you to talk together about it now and decide on this one meal that you would all enjoy. Remember, it can only have one meat, two vegetables, one drink, and one dessert. You must end up agreeing on this one meal that everyone will enjoy. All right now, turn off the machine and go ahead with your discussion. When you're ready to go on to the next question, turn on the machine once again please.

2. All right now, we're ready for the next question. In every family things happen that cause a fuss now and then. We'd like you to discuss and talk together about an argument you've had, a fight or argument at home that you can remember. We'd like you to talk together about it. You can cover what started it, who was in on it, what went on, and how it turned out. See if you can remember what it was all about. We'd like you to take your time and discuss it at length. You can turn off the machine and go ahead.

3. We're ready now for the next question. For this one, we'd like each of you to tell about the things everyone does in the family: the things that please you the most and make you feel good but also the things each one does that make you unhappy or mad. Everyone try to give his or her own ideas about this. You can go ahead and turn off the machine now.

4. Here is the next question. On the table you will find a folder with two picture cards in it. Each of these pictures shows a family

scene. We'd like you to make up a story together about each of the pictures. We'd like you to tell what is happening in the picture, what you think led up to this scene, and what the people are thinking and feeling. Then make up an ending for the story. First make up a story for picture one, and when you're finished with that, make up a story for picture two. Remember, discuss the pictures and make up the stories together. You may now turn off the tape recorder and go ahead.

5. We are now ready for the last question. We have something we want you to make together. On the easel we have made a model for you to copy. In the folder in front of you there are enough pieces for you to put it together. The pieces are divided into bunches. There is one bunch for each of you to start with. Make your copy on the table and stay seated. Remember, it's for the whole family to work on together. We're now ready; you may turn off the machine and go ahead with your model.

Preparation

1. Family members are asked to seat themselves as they wish at the table as long as all are facing the camera, full or profile.

2. On the table is placed the tape recorder containing the Family Task cassette, a folder with the picture cards, and a folder with the color-forms model pieces in envelopes. The model to be copied is taped to the wall facing the family.

3. Number of family members: All of our tasks have been done with no more than three children, the index patient plus two siblings. The pieces for task no. 5 are divided for three children. If the family has only one or two children, distribute the extra pieces among the other family members' envelopes prior to the task.

Verbal Instructions

1. Explain about the videotape, cameras, microphones, and one-way mirror. Tell them you will be watching.

2. "We have some things for you to do today, for you to do together as a family. The instructions for each of these things are on this tape recorder."

Explain the mechanical use of the tape recorder, how to turn on the play button, how to stop it, etc. MAKE SURE YOU LOOK AT ALL FAMILY MEMBERS WHEN EXPLAINING.

"First listen to the direction for the first thing to do. After you have finished the first task, go on to the second, and so on. Any questions?"

The experimenter leaves the room.

3. If the discussion for task nos. 2 or 3 lasts excessively long and seems interminable, as will happen on occasion, go in and suggest that the family proceed to the next item. In these cases the task has usually been more or less completed, but the discussion goes ruminatively on and on.

4. If for the last task the family does not grasp about copying the model and starts making up their own creation, you may go in and tell them to copy the model. Give them a couple of minutes first, because sometimes someone from the family will call this problem to the attention of the others and then they will shift to copy the model. However, if it is clear there is no internal disagreement about the task and everyone has the wrong idea, or the one who thinks that they should make his own version "wins," then you can go in and set them straight.

Research in Endocrine Adaptation

APPENDIX B

Our research on anorectic inpatients always had a dual purpose: investigation into psychological and physiological mechanisms, and investigation into more effective modes of therapy. The conceptual model of psychosomatic disease was achieved by this dual approach. In patients with anorexia nervosa, we also pursued studies regarding the endocrine adaptation to chronic starvation, with particular emphasis on thyroid and pituitary function. The endocrine abnormalities seen in these patients turned out to be secondary events, not part of an originating or causal process.

Physiological studies were carried out concerning thyroid function and pituitary function in patients with anorexia nervosa. Anorectic patients generally demonstrate normal thyroxine levels, but we found that the circulating triiodothyroine levels (T_3) were low. These data were interpreted as an adaptive responsive of the metabolically active thyroid hormone level in the face of chronic starvation, thereby filling the need to conserve energy and body mass. It is very likely that the low T_3 levels were achieved by an increase in the concentration of reverse T_3, a metabolically inactive product of thyroid hormone. These data are published in *J. Clin. Endo. & Metab.* 40 (1975): 468.

We looked at the patterns of response of various pituitary hormones in patients with anorexia nervosa (voluntary starvation) and patients with inflammatory bowel disease (anorexia and weight loss secondary to organic bowel disease). We found that there was an increase in the concentration of cortisol in both groups involving both the A.M. and P.M. specimens, when compared to normals. A variety of patterns was seen with regard to LH and FSH. These varied from a prepubertal type of secretion to nocturnal spurts of the hormone, while others showed normal adolescent patterns. The prolactin response to TSH was also considered normal.

Indeed, the only consistently abnormal findings in patients with anorexia nervosa with regard to their pituitary hormones involved TSH (thyroid stimulating hormone) and GH (growth hormone). The TSH response to TRF (thyrotropin releasing factor) in patients with anorexia nervosa is abnormal, with a peak which was much lower than that seen in normal females and delayed in terms of the time of its appearance.

The response of growth hormone was studied by means of a propranalol-glucagon stimulation test. In normal individuals, the administration of propranalol causes a rise in growth hormone concentration from a mean of 4 ng/ml to 10 ng/ml. Glucagon administration at that time results in a further rise in GH to a mean of 15 ng/ml four hours later. In patients with inflammatory bowel disease, an elevated concentration of GH was seen (mean = 6 ng/ml), with a further rise following propranalol to 15 ng/ml. Administration of glucagon to these patients caused a profound rise to levels of 45 ng/ml. In contrast to these two patterns, children with anorexia nervosa showed depressed fasting levels of GH (mean = 2 ng/ml). Administration of propranalol caused a rise to 7 ng/ml, but the administration of glucagon did not cause a change in the shape of the curve. There was a rise to a mean of 10 four hours following the administration of glucagon, but the rate of rise from the starting level and following the administration of propranalol appeared unaltered. We have interpreted these data to indicate that in patients with anorexia nervosa there are strong hypothalamic consequences which lead to increased beta-adrenergic stimulation. This results in a depressed response of TSH to the administration of TRF, while a normal prolactin response to TRF is seen. It also is reflected in the abnormally low fasting levels of GH, with a significant rise after the administration of the beta-adrenergic blocking agent propranalol. It is intriguing to note that the GH responses during sleep in patients with anorexia nervosa are completely normal. This difference in the GH pattern between the sleeping the waking state raises the question as to whether the increased beta-adrenergic tone noted during the day is not a direct physiological consequence of the emotional arousal in these patients. These data are being prepared for publication.

Notes

1. Perspectives on Anorexia Nervosa

1. K. Tolstrup, "The Treatment of Anorexia Nervosa in Childhood and Adolescence," *J. Child Psychology and Psychiatry* 16 (1975): 75–78.

2. Bernice Rosman, Salvador Minuchin, and Ronald Liebman, "Family Lunch Session: An Introduction to Family Therapy in Anorexia Nervosa," *Amer. J. Orthopsychiatry* 45, no. 5 (October 1975): 846–853.

3. A. H. Crisp, R. S. Kalucy, J. H. Lacey, and B. Harding, "The Long-Term Prognosis in Anorexia Nervosa: Some Factors Predictive of Outcome," in R. A. Vigersky, ed., *Anorexia Nervosa* (New York: Raven Press, 1977), pp. 55–65.

4. R. Morton, *Phthisiologica: Or a Treatise of Consumptions* (London, 1689).

5. W. W. Gull, "Anorexia Nervosa," *Lancet* 1 (1888): 516–517.

6. E. C. Lasègue, "On Hysterical Anorexia," *Medical Times Gazette* 2 (1873): 265.

7. J. Naudeau, "Observations sur une maladie nerveuse accompagnée d'un degôut extraordinaire pour les aliments," *J. méd. chir. et pharmacol.* 80 (1789): 197.

8. Lasègue, "On Hysterical Anorexia."

9. Robert A. Vigersky, ed., *Anorexia Nervosa* (New York: Raven Press, 1977), pp. 277–382.

10. Theodore Lidz, "General Concepts of Psychosomatic Medicine," in Silvano Arieti, ed., *American Handbook of Psychiatry* (New York: Basic Books, 1959), pp. 647–658.

11. Edward Weiss and O. S. English, *Psychosomatic Medicine*, 3rd ed. (Philadelphia-London: W. B. Saunders, 1957), p. 324.

12. W. B. Cannon, *The Wisdom of the Body* (New York: Norton, 1932); H. Selye, "The General Adaptation Syndrome and the Diseases of

Adaptation," *J. Clin. Endocrinology* 6 (1946): 117; H. G. Wolff, "Life Stress and Bodily Disease—A Formulation," *Proceedings of the Association for Research in Nervous and Mental Diseases* 29 (1950): 1059.

13. H. F. Dunbar, *Psychosomatic Diagnosis* (New York: Hoeber, 1943).

14. Franz Alexander, *Psychosomatic Medicine* (New York: Norton, 1932).

15. Roy R. Grinker, *Psychosomatic Research* (New York: Norton, 1953), p. 153.

16. W. Patterson Brown, in M. Ralph Kaufman and M. Heiman, eds., *Evolution of Psychosomatic Concepts: Anorexia Nervosa, a Paradigm* (New York: International University Press, 1964).

17. J. V. Waller, R. M. Kaufman, and Felix Deutsch, in Kaufman and Heiman, eds., *Evolution of Psychosomatic Concepts: Anorexia Nervosa, a Paradigm.*

18. J. H. Masserman, in Kaufman and Heiman, eds., *Evolution of Psychosomatic Concepts: Anorexia Nervosa, a Paradigm.*

19. Helmut Thoma, *Anorexia Nervosa* (New York: International University Press, 1967).

20. E. I. Falstein, S. C. Feinstein, and I. Judas, "Anorexia Nervosa in the Male Child," *Amer. J. Orthopsychiatry* 26 (1956): 751–772.

21. Salvador Minuchin, Lester Baker, Bernice Rosman, Ronald Liebman, Leroy Milman, and Thomas Todd, "A Conceptual Model of Psychosomatic Illness in Children: Family Organization and Family Therapy," *Archives of General Psychiatry* 32 (August 1975): 1031–1038.

22. G. L. Engel, "Training in Psychosomatic Research," *Advances in Psychosomatic Medicine* 5 (1967): 16.

23. G. L. Engel, "A Unified Concept of Health and Disease," *Perspectives in Biology and Medicine* 3 (1960): 459.

24. I. A. Mirsky, "The Psychosomatic Approach to the Etiology of Clinical Disorders," *Psychosomatic Medicine* 19 (1957): 424.

25. Grinker, *Psychosomatic Research*, p. 161.

26. Hilde Bruch, *Eating Disorders: Obesity, Anorexia, and the Person Within* (New York: Basic Books, 1973), p. 44.

27. Ibid., p. 56.

28. Ibid., p. 47.

29. J. R. Blitzer, Nancy Rollins, and Amelia Blackwell, "Children Who Starve Themselves: Anorexia Nervosa," *Psychosomatic Medicine* 23, no. 5 (1961): 369–383; W. Warren, "A Study of Anorexia Nervosa in Young Girls," *J. Child Psychology and Psychiatry* 9 (1968): 27–40; S. Gifford, B. J. Murawski, and M. L. Pilot, "Anorexia Nervosa in One of Identical Twins," in Christopher V. Rowland, Jr., ed., *Anorexia and Obesity* (Boston: Little Brown, 1970), pp. 139–228; Mohammed Shafii,

Carlos Salguero, and Stuart M. Finch, "Anorexia à Deux: Psychopathology and Treatment of Anorexia Nervosa in Latency Age Siblings," paper presented at Annual Meeting of the American Academy of Child Psychiatry, October 1972, New Orleans.

30. Leonard P. Ullman, "The Major Concepts Taught to Behavior Therapy Trainees," in Anthony M. Graziano, ed., *Behavior Therapy with Children* (Chicago: Aldine, 1971), pp. 368–370.

31. John Paul Brady and Wolfram Rieger, "Behavioral Treatment in Anorexia Nervosa," in Travis Thompson and William S. Dockens, III, eds., *Applications of Behavior Modification* (New York: Academic Press, 1975), pp. 45–63.

32. Thomas S. Kuhn, *The Structure of Scientific Revolutions*, 2nd ed., International Encyclopedia of Unified Science, vol. 2, no. 2 (Chicago: University of Chicago Press, 1970), pp. 5–6, 177.

2. The Psychosomatic Family

1. Salvador Minuchin and Avner Barcai, "Therapeutically Induced Family Crisis," in *Science and Psychoanalysis*, vol. 14 (New York: Grune & Stratton, 1969).

2. M. D. Bogdonoff and C. R. Nichols, "Psychogenic Effect on Lipid Mobilization," *Psychosomatic Medicine* 26 (1964): 710.

3. Lester Baker, Salvador Minuchin, and Bernice Rosman, "The Use of Beta-adrenergic Blockade in the Treatment of Psychosomatic Aspects of Juvenile Diabetes Mellitus," in *Advances in Beta-adrenergic Blocking Therapy*, vol. 5, ed. A. Snart (Princeton: Excerpta Medica, 1974), V, 67–80.

4. Ibid., p. 71.

5. Salvador Minuchin, Braulio Montalvo, B. G. Guerney, Jr., B. L. Rosman, and F. Schumer, *Families of the Slums: An Exploration of Their Structure and Treatment* (New York: Basic Books, 1967).

6. This report is being prepared for publication.

3. The Anorectic Family

1. Salvador Minuchin, *Families and Family Therapy* (Cambridge: Harvard University Press, 1974), p. 22.

2. Ibid., p. 52.

3. Gregory Bateson, "The Cybernetics of Self: A Theory of Alcoholism," *Psychiatry* 34 (1971): 1–18.

4. Mohammed Shafii, Carlos Salguero, and Stuart M. Finch, "Anorexia à Deux: Psychopathology and Treatment of Anorexia Nervosa in Latency Age Siblings," paper presented at Annual Meeting of the American Academy of Child Psychiatry, October 1972, New Orleans.

4. Blueprints for Therapy

1. Thomas S. Kuhn, *The Structure of Scientific Revolutions* (Chicago: University of Chicago Press, 1970).

2. Edgar A. Levenson, *The Fallacy of Understanding* (New York: Basic Books, 1972), p. 38.

3. Don D. Jackson, "The Individual and the Larger Contexts," *Family Process* 6, no. 2 (September 1967): 139–154.

4. Levenson, *The Fallacy of Understanding,* p. 59.

5. Ibid., p. 64.

6. Ibid., p. 70.

7. Hilde Bruch, *Eating Disorders: Obesity, Anorexia, and the Person Within* (New York: Basic Books, 1973), p. 5.

8. Gerard Chrzanowski, "Participant Observation," *Contemporary Psychoanalysis* 13, no. 3 (July 1977): 351–355.

9. Jean Guillaumin, "A Discussion of the Paper by Henry Edelheit on Complementarity as a Rule in Psychological Research," *Intnl. J. Psychoanalysis* 57, no. 31 (1976): 31–36.

10. Gregory Bateson, "The Cybernetics of Self: A Theory of Alcoholism," *Psychiatry* 34 (1971): 1.

11. Jay Haley, "Family Therapy: A Radical Change," in Jay Haley, ed., *Changing Families* (New York: Grune & Stratton, 1971), pp. 272–284.

12. Murray Bowen, "Theory in the Practice of Psychotherapy," in Philip Guerin, ed., *Family Therapy, Theory and Practice* (New York: Gardner Press, 1976), pp. 42–90.

13. R. D. Laing, *The Politics of the Family* (New York: Pantheon, 1971).

14. Mara Selvini-Palazzoli, *Self-Starvation: From the Intrapsychic to the Transpersonal Approach to Anorexia Nervosa,* trans. Arnold Pomerans, Human Context Books (London: Chaucer, 1974).

15. Ibid., p. 92.

16. Ibid., p. 88.

17. Ibid., p. 92.

18. Joseph Wolpe, Letters to the Editor, *JAMA* 233, no. 4 (July 28, 1975): 317.

19. Hilde Bruch, "Perils of Behavior Modification in Treatment of Anorexia Nervosa," *JAMA* 230, no. 10 (Dec. 9, 1974): 1421.

20. Wolpe, Letters to the Editor, p. 317.

21. Bruch, *Eating Disorders,* pp. 337–338.

22. Selvini-Palazzoli, *Self-Starvation,* p. 109.

23. Bruch, *Eating Disorders,* p. 343.

24. Ibid., p. 345.

25. Leonard P. Ullman, "The Major Concepts Taught to Behavior

Therapy Trainees," in Anthony M. Graziano, ed., *Behavior Therapy with Children* (Chicago: Aldine-Atherton, 1971), pp. 367–375.

26. Mohammed Shafii, Carlos Salguero, and Stuart M. Finch, "Anorexia à Deux: Psychotherapy and Treatment of Anorexia Nervosa in Latency Age Siblings," paper presented at Annual Meeting of the American Academy of Child Psychiatry, October, 1972, New Orleans.

27. John Paul Brady and Wolfram Rieger, "Behavioral Treatment in Anorexia Nervosa," in Travis Thompson and William S. Dockens, III, eds., *Applications of Behavior Modification* (New York: Academic Press, 1975), pp. 59–60.

28. Arthur Schlesinger, Jr., "Lessons in History," in H. O. Hess, ed., *The Nature of a Humane Society* (Philadelphia: Fortress Press, 1976), pp. 1–43.

29. Ricardo Avenburg and Marcus Guiter, "The Concept of Truth in Psychoanalysis," *Intnl. J. Psychoanalysis* 57, no. 11 (1976): 11–21.

30. Selvini-Palazzoli, *Self-Starvation*, p. 232.

6. The Opening Moves

1. A. R. Lucas, J. W. Duncan, and V. Piens, "The Treatment of Anorexia Nervosa," *Am. J. Psychiatry* 133 (1976): 1034–1037; J. A. Silverman, "Anorexia Nervosa: Clinical and Metabolic Observations in a Successful Treatment Plan," in R. A. Vigersky, ed., *Anorexia Nervosa* (New

2. W. S. Langford, *Pediatrics*, 15th ed., ed. H. L. Barnett and A. H. Einhorn (New York: Appleton-Century-Crofts, 1972), pp. 270–273. York: Raven Press, 1977).

3. B. J. Blinder, D. M. Freeman, and A. J. Stunkard, "Behavior Therapy of Anorexia Nervosa: Effectiveness of Activity as a Reinforcer of Weight Gain," *Am. J. Psychiatry* 126 (1970): 1093–1098.

4. R. Galdston, "Mind over Matter," *J. Amer. Acad. of Child Psychiatry* 13, no. 2 (1974): 246–263.

5. Lucas et al., "The Treatment of Anorexia Nervosa."

6. Silverman, "Anorexia Nervosa."

7. Salvador Minuchin, "The Use of an Ecological Framework in the Treatment of a Child," in E. James Anthony and Cyrille Koupernik, eds., *The Child in His Family* (New York: Wiley, 1970), pp. 41–57, Case 18 in Table 3.

8. "Between You and Me," a videotape available from the Philadelphia Child Guidance Clinic. See also Case 22 in Table 3.

9. Bernice Rosman, Salvador Minuchin, and Ronald Liebman, "Family Lunch Session: An Introduction to Family Therapy in Anorexia Nervosa," *Amer. J. Orthopsychiatry* 45, no. 5 (October 1975): 846–853.

7. The Outcome

1. Hilde Bruch, "Perils of Behavior Modification in Treatment of Anorexia Nervosa," *JAMA* 230, no. 10 (Dec. 9, 1974): 1419–1422.

2. M. J. Pertshuk, "Behavior Therapy: Extended Follow-up," in R. A. Vigersky, ed., *Anorexia Nervosa* (New York: Raven Press, 1977).

3. R. Bruce Sloan, Fred R. Staples, Allan H. Cristol, Neil J. Yorkston, and Katherine Whipple, *Psychotherapy Versus Behavior Therapy* (Cambridge: Harvard University Press, 1975), p. 223.

4. A. H. Crisp, R. S. Kalucy, J. H. Lacey, and B. Harding, "The Long-Term Prognosis in Anorexia Nervosa: Some Factors Predictive of Outcome," in Vigersky, ed., *Anorexia Nervosa*, pp. 55–65.

5. K. Tolstrup, "The Treatment of Anorexia Nervosa in Childhood and Adolescence," *J. Child Psychology and Psychiatry* 16 (1975): 75–78.

6. W. S. Langford, *Pediatrics*, 15th ed., ed. H. L. Barnett and A. H. Einhorn (New York: Appleton-Century-Crofts, 1972), pp. 270–273.

7. Bernice Rosman, Salvador Minuchin, Ronald Liebman, and Lester Baker, "Input and Outcome of Family Therapy in Anorexia Nervosa," in *Adolescent Psychiatry*, vol. 5, ed. S. C. Feinstein and P. L. Giovacchini (New York: Jason Aronson, 1977), pp. 319–322.

8. L. I. Lesser, B. J. Ashenden, M. Debuskey, and L. Eisenberg, "Anorexia Nervosa in Children," *Amer. J. Orthopsychiatry* 30 (1960): 572–580.

9. Hilde Bruch, *Eating Disorders: Obesity, Anorexia Nervosa, and the Person Within* (New York: Basic Books, 1973).

10. Lesser et al., "Anorexia Nervosa in Children."

11. J. R. Blitzer, Nancy Rollins, and Amelia Blackwell, "Children Who Starve Themselves: Anorexia Nervosa," *Psychosomatic Medicine* 23 (1961): 369–383.

12. W. Warren, "A Study of Anorexia Nervosa in Young Girls," *J. Child Psychology and Psychiatry* 9 (1968): 27–40.

13. A. R. Lucas, J. W. Duncan, and V. Piens, "The Treatment of Anorexia Nervosa," *Am. J. Psychiatry* 133 (1976): 1034–1037.

14. R. Galdston, "Mind over Matter: Observations on Fifty Patients Hospitalized with Anorexia Nervosa," *J. Am. Acad. Child Psychiatry* 13 (1974): 246–263.

15. Lucas et al., "The Treatment of Anorexia Nervosa."

16. J. B. Reinhart, M. D. Kenna, and R. A. Succop, "Anorexia Nervosa in Children: Outpatient Management," *J. Am. Acad. Child Psychiatry* 11 (1972): 114–131.

17. P. L. Goetz, R. A. Succop, J. B. Reinhart, and A. Miller, "Anorexia in Children: A Follow-up Study," *Am. J. Orthopsychiatry* 47 (1977): 597–603.

18. J. A. Silverman, "Anorexia Nervosa: Clinical and Metabolic Ob-

servations in a Successful Treatment Plan," in Vigersky, ed., *Anorexia Nervosa*.

12. Psychotherapy for a Small Planet

1. Mara Selvini-Palazzoli, *Self-Starvation: From the Intrapsychic to the Transpersonal Approach to Anorexia Nervosa*, trans. Arnold Pomerans, Human Context Books (London: Chaucer, 1974), p. 25.

2. Ludwig Binswanger, "The Case of Ellen West: An Anthropological-Clinical Study," in Rollo May, Ernest Angel, and Henri F. Ellenberger, eds., *Existence: A New Dimension in Psychiatry and Psychology* (New York: Basic Books, 1958), pp. 237–364.

3. Edgar Z. Friedenberg, *R. D. Laing* (New York: Viking Press, 1973), p. 70.

4. E. F. Schumacher, *Small Is Beautiful* (New York: Harper & Row, 1973), p. 14.

5. Loren Eisley, *The Immense Journey* (New York: Random House, 1957), p. 25.

6. Roy R. Grinker, *Psychosomatic Research* (New York: W. W. Norton, 1953), pp. 152–162.

Index